Serono Symposia, USA
Norwell, Massachusetts
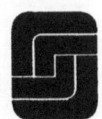

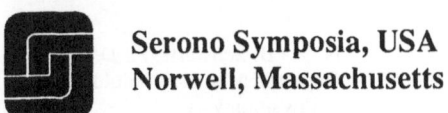

Serono Symposia, USA
Norwell, Massachusetts

Mary Hunzicker-Dunn   Neena B. Schwartz
Editors

Follicle Stimulating Hormone

Regulation of Secretion and Molecular Mechanisms of Action

With 132 Figures

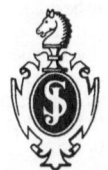

Springer-Verlag
New York Berlin Heidelberg London Paris
Tokyo Hong Kong Barcelona Budapest

Mary Hunzicker-Dunn, Ph.D.
Department of Cell, Molecular, and
    Structural Biology
Northwestern University Medical School
Chicago, IL 60611
USA

Neena B. Schwartz, Ph.D.
Department of Neurobiology and
    Physiology
Northwestern University
Evanston, IL 60201
USA

Proceedings of the Symposium on the Regulation and Actions of Follicle Stimulating Hormone, sponsored by Serono Symposia, USA, held October 25 to 28, 1990, in Evanston, Illinois.

For information on previous volumes, please contact Serono Symposia, USA.

Library of Congress Cataloging-in-Publication Data
Symposium on the Regulation and Action of Follicle Stimulating Hormone
    (1990: Evanston, Ill.)
    Follicle stimulating hormone: regulation of secretion and molecular mechanisms of action/ edited by Mary Hunzicker-Dunn, Neena Schwartz.
        p. cm.
    "Proceedings of the Symposium on the Regulation and Action of Follicle Stimulating Hormone, sponsored by Serono Symposia, USA, held October 25 to 28, 1990, in Evanston, Illinois"—T.p. verso.
    Includes bibliographical references and index.
    ISBN-13: 978-1-4684-7105-2
    1. Follicle-stimulating hormone—Secretion—Regulation—Congresses.   2. Follicle-stimulating hormone—Mechanism of action—Congresses.   I. Hunzicker-Dunn, Mary.
II. Schwartz, Neena B.   III. Serono Symposia, USA.   IV. Title.
    [DNLM: 1. FSH—congresses.   2. Ovulation Induction—congresses.
WK 515 S9896f 1990]
QP572.F6S96   1992
599'.016—dc20
DNLM/DLC
for Library of Congress
                                                                                                            91-5018

Printed on acid-free paper.

Production coordinated by Technical Texts and managed by Francine Sikorski.
Production and typesetting services by Technical Texts, Scituate, MA.

9 8 7 6 5 4 3 2 1

ISBN-13: 978-1-4684-7105-2   e-ISBN-13: 978-1-4684-7103-8
DOI: 10.1007/978-1-4684-7103-8

SYMPOSIUM ON THE REGULATION AND ACTIONS OF FOLLICLE STIMULATING HORMONE

Scientific Committee

Mary Hunzicker-Dunn, Ph.D., Cochairman
Northwestern University

Neena B. Schwartz, Ph.D., Cochairman
Northwestern University

James Hammond, M.D.
Pennsylvania State University

Jo Anne Richards, Ph.D.
Baylor College of Medicine

Robert Ryan, M.D.
Mayo Medical School

Wylie Vale, Ph.D.
Salk Institute

Organizing Secretary

L. Lisa Kern, Ph.D.
Serono Symposia, USA
100 Longwater Circle
Norwell, Massachusetts

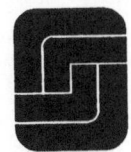

Preface

The chapters in this book represent presentations at the first meeting ever held on the regulation and actions of follicle stimulating hormone. The meeting took place on the campus of Northwestern University, Evanston, Illinois, from October 25 to 28, 1990. The idea for this meeting was conceived by Neena B. Schwartz, and the valuable advice of the organizing committee contributed greatly to its scientific success.

We gratefully acknowledge the funding and coordination of this meeting by Serono Symposia, USA. We also wish to acknowledge the financial contributions made by Northwestern University. We especially thank the invited speakers, poster presenters, and discussion participants who provided the science, interest, and enthusiasm that made this meeting on FSH a success.

MARY HUNZICKER-DUNN
NEENA B. SCHWARTZ

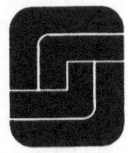

Contents

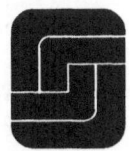

Contributors

N.A. AHMED-ELABBIARY, Department of Obstetrics and Gynaecology, University of Sheffield, United Kingdom.

K. AISAKA, Department of Obstetrics and Gynecology, San-ikukai Hospital, Sumida-Ku, Tokyo, Japan.

MARK F. ALBRECHT, Pacific Biotechnology Ltd., Edgecliff, Australia.

BOGI ANDERSEN, Department of Pharmacology, School of Medicine, Case Western Reserve University, and Department of Medicine, Cleveland Metro General Hospital, Cleveland, Ohio, USA.

CATHERINE TANANIS ANTHONY, Department of Pharmacology, School of Medicine, Vanderbilt University, Nashville, Tennessee, USA.

MARIO ASCOLI, Department of Pharmacology, The University of Iowa, Iowa City, Iowa, USA.

ANDRZEJ BARTKE, Department of Physiology, School of Medicine, Southern Illinois University, Carbondale, Illinois, USA.

M.W. BECKMANN, Department of Obstetrics and Gynecology, The University of Chicago, Chicago, Illinois, USA.

P. BERGER, Immunoendocrinology Research Unit of the Austrian Academy of Sciences, University of Innsbruck, Innsbruck, Austria.

LEONORA A. BISHOP, Pacific Biotechnology Ltd., Edgecliff, and Garvan Institute of Medical Research, St. Vincents Hospital, Darlinghurst, Australia.

IRVING BOIME, Department of Pharmacology, Washington University School of Medicine, St. Louis, Missouri, USA.

DARRELL W. BRANN, Department of Physiology and Endocrinology, Medical College of Georgia, Augusta, Georgia, USA.

THOMAS BRAUN, Laboratory of Molecular Neuroendocrinology, Center for Molecular Biology (ZMBH) University Heidelberg, Heidelberg, Germany.

WILLIAM J. BREMNER, Veterans Affairs Medical Center, Population Center for Research in Reproduction, Department of Medicine, University of Washington School of Medicine, Seattle, Washington, USA.

P.G. BURGON, Departments of Anatomy and Biochemistry, Monash University, Melbourne, Victoria, Australia.

TAMARA A. CAMP, Department of Biochemistry, Molecular Biology, and Cell Biology, Northwestern University, Evanston, Illinois, USA.

SANDRA F. CANNING, Division of Endocrinology, M.S. Hershey Medical Center, Pennsylvania State University, Hershey, Pennsylvania, USA.

JANET M. CARTER, Department of Obstetrics and Gynecology, University of Cincinnati College of Medicine, Cincinnati, Ohio, USA.

ANNE CERPA-POLJAK, Pacific Biotechnology Ltd., Edgecliff, and Garvan Institute of Medical Research, St. Vincents Hospital, Darlinghurst, Australia.

ROBERT T. CHATTERTON, JR., Department of Obstetrics and Gynecology, Northwestern University Medical School, Chicago, Illinois, USA.

LISA A. CONAGHAN, Department of Neurobiology and Physiology, Northwestern University, Evanston, Illinois, USA.

I.D. COOKE, Department of Obstetrics and Gynaecology, University of Sheffield, United Kingdom.

ALAN C. DALKIN, Divisions of Endocrinology and Metabolism, Departments of Internal Medicine and Pediatrics, University of Michigan, Ann Arbor, Michigan, USA.

ROBERT DEKROON, Garvan Institute of Medical Research, St. Vincents Hospital, Darlinghurst, Australia.

DEBORAH. A. DEMANNO, Department of Cell, Molecular, and Structural Biology, Northwestern University Medical School, Chicago, Illinois, USA.

L. DE MARINIS, Institute of Endocrinology, The Catholic University School of Medicine, Rome, Italy.

S. DIRNHOFER, Institute for General and Experimental Pathology, University of Innsbruck, Innsbruck, Austria.

ROBIN E. DODSON, Department of Biochemistry, Molecular Biology, and Cell Biology, Northwestern University, Evanston, Illinois, USA.

JAMES DOUGLASS, Vollum Institute for Advanced Biomedical Research, Oregon Health Sciences University, Portland, Oregon, USA.

D.M. DRISCOLL, Department of Pathology, The University of Chicago, Chicago, Illinois, USA.

JOANNA C. DYKEMA, Department of Biochemistry, Molecular Biology, and Cell Biology, Northwestern University, Evanston, Illinois, USA.

M.L. FABRIZI, Institute of Endocrinology, The Catholic University School of Medicine, Rome, Italy.

F.A.M. FARES, Department of Pharmacology, Washington University School of Medicine, St. Louis, Missouri, USA.

SUSAN L. FITZPATRICK, Department of Cell Biology, Baylor College of Medicine, Houston, Texas, USA.

C. FIUMARA, Institute of Endocrinology, The Catholic University School of Medicine, Rome, Italy.

BRIAN K. FOLLETT, AFRC Group on Photoperiodism and Reproduction, Department of Zoology, School of Biological Sciences, University of Bristol, Bristol, United Kingdom.

R. FRANK, European Molecular Biology Laboratory, Biochemical Instrumentation, Heidelberg, Germany.

H. FUJINAGA, Department of Obstetrics and Gynecology, Wakayama Medical College, Wakayama, Japan.

A. BRENDA GALWAY, Department of Reproductive Medicine, University of California-San Diego, La Jolla, California, USA.

SEEMA V. GARDE, Institute for Research in Reproduction (ICMR), Parel, Bombay, India.

G.S. GETZ, Department of Pathology, The University of Chicago, Chicago, Illinois, USA.

G. TIMOTHY GOODMAN, Divisions of Endocrinology and Metabolism, Departments of Internal Medicine and Pediatrics, University of Michigan, Ann Arbor, Michigan, USA.

RANDALL W. GRIMES, Division of Endocrinology, M.S. Hershey Medical Center, Pennsylvania State University, Hershey, Pennsylvania, USA.

MICHAEL D. GRISWOLD, Department of Biochemistry and Biophysics, Washington State University, Pullman, Washington, USA.

DANIEL R. HAGEN, Department of Dairy and Animal Science, Pennsylvania State University, University Park, Pennsylvania, USA.

DANIEL J. HAISENLEDER, Divisions of Endocrinology and Metabolism, Departments of Internal Medicine and Pediatrics, University of Michigan, Ann Arbor, Michigan, USA.

DEBORA L. HAMERNIK, Department of Pharmacology, School of Medicine, Case Western Reserve University, Cleveland, Ohio, USA.

GEOFFREY L. HAMMOND, Director, Cancer Research Laboratories, London Regional Cancer Centre, Member M.R.C. Group in Fetal and Neonatal Health and Development, University of Western Ontario, London, Ontario, Canada.

JAMES M. HAMMOND, Division of Endocrinology, M.S. Hershey Medical Center, Pennsylvania State University, Hershey, Pennsylvania, USA.

M.T.W. HEARN, Departments of Anatomy and Biochemistry, Monash University, Melbourne, Victoria, Australia.

LESLIE HECKERT, Department of Biochemistry and Biophysics, Washington State University, Pullman, Washington, USA.

YVONNE J. HORT, Pacific Biotechnology Ltd., Edgecliff, Australia.

AARON J.W. HSUEH, Department of Reproductive Medicine, University of California-San Diego, La Jolla, California, USA.

MARY HUNZICKER-DUNN, Department of Cell, Molecular, and Structural Biology, Northwestern University Medical School, Chicago, Illinois, USA.

T. IACONA, Institute of Endocrinology, The Catholic University School of Medicine, Rome, Italy.

ANDRZEJ JAKUBOWIAK, Department of Obstetrics, Gynecology, and Reproductive Sciences, University of Texas Medical School at Houston, Houston, Texas, USA.

ANDRŽEJ JANECKI, Department of Obstetrics, Gynecology, and Reproductive Sciences, University of Texas Medical School at Houston, Houston, Texas, USA.

S. KANEDA, Department of Obstetrics and Gynecology, San-ikukai Hospital, Sumida-Ku, Tokyo, Japan.

ALAN H. KAYNARD, Divisions of Neuroscience and Reproductive Biology and Behavior, Oregon Regional Primate Research Center, Beaverton, Oregon, USA.

J. KEENE, Department of Pharmacology, Washington University School of Medicine, St. Louis, Missouri, USA.

ROBERT P. KELCH, Divisions of Endocrinology and Metabolism, Departments of Internal Medicine and Pediatrics, University of Michigan, Ann Arbor, Michigan, USA.

GIULIA C. KENNEDY, Department of Pharmacology, School of Medicine, Case Western Reserve University, Cleveland, Ohio, USA.

RUTH A. KERI, Department of Pharmacology, School of Medicine, Case Western Reserve University, Cleveland, Ohio, USA.

JUNG GU KIM, Department of Obstetrics and Gynecology, University of Cincinnati College of Medicine, Cincinnati, Ohio, USA.

R. KLIEBER, Immunoendocrinology Research Unit of the Austrian Academy of Sciences, University of Innsbruck, Innsbruck, Austria.

K. KOKUHO, Department of Obstetrics and Gynecology, San-ikukai Hospital, Sumida-Ku, Tokyo, Japan.

JON M. KORNHAUSER, Institute for Neuroscience, Department of Biochemistry, Molecular Biology, and Cell Biology, Northwestern University, Evanston, Illinois, USA.

WLODZIMIERZ KOWALSKI, Department of Obstetrics and Gynecology, Northwestern University Medical School, Chicago, Illinois, USA.

RICHARD C. KURTEN, Department of Cell Biology, Baylor College of Medicine, Houston, Texas, USA.

ANDREW R. LABARBERA, Department of Obstetrics and Gynecology, University of Cincinnati College of Medicine, Cincinnati, Ohio, USA.

PHILIP S. LAPOLT, Department of Reproductive Medicine, University of California-San Diego, La Jolla, California, USA.

JOHN K. LEIGHTON, Division of Endocrinology, M.S. Hershey Medical Center, Pennsylvania State University, Hershey, Pennsylvania, USA.

E.A. LENTON, Department of Obstetrics and Gynaecology, University of Sheffield, United Kingdom.

JON E. LEVINE, Department of Neurobiology and Physiology, Northwestern University, Evanston, Illinois, USA.

ULRIKE LUDERER, Department of Neurobiology and Physiology, Northwestern University, Evanston, Illinois, USA.

S. MADERSBACHER, Immunoendocrinology Research Unit of the Austrian Academy of Sciences, University of Innsbruck, Innsbruck, Austria.

VIRENDRA B. MAHESH, Department of Physiology and Endocrinology, Medical College of Georgia, Augusta, Georgia, USA.

SUBEER S. MAJUMDAR, Department of Physiology, School of Medicine, Southern Illinois University, Carbondale, Illinois, USA.

A. MANCINI, Institute of Endocrinology, The Catholic University School of Medicine, Rome, Italy.

JOHN C. MARSHALL, Divisions of Endocrinology and Metabolism, Departments of Internal Medicine and Pediatrics, University of Michigan, Ann Arbor, Michigan, USA.

ALVIN M. MATSUMOTO, Veterans Affairs Medical Center, Population Center for Research in Reproduction, Department of Medicine, University of Washington School of Medicine, Seattle, Washington, USA.

KELLY E. MAYO, Institute for Neuroscience, Department of Biochemistry, Molecular Biology, and Cell Biology, Northwestern University, Evanston, Illinois, USA.

CYNTHIA T. MCMURRAY, Vollum Institute for Advanced Biomedical Research, Oregon Health Sciences University, Portland, Oregon, USA.

MICHAEL H. MELNER, Divisions of Neuroscience and Reproductive Biology and Behavior, Oregon Regional Primate Research Center, Beaverton, Oregon, USA.

E. MENINI, Institute of Biochemistry, The Catholic University School of Medicine, Rome, Italy.

JUDITH S. MONDSCHEIN, Division of Endocrinology, M.S. Hershey Medical Center, Pennsylvania State University, Hershey, Pennsylvania, USA.

N.R. MOUDGAL, Center for Advanced Research in Reproductive Biology, Department of Biochemistry, Indian Institute of Science, Bangalore, India.

R. NAKANO, Department of Obstetrics and Gynecology, Wakayama Medical College, Wakayama, Japan.

DWIGHT E. NELSON, Institute for Neuroscience, Department of Neurobiology and Physiology, Northwestern University, Evanston, Illinois, USA.

JOHN H. NILSON, Department of Pharmacology, School of Medicine, Case Western Reserve University, Cleveland, Ohio, USA.

K. NISHIMORI, Department of Obstetrics and Gynecology, Wakayama Medical College, Wakayama, Japan.

M. NOJIMA, Department of Obstetrics and Gynecology, San-ikukai Hospital, Sumida-Ku, Tokyo, Japan.

JOHN N. NORTON, Department of Pharmacology, School of Medicine, Vanderbilt University, Nashville, Tennessee, USA.

L.M. OLSON, Department of Pathology, The University of Chicago, Chicago, Illinois, USA.

RIA B. OONK, Department of Cell Biology, Baylor College of Medicine, Houston, Texas, USA.

OK-KYONG PARK, Department of Biochemistry, Molecular Biology, and Cell Biology, Northwestern University, Evanston, Illinois, USA.

SANDER J. PAUL, Divisions of Endocrinology and Metabolism, Departments of Internal Medicine and Pediatrics, University of Michigan, Ann Arbor, Michigan, USA.

LIN PEI, Department of Biochemistry, Molecular Biology, and Cell Biology, Northwestern University, Evanston, Illinois, USA.

TONY M. PLANT, Department of Physiology, University of Pittsburgh School of Medicine, Pittsburgh, Pennsylvania, USA.

CARLA D. PUTNAM, Department of Physiology and Endocrinology, Medical College of Georgia, Augusta, Georgia, USA.

ROBERT W. REBAR, Department of Obstetrics and Gynecology, University of Cincinnati College of Medicine, Cincinnati, Ohio, USA.

JOANNE S. RICHARDS, Department of Cell Biology, Baylor College of Medicine, Houston, Texas, USA.

CATHERINE RIVIER, The Clayton Foundation Laboratories for Peptide Biology, La Jolla, California, USA.

D.M. ROBERTSON, Departments of Anatomy and Biochemistry, Monash University, Melbourne, Victoria, Australia.

ZEV ROSENWAKS, The Center for Reproductive Medicine and Infertility, The New York Hospital–Cornell Medical Center, New York, New York, USA.

SUSAN E. SAMARAS, Division of Endocrinology, M.S. Hershey Medical Center, Pennsylvania State University, Hershey, Pennsylvania, USA.

L. SAMMARTANO, Institute of Endocrinology, The Catholic University School of Medicine, Rome, Italy.

V.M. SCHMIT, Department of Obstetrics and Gynecology, The University of Chicago, Chicago, Illinois, USA.

PETER R. SCHOFIELD, Pacific Biotechnology Ltd., Edgecliff, Australia.

J.R. SCHREIBER, Department of Obstetrics and Gynecology, The University of Chicago, Chicago, Illinois, USA.

NEENA B. SCHWARTZ, Department of Neurobiology and Physiology, Northwestern University, Evanston, Illinois, USA.

DEBORAH L. SEGALOFF, Department of Physiology and Biophysics, The University of Iowa, Iowa City, Iowa, USA.

ANIL R. SHETH, Institute for Research in Reproduction (ICMR), Parel, Bombay, India.

T. SHIKONE, Department of Obstetrics and Gynecology, Wakayama Medical College, Wakayama, Japan.

CYNTHIA K. SITES, Department of Obstetrics and Gynecology, University of Cincinnati College of Medicine, Cincinnati, Ohio, USA.

MICHAEL K. SKINNER, Department of Pharmacology, School of Medicine, Vanderbilt University, Nashville, Tennessee, USA.

GLENN M. SMITH, Pacific Biotechnology Ltd., Edgecliff, Australia.

DINA Y. SONG, Department of Obstetrics and Gynecology, University of Cincinnati College of Medicine, Cincinnati, Ohio, USA.

ROLF SPRENGEL, Laboratory of Molecular Neuroendocrinology, Center for Molecular Biology (ZMBH) University Heidelberg, Heidelberg, Germany.

P.G. STANTON, Departments of Anatomy and Biochemistry, Monash University, Melbourne, Victoria, Australia.

ANNA STEINBERGER, Department of Obstetrics, Gynecology, and Reproductive Sciences, University of Texas Medical School at Houston, Houston, Texas, USA.

FRANK J. STROBL, Department of Neurobiology and Physiology, Northwestern University, Evanston, Illinois, USA.

MARGARET C. STUART, Garvan Institute of Medical Research, St. Vincents Hospital, Darlinghurst, and School of Biological Sciences, Macquarie University, Australia.

WALTER E. STUMPF, Department of Cell Biology and Anatomy, University of North Carolina, Chapel Hill, North Carolina, USA.

JOSEPH S. TAKAHASHI, Institute for Neuroscience, Department of Neurobiology and Physiology, Northwestern University, Evanston, Illinois, USA.

Y. TORIYA, Department of Obstetrics and Gynecology, San-ikukai Hospital, Sumida-Ku, Tokyo, Japan.

H. TSUZUKI, Department of Obstetrics and Gynecology, San-ikukai Hospital, Sumida-Ku, Tokyo, Japan.

FRED W. TUREK, Department of Neurobiology and Physiology, Northwestern University, Evanston, Illinois, USA.

MAHIMA Y. VAISHNAV, Center for Advanced Research in Reproductive Biology, Department of Biochemistry, Indian Institute of Science, Bangalore, India.

WYLIE VALE, The Clayton Foundation Laboratories for Peptide Biology, La Jolla, California, USA.

HAIYUN WANG, Department of Physiology and Biophysics, The University of Iowa, Iowa City, Iowa, USA.

B. WHITE, Departments of Anatomy and Biochemistry, Monash University, Melbourne, Victoria, Australia.

G. WICK, Institute for General and Experimental Pathology, University of Innsbruck, Innsbruck, Austria.

WINONA L. WONG, Department of Cell Biology, Baylor College of Medicine, Houston, Texas, USA.

D. WRIGHT, Department of Statistics, University of Sheffield, United Kingdom.

GREG WRIGHT, Garvan Institute of Medical Research, St. Vincents Hospital, Darlinghurst, Australia.

K. L. WYNE, Department of Pathology, The University of Chicago, Chicago, Illinois, USA.

M. YAMOTO, Department of Obstetrics and Gynecology, Wakayama Medical College, Wakayama, Japan.

K. YOSHIDA, Department of Obstetrics and Gynecology, San-ikukai Hospital, Sumida-Ku, Tokyo, Japan.

P. ZUPPI, Institute of Endocrinology, The Catholic University School of Medicine, Rome, Italy.

Serono Symposia, USA
Norwell, Massachusetts

Follicle Stimulating Hormone

1

An Overview of FSH Regulation and Action

Ulrike Luderer and Neena B. Schwartz

Follicle stimulating hormone (FSH) and luteinizing hormone (LH) are the two anterior pituitary hormones that control gonadal function. Of the two, LH has been much more extensively studied, due in large part to the earlier development of a sensitive radioimmunoassay (RIA) for LH. Much of what is known about the regulation of FSH synthesis and secretion has been extrapolated from studies of LH. This approach was initially considered valid because both hormones are synthesized and secreted by the same pituitary cells (1, 2) and because a single hypothalamic hormone, gonadotropin releasing hormone (GnRH), has been shown to influence both (3, 4). Despite these important similarities, our understanding of gonadotropin regulation might have been quite different today if we had based it on an equally intensive study of FSH.

CNS Regulation of FSH Secretion

Hypothalamic Regulation

Although GnRH is capable of stimulating both LH and FSH release and synthesis, it exerts much tighter control over LH than FSH secretion and synthesis, thus lending credence to speculation about the existence of a separate FSH releasing factor (FSHRF). There are still two schools of thought on this matter, although evidence that GnRH is the only hypothalamic releasing hormone controlling gonadotropin secretion is mounting.

Early studies showed that exogenous GnRH stimulates both LH and FSH release in vivo (5, 6); however, different GnRH infusion patterns favor one or the other gonadotropin. Slow infusion of GnRH favors FSH release over LH release (7–9); indeed, in rats very slow infusion can selectively stimulate FSH release (10). When endogenous GnRH secretion is elicited by electrical stimulation of the medial preoptic area (MPOA), high-intensity, high-frequency stimulation, which activates more MPOA tissue, favors LH pulses, and low-intensity, low-frequency stimulation favors FSH (10). Similarly, low-frequency exogenous GnRH pulses administered to hypothalamic-lesioned ovariectomized female monkeys increase FSH secretion selectively (11). Further evidence that FSH is less GnRH dependent than LH derives from experiments using NMA (N-methyl-D-aspartate), an analog of the excitatory amino acid aspartate. NMA stimulates GnRH secretion and thus elicits LH, but not FSH, release in intact male and female rats (12, 13), while it stimulates both in monkeys (14).

GnRH also elicits FSH release and synthesis in vitro, but LH is stimulated to a much greater extent. Increasing concentrations of GnRH stimulate FSH release up to 5-fold and LH up to 100-fold (15, 16). Hourly stimulation of pituitary fragments in a dynamic perfusion system with pulses of GnRH elicits pulses of FSH and LH from pituitaries of intact and gonadectomized male and female rats in a dose-dependent manner (17, 18).

LH and FSH responses to GnRH antagonists and antisera also differ. GnRH antagonists or antisera maximally reduce immunoreactive FSH by only 30%–60% in castrates of both sexes after 12 h, while LH drops by 80% within 2 h and by 90% within 5 h (19–24). Superimposing inhibin on GnRH antagonist treatment further suppresses FSH to intact levels (25). Certain circulating isoforms of FSH, which are induced by GnRH antagonist administration, have been found to possess anti-FSH activity (26). Superimposing testosterone (T) or dihydrotestosterone (DHT), but not estradiol (E), on long-term GnRH antagonist treatment in intact and orchidectomized rats prevents or slows the declines in serum and pituitary FSH caused by antagonist alone, indicating a stimulatory effect of T on FSH synthesis that is independent of GnRH (27, 28).

Further evidence that FSH is not dependent upon minute-to-minute regulation by GnRH pulses comes from studies measuring pulsatile hormone secretion. LH is released in a pulsatile manner in intact and gonadectomized rats, with pulse frequency and amplitude increasing after gonadectomy (29–32). FSH secretion in intact rats also appears to be pulsatile; however, the pulses are much more variable in amplitude and frequency (33, 34). After gonadectomy the FSH pulse frequency does not attain the high values that LH pulse frequency reaches (Fig. 1.1) (33–35).

Assuming that each LH pulse reflects a preceding GnRH pulse, these data imply that a GnRH pulse frequently is not followed by an FSH pulse. Use of the push-pull perfusion technique to measure GnRH output from the hypothalamus demonstrates a high correlation between GnRH pulses and serum LH, but not FSH, pulses in male rats (33). Lumpkin et al. (35) found that 83% of FSH pulses in ovariectomized rats coincided with LH pulses; however, they also noted that since many more LH than FSH pulses were detected, many GnRH pulses were not followed by an FSH pulse. Only one group (36), working with orchidectomized rats, has found a high correlation between GnRH, LH, and FSH pulses. Differences in protocols, such as postcastration time of sampling or the sampling interval used, may explain these contradictions.

One aspect of FSH secretion in which GnRH unquestionably plays a role is the preovulatory primary FSH surge. Pretreatment with GnRH antisera and antagonists blocks both the LH and primary FSH surges (37, 38). NMA receptor blockers administered before the gonadotropin surge to estrogen-treated, ovariectomized rats block the LH surge, but not the FSH or prolactin (PRL) surges (39). GnRH is not involved in the sustained FSH elevation, known as the secondary FSH surge, which is maintained after LH levels have dropped (21, 40). The secondary surge can be restored by exogenous LH or FSH administration in these rats (41, 42), indicating that the primary surge itself provides the stimulus for the secondary surge. The site of this action is not known at present.

GnRH also regulates gonadotropin synthesis. Some studies suggest that GnRH, when added to pituitary cultures, increases only the glycosylation of LH, but not the incorporation of amino acids, while other studies have demonstrated that GnRH does increase amino acid incorporation as well (reviewed in 43). The in vitro studies of GnRH effects on gonadotropin mRNA levels or synthesis have been similarly equivocal, with some demonstrating stimulatory effects and others not (43). In vivo experiments using pulsatile GnRH administration in animals with disrupted hypothalamo-pituitary contact have universally demonstrated stimulation of gonadotropin subunit mRNA levels. As with the effect of GnRH pulses on LH and FSH secretion, lower GnRH frequency favors FSHβ mRNA levels over α and LHβ (43). Similarly, the postcastration gonadotropin subunit mRNA rise can be prevented by GnRH antagonist or antiserum pretreatment (43), but GnRH antagonist suppresses FSHβ less than LHβ mRNA (44).

CNS Regulation of Hypothalamic GnRH

Electrical stimulation of the preoptic area-suprachiasmatic nucleus elicits a proestrouslike surge of LH and FSH (45). Selective FSH release in the rat can be elicited by electrical stimulation of, or prostaglandin-E_2 application to, the dorsal anterior hypothalamic area (DAHA) during proestrus (45). Bilateral DAHA lesions cause reduced FSH levels during proestrus (45). Catecholamines, serotonin, GABA, histamines, and neuropeptides, such as neuropeptide-Y (NPY), somatostatin, and opiates, have all been implicated in the regulation of gonadotropin secretion; however, a clear picture has not yet emerged. Most of this vast literature concentrates on the regulation of LH secretion (46).

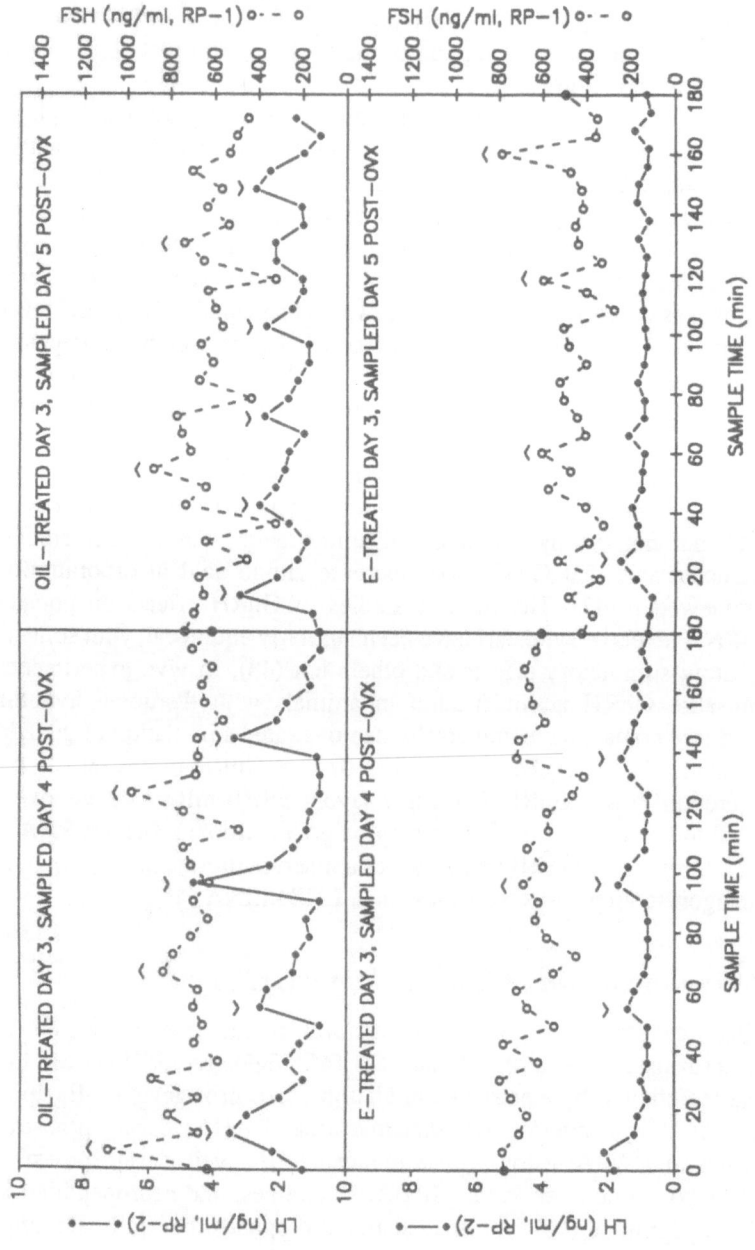

Catecholamines are perhaps the most widely studied of the neural agents that affect gonadotropin secretion (reviewed in 47). The major noradrenergic input to the hypothalamus is from the ventral tegmental pathway (cell groups A1, A5, and A7), which originates in the midbrain. These inputs inhibit intrahypothalamic dopaminergic neurons and/or inhibitory interneurons in the MPOA, which then disinhibits GnRH-containing neurons of the MPOA and the arcuate-median eminence region. Studies using pharmacologic agents have shown that α-adrenergic blockade and depletion of cat-echolamines or inhibition of their synthesis block both the LH surge and ovulation (47). Despite the obvious role of noradrenergic inputs to the hypothalamus in gonadotropin secretion, it is nonetheless true that cyclic LH release and ovulation continue to occur in the completely hypothalamo-pituitary deafferented monkey (47). Rats that have had the ascending nora-drenergic pathways surgically or pharmacologically disrupted initially cease to cycle, but resume normal estrous cycles by 23 days (47).

Based on the relatively few studies that also examined FSH secretion, FSH does not appear to be as dependent upon catecholamines as LH. Barbiturates, which block the increased norepinephrine turnover in the median eminence on proestrous afternoon, have divergent effects. Both pentobarbital (48) and phenobarbital (49) block the LH surge and ovula-tion, but only phenobarbital blocks the primary and secondary FSH surges as well. More recent studies have shown that pharmacologic depletion of CNS norepinephrine and dopamine causes loss of LH pulsatility without affecting FSH secretion (22, 23).

NPY has recently been shown to have different effects on LH and FSH release depending upon the steroidal milieu and the site of action in the hypothalamo-pituitary axis. In ovariectomized rats, NPY administration into the third ventricle causes a dose-dependent reduction of LH pulse frequency, amplitude, and mean levels, without affecting FSH pulsatility (50, 51). Following this inhibition of LH, there is a 10-fold increase in the LH response to GnRH administration (51). In ovariectomized estrogen-primed

---

◄ FIGURE 1.1. Representative plasma LH and FSH profiles from samples obtained from atrially catheterized, ovariectomized (ovx) rats. At 0900 h on day 3 post-ovx, each animal received an implant containing 150-μg 17β-estradiol/mL oil (E) or oil alone. The capsules were removed at 0900 h on day 4. Serial blood sampling occurred at 6-min intervals from 0900 to 1200 h on the day indicated. Significant LH and FSH pulses are denoted by downward- and upward-pointing arrowheads, respec-tively. Only 42% of the FSH peaks occurred within one sampling interval of an LH peak, and overall, there were only 38% as many FSH as LH peaks. E-treatment for 24 h suppressed LH mean plasma levels ($P < 0.05$) and pulse frequency ($P < 0.002$) for 3–5 days after E-capsules were removed, compared to oil-treated controls, with-out altering FSH pulsatility.

animals, NPY injected into the third ventricle exerts an opposite, transient, stimulatory effect on LH release (52). NPY also enhances GnRH secretion from hypothalami of steroid-primed ovariectomized females in vitro (51). NPY directly stimulates pituitary LH and FSH secretion in vitro (50). It also enhances FSH and LH secretion in response to GnRH in cultured dispersed pituitary cells (53). Thus, the effects of NPY appear to be exerted at both the hypothalamic and pituitary levels.

Feedback Regulation of FSH Synthesis and Secretion

Regulation of Serum and Pituitary Gonadotropin Levels

The predominant negative feedback hormones are the steroids, T in the male and E and progesterone (P) in the female, and the peptides, inhibin and follistatin (reviewed in 54–57). The removal of all of these negative feedback signals by gonadectomy results in increased gonadotropin secretion. In rats FSH increases rapidly in both sexes, while LH rises rapidly in the male, but only after a 4- to 7-day lag in the female (58). Replacement of the sex-appropriate steroid (reviewed in 57) can prevent the postgonadectomy LH increase. By itself, T can also restore FSH to precastration levels in male rats (59) and monkeys (60), but the addition of porcine follicular fluid (pFF, a source of inhibin and follistatin) further suppresses FSH (59). In contrast, in ovariectomized females E suppresses FSH, but intact levels can only be attained through the addition of pFF (61). We have recently shown that LH pulse amplitude and frequency in ovariectomized female rats remain suppressed for several days after removal of E implants, but that FSH pulsatility in the E-treated animals is indistinguishable from that of untreated ovariectomized animals (Fig. 1.1) (34).

Inhibin is a gonadal peptide composed of an α- and a β-subunit that selectively suppresses FSH without altering LH secretion (55, 56). Serum inhibin levels in intact female rats are inversely correlated with serum FSH levels: They are highest on the morning of proestrus, begin to fall after the gonadotropin surge and reach their nadir during the night of proestrus and early estrous morning (62, 63). Most studies of inhibin replacement in gonadectomized animals have used pFF as the source of inhibin due to lack of availability of the purified protein (reviewed in 64, 55, 56). In castrates of both sexes, pFF suppresses FSH specifically, but only in acutely ovariectomized females is it capable of suppressing FSH to intact levels (25, 59, 61). Also, pFF further suppresses FSH to intact levels in GnRH antagonist-treated animals (25). Recently, the importance of endogenous inhibin has been studied in male rats and monkeys using inhibin antisera. In prepubertal, but not adult, male rats, inhibin antiserum administration results in increases in serum FSH levels (65), while in monkeys inhibin appears to be an important regulator of FSH levels in adult males as well (67). Inhibin antiserum, however, is capable of increasing FSH secretion in adult male rats in which the Leydig cells have been selectively destroyed (66).

Unilateral gonadectomy provides another example of divergent FSH and LH secretion (54). In females compensatory ovulation occurs. First, FSH rises transiently and progesterone falls; then, 24 h later, a new crop of follicles has been recruited. Injection of pFF, but not P, blocks this ovulation (68, 69). In males such compensatory hypertrophy occurs in young, but not in mature, males (70).

Follistatin, or FSH-suppressing protein, a 35-kD gonadal protein that is *not* structurally homologous to inhibin or activin (55), suppresses in vitro pituitary basal FSH secretion and cell content in a dose-dependent manner (71). It has similar, although much smaller, effects on LH (71). Follistatin also antagonizes GnRH-stimulated FSH and, again, to a lesser extent, LH release (71). Inhibin antiserum does not neutralize follistatin actions, and the effects of inhibin and follistatin are additive (71).

Positive steroidal feedback from the gonads (reviewed in 57) has long been known to be crucial in the development of the preovulatory gonadotropin surge. Briefly, the primary surge is triggered by high estradiol levels on diestrus and proestrus. Estrogen given to ovariectomized rats triggers afternoon surges of LH and FSH for 3–5 days (72). Progesterone given at noon to E-primed ovariectomized rats advances the time of the surge (73), but P also turns off the E-triggered repetitive surges on the following days (74), as it does during the cycle.

The secondary FSH surge is a prolonged elevation of FSH secretion during the morning of estrus after LH levels have fallen back to nonsurge levels, which is seen in rats, horses, rabbits, and hamsters. The purpose of the secondary surge is to recruit the cohort of follicles that will ovulate at the next estrus in these animals with extremely short estrous cycles (75, 42). The mechanism of the secondary surge is not yet completely understood; however, it appears to require both the low inhibin (62, 63) and high P-levels (76) that occur after the primary surge.

Activin is a recently discovered gonadal factor, the physiological importance of which is not yet understood. It is found primarily in the interstitial cells of the testis (77) and in the ovary (78) and consists of a dimer of the inhibin β-subunit (79). Activin stimulates FSH secretion after 4 h of exposure to pituitary tissue without reducing pituitary FSH content (78).

Regulation of Gonadotropin Transcription by Gonadal Feedback

The recent application of molecular techniques to the study of gonadotropin synthesis has provided evidence that FSH secretion rate is more highly dependent on synthesis than is LH secretion rate. Previously, synthesis could only be indirectly estimated by measurements of pituitary hormone content.

Pituitary FSH content rises in females, but falls in males during the first 5 days after gonadectomy and then rises in both sexes (58). Inhibin suppresses pituitary FSH content (80). Similarly, common α, LHβ and FSHβ subunit mRNA levels increase gradually following gonadectomy. In female rats LHβ levels first increase significantly by 7 days postovariectomy and eventually reach 10- to 20-fold intact levels; α-levels increase 4-fold by 7 days and remain at that level; FSHβ levels are already increased significantly by 3 days and reach 4- to 10-fold intact levels by 21 days (81–85). In males mRNA levels of all three subunits increase significantly by 3 days postcastration (81, 82). LHβ gradually attains 8- to 10-fold, and α reaches 3- to 5-fold intact levels (82–86). FSHβ increases 4- to 7-fold within 7 days after orchidectomy, then declines to 1.5-fold intact levels by 28 days and finally increases again to 4- to 5-fold intact levels by 90 days (81, 84, 85, 87). Similar results have been reported in sheep (88–90). The increases in gonadotropin subunit mRNA levels can be attributed to rising mRNA transcription rates postgonadectomy. In females at 7 days postovariectomy, transcription rates are increased 2.5-fold for α-subunit, 10-fold for LHβ, and 2-fold for FSHβ (91). Thus, the rapid increases in serum FSH levels following gonadectomy are associated with rapid increases in FSHβ mRNA levels.

Not surprisingly, the various gonadal factors have profound effects on gonadotropin synthesis as well as on secretion. Estrogen suppresses α, LHβ, and FSHβ mRNA in vivo in ovariectomized rats within 4 h of treatment onset and suppresses them further to near-intact and intact levels after 24-h and 7-day treatments (91, 81). As little as 4 h in vivo E-treatment also suppresses the mRNA transcription rates of all three subunits in ovariectomized rats (91). In long-term castrate male rats and sheep, E also suppresses α, FSHβ, and LHβ subunit mRNA levels to intact values (88–90). In vitro E-treatment of pituitaries from long-term castrate male sheep also suppresses pituitary FSH content (92), α and FSHβ subunit mRNA levels, and transcription rates from these animals in a dose-dependent manner (88, 93). In rats, however, in vitro E-treatment of pituitaries from intact or ovariectomized rats does not alter common α or FSHβ, while it enhances LHβ mRNA levels and transcription rates (94).

In vivo studies of the rat estrous cycle reveal that α and LHβ mRNA levels peak just before the serum LH peak, while FSHβ peaks immediately after the surge (43). Similarly, in sheep α and LHβ mRNA increase during the LH surge, but FSHβ mRNA are at their lowest (43). In the ovariectomized, E-treated rat model, however, only α but not LHβ mRNA increases with the LH surge (43). Estrogen given to anestrous ewes to produce gonadotropin surges also increases α-mRNA, while it decreases FSHβ mRNA and does not alter LHβ mRNA (95).

Testosterone and DHT administered for 7 days in vivo suppress LHβ and α-subunit mRNA towards intact levels in castrated adult males, but there is no regulation of FSHβ by androgens in vivo (81, 87). In pituitary cultures from male and female rats, however, androgens increase FSHβ mRNA levels without altering α or LHβ levels (43).

The effects of P on gonadotropin subunit synthesis in rats and sheep are still controversial. In sheep, one in vivo study demonstrated no effect on any of the gonadotropin subunit levels (43), while in two in vitro studies, α and FSHβ mRNA levels and transcription rates were decreased (96, 93). Similarly, conflicting data has been reported in the rat (43). Most recently, the effect of P on FSH synthesis during E-induced gonadotropin surges has been studied. When P was given 24 h after E-implants were inserted, serum FSH and FSHβ mRNA levels were greatly enhanced at 1700 h, but mRNA levels were suppressed at 0900 h the next day, relative to animals receiving E alone (97).

In male pituitary cell cultures, inhibin application of 4 h or longer suppresses FSHβ to undetectable levels and also significantly suppresses α-mRNA, as well as FSH secretion (24 h application required), into the medium in a dose-responsive manner, but does not affect LHβ (98, 99).

Activin increases FSHβ mRNA and FSH secretion from male dispersed pituitaries within 4 h of application in a dose-dependent manner, while not affecting α or LHβ mRNA. Inhibin is able to overcome 20-ng/mL activin completely at a dose of 10 ng/mL (99).

Like inhibin, follistatin reduces FSHβ mRNA and FSH secretion in male dispersed pituitaries in a dose-dependent manner without affecting LHβ mRNA levels; however, unlike inhibin, follistatin does not also suppress common α-subunit mRNA levels (99). Activin can overcome the effects of follistatin only in equimolar concentrations (99).

Biochemistry of FSH

FSH is a globular glycosylated protein with a molecular weight of 28,000–30,000 D, consisting of an α- and a β-subunit (reviewed by 43, 45, 100). It shares a common α-subunit with LH, CG, and TSH. Neither subunit has any biological activity individually. The four β-subunits have significant amino acid homology with one another and probably evolved from a common precursor. Both LH and FSHβ subunits are found in the same cells within the anterior pituitary (101–103). The amino acid sequence determination for the α-subunit was reviewed by Sairam (104). The α-subunit is stabilized by 5 disulfide bonds. Heterogeneity of the amino acid sequence within a species is often found at the N-terminus due to loss of amino acid residues by additional proteolysis after the removal of the signal peptide of new α-subunit. Oligosaccharides are N-linked at the 2 asparagine residues. There is a single α-gene with 4 exons and 3 introns, which varies considerably between species in the first intron, that interrupts the 5'-untranslated region (43). Introns 2 and 3 both interrupt the coding sequence of the peptide.

There is high homology among the nucleotide and amino acid sequences of the FSHβ genes and subunits of different species. The FSHβ subunit contains 6 disulfide bonds. Like the α-subunit, oligosaccharides are N-linked at 2 asparagine residues. Neuraminic acid is always the terminal oligosaccharide, and there are no N-acetylgalactosamine residues. The FSHβ gene contains 3 exons and 2 introns (43). The first exon contains the 5'-untranslated region; the second contains the signal peptide and 34–41 amino acids of the mature peptide; and the third contains the rest of the mature peptide and the 3'-untranslated region. A single gene encodes this subunit in all species studied (43).

Once synthesized and secreted, the FSH molecule has a plasma half-life averaging 149 min (ranging from 95 to 250 min), which is about 5 times longer than the approximately 30 min for LH (105, 106). Removal of sialic (neuraminic) acid residues from the proteins reduces their plasma half-lives because the liver binds asialoglycoproteins and removes them from the circulation (107). Metabolic clearance is decreased by only one-third following bilateral nephrectomy (108), further indicating that the liver is the major site of clearance. The implication of its slow clearance rate in vivo for serum FSH levels is that they can neither increase nor decrease as rapidly as those of LH: It takes one half-life for the equilibrium concentration of a molecule to be attained after its secretion rate has increased or decreased abruptly. This difference between LH and FSH clearance rate in vivo may explain why GnRH stimulation is incapable of eliciting pulses of FSH in vivo, while it does stimulate FSH pulses in vitro.

Microheterogeneity of FSH and Variability in B:I Ratio

Recently, it has become clear that RIA and bioassay measurements of FSH frequently do not coincide because numerous, slightly varying forms of FSH exist that vary in their bioactivity:immunoactivity (B:I) ratios. The most commonly used and best-characterized FSH bioassays are assays that measure Sertoli or granulosa cell (GC) aromatase activity. FSH induction of aromatase activity can be enhanced with the addition of estrogens, androgens, insulin or IGF-I, a phosphodiesterase inhibitor, and hCG. Polyethylene glycol is used to separate FSH from other serum proteins that may inhibit bioactivity (109). This variability results from different carbohydrate moieties being covalently linked to asparagine residues at positions 52 and 78 of the α-subunit and positions 13 and 30 of the β-subunit (45, 109). The most important of these residues in terms of bioactivity are sialic acid residues. Removal of sialic acid residues decreases the overall in vivo bioactivity by increasing clearance rate (45, 109, 110); however, the FSH receptor binding activity and the in vitro bioactivity increase with the removal of sialic acid residues (111). The removal of other sugar moieties internal to sialic acid reduces the protein's ability to increase cAMP levels in target cells (112). Several different subpopulations of FSH have been detected in the circulation using two separation techniques (45), and the term *microheterogeneity* is used to refer to this phenomenon. Two sub-groups of FSH are revealed by Concanavalin A (Con A) affinity chroma-tography. The Con A unbound:Con A bound ratio increases dramatically just before the proestrous surge and then declines during the afternoon (45). This is blocked by phenobarbital treatment (45). Polyacrylamide gel isoelectric focusing (PAGE-IEF) further breaks these two groups down to 6 species, 4 of which bind to Con A (pI = 6.0, 5.7, 5.1, and 4.7) and 2 of which do not (pI = 5.4 and 4.2–3.8). The species with the lowest pI also have the greatest number of sialic acid residues (45). These species also have little binding activity in a seminiferous tubule radioreceptor assay (RRA). The results with an in vitro granulosa cell bioassay are very simi-lar, with the more alkaline species having the greatest bioactivity (45). Treatment of the most acidic FSH species with neuraminidase produces the other 5 forms of the hormone, each with an isoelectric point and RRA:RIA ratio identical to the endogenously produced versions (45).

The relative amounts of the different forms of FSH change during sexual maturation, during the estrous cycle, after gonadectomy, and after GnRH antagonist or steroid treatment. In female rats before vaginal opening (VO), all 6 of the FSH species are present; however, 60%–70% of these are the more acidic isoforms (45). At VO, these low-bioactive forms appear to be transformed to the more alkaline, highly bioactive forms (45). Similar changes occur at puberty in male hamsters (45). The overall B:I ratio de-clines in female humans between birth and puberty due mainly to declining bioactivity, while it remains constant in males (109). During the estrous cycles of the hamster (45) and the rat (113), the acidic forms predominate and increase prior to the proestrous surge; then, during the surge the propor-tion of the more basic forms increases. The more acidic, less bioactive in vitro, less rapidly cleared FSH isoforms also predominate (~90%) in ovariectomized and castrated rats, hamsters, and monkeys (45); however, the overall in vivo bioactivity is higher due to the longer half-life (45). Treat-ment of ovariectomized females with E not only suppresses gonadotropin levels, but also decreases the relative proportions of the acidic forms, while increasing those of the more basic, more bioactive in vitro, more rapidly cleared forms (45). In contrast, T-treatment of intact and castrate male rats has been shown to increase the in vivo bioactivity, the plasma half-life, and the percentage of more acidic isoforms of FSH (114–116). GnRH treatment also results in the secretion of the more basic isoforms (45). GnRH antagonist suppresses immunoactive FSH in women by only 20%–40%, but suppresses bioactive FSH, and thus the B:I ratio, more profoundly (109). In hypogonadal women, GnRH antagonist greatly increases the least bioactive of 4 isohormone peaks. These isoforms actually inhibit FSH-stimulated E-production in the granulosa cell bioassay (26). Gonadal steroids and GnRH probably influence pituitary neuraminidase and sialyltransferase activity to generate these changes in isoforms (45).

FSH Receptor

The FSH receptor (FSH-R) is located primarily on Sertoli cell membranes in the testis and on granulosa cell membranes in the ovary (117). Photoaffinity labelling and chemical crosslinking studies performed by Shin and Ji (118, 119) and Reichert and coworkers (120, 121) led both groups to the conclusion that the FSH-R is composed of three different subunits; however, the groups differed on the molecular weights of the subunits. Later, using stable, solubilized, highly purified FSH-R from calf testis, a single band was found with apparent M_r of 240,000 on autoradiography after SDS-PAGE (122). When SDS-PAGE was repeated in the presence of reducing agents, the 240,000 band disappeared, and a single band with M_r of 60,000 appeared (122). Based on these results, the FSH-R seemed to be oligomeric, consisting of 4 disulfide-linked monomers of 60,000 M_r each (122). Most recently, the cDNA for the FSH receptor has been cloned (123), demonstrating significant amino acid homology with the LH/CG (124) and TSH receptors: It is a single polypeptide that is predicted to contain 675 amino acids with M_r of 75,000 and that contains a large hydrophilic N-terminal domain attached to a region homologous with other G-protein-coupled receptors (123, 124). Since the LH-R has been shown to be readily proteolyzed into fragments, it is likely that the FSH-R is similarly labile, thus accounting for the many discrepancies among earlier studies as to its structure (123). It has been hypothesized for all three receptors, and demonstrated for LH/CG (125), that the large N-terminal hydrophilic domain is glycosylated and located extracellularly and that the C-terminal portion of the receptor spans the membrane 7 times and ends with a cytoplasmic tail that may be important in coupling to G_s.

The FSH membrane receptor—like the LH, TSH, and various neurotransmitter and rhodopsin receptors—probably exists, complexed with a guanine nucleotide-binding protein (G-protein). Functional receptor/G-protein/adenylate cyclase complexes have been reconstituted in lysosomes (126). Specifically, guanyl nucleoside triphosphates augment FSH-stimulated adenylate cyclase activity, and the GTPase activity of the G-protein

α-subunit terminates the signal (122). FSH enhances the exchange of bound GDP for GTP (126). Bovine calf testis contains both high-affinity:low-capacity and low-affinity:high-capacity GTP binding sites. GTP binding to either site can modulate FSH binding with the receptor by decreasing the affinity of the receptors for FSH (126, 127). Since cholera toxin, but not pertussis toxin, plus NAD eliminates the inhibitory effect on FSH binding, this is probably a G_s-protein (127); however, in both females (128) and males (127), the FSH receptor-associated G_s-protein possesses unique properties that distinguish it from those of other adenyl cyclase systems. FSH does not have a direct effect on the phosphatidylinositide system (122).

Removal of sialic acid residues from membrane preparations by neuraminidase treatment has been found to increase FSH binding to rat testis membranes (122) and porcine GCs (129). Phospholipase A- and C-, but not D-, treatment abolished FSH-specific binding to cell-free membrane preparations, but not to detergent-solubilized receptors, suggesting a permissive role for receptor or parareceptor phospholipids in situ (122). In another study, however, neither 24-h coincubation with neuraminidase nor phospholipase altered binding of FSH in cell-free membrane preparations of porcine GCs (130).

FSH itself increases FSH binding in GCs in vitro (131) and in vivo (132) in a time-, dose-, and temperature-dependent manner, due to a 2.3-fold increase in receptor number and a 5.4-fold increase in affinity (130). The increase in binding appears to be due to unmasking of cryptic FSH binding sites (130). Two classes of binding sites also occur in purified rat testis tubule membranes: high affinity ($Kd = 7 \times 10^{-11}$ M_r) and low capacity ($B_0 = 100$ fmol/mg); and low affinity ($Kd = 2.6 \times 10^{-9}$ M_r) and high capacity ($B_0 = 630$ fmol/mg). Highly purified receptor from bovine testis shows a single class of high-affinity binding sites ($Ka = 10^{-10}$ M_r; $B_0 = 200$ fmol/mg) (122). Large doses of FSH induce loss of receptors from rat Sertoli cells in vivo and in vitro, probably through endocytosis (122). Fifty percent of radioactively labeled FSH is removed from the cell surface within 15 min and is broken down into amino acids, probably in lysosomes (122). However, in porcine GCs, it has been noted that the cAMP response to FSH attenuates very slowly in the presence of physiological and supraphysiological concentrations of FSH (131), but this attenuation of responsiveness seems to be inversely related to the above-mentioned ability of FSH to increase FSH binding to GCs (130). Taken together, these results may indicate that in the ovary, down-regulation of its receptors by FSH may not be an important regulatory mechanism. This might result in the prolongation of FSH action necessary for differentiation.

Mn^{++}, Mg^{++}, and Ca^{++} stimulate FSH-R binding. Co^{++} and Ni^{++} inhibit it by changing receptor affinity (122).

Actions of FSH

In the ovary FSH binds to receptors located on GCs and acts via the cAMP-dependent protein kinase pathway. FSH binding enhances early follicle cell development, as shown by the dramatic reduction of secondary follicles after immunoneutralization of FSH (133, 134) and hypophysectomy (135–137). The mechanisms of FSH action have begun to be understood more recently with the development of molecular techniques (reviewed in 138). FSH is important in the development of preovulatory follicles (PFs). The enhanced FSH responsiveness of PFs appears to result from an increase in the content of the stimulatory G-protein of the adenyl cyclase system (138). FSH is necessary for the induction of LH receptors in PFs (138). FSH binding to antral and preovulatory follicles increases aromatase activity (139) subsequent to LH-stimulated increases in follicular 17α-hydroxylase cytochrome P450 ($P450_{17\alpha}$) activity and mRNA content that leads to the production of androgens, which are then rapidly aromatized to estradiol by aromatase cytochrome P450 ($P450_{arom}$) (138). Estrogen and FSH then synergize to further increase aromatase activity, and $P450_{arom}$ mRNA content is greatly enhanced in the corpora lutea of pregnancy (138). FSH in PFs increases the protein and mRNA content of the inhibitory regulatory subunit of the cAMP-dependent protein kinase type II (RII_β or RII_{51}). This stimulatory action on RII_{51} of FSH is much enhanced in the presence of E (138). The role of this increase is not yet clear. FSH binding in the presence of androgen also stimulates progesterone biosynthesis (140), of which cholesterol side-chain cleavage (scc) is the rate-limiting step (141, 142). FSH plus E is 5–10 times more effective than FSH alone at increasing $P450_{scc}$ activity and mRNA levels, while E alone is ineffective (138). The stimulatory effects of FSH on LH receptors, RII_{51} and $P450_{17\alpha}$ are abolished by the LH surge, while the effects on $P450_{scc}$ are enhanced by the LH surge and remain enhanced throughout gestation if pregnancy occurs (138). The paracrine effects of activin and follistatin on GCs also require the presence of FSH. Activin increases FSH-induced aromatase activity and P and inhibin production, while follistatin inhibits aromatase activity and inhibin production and also stimulates P synthesis (143).

In males FSH binds to receptors on Sertoli cells of the testis, causing a variety of effects that are mediated, as in the ovary, by adenylate cyclase activation (117). The specific ways in which Sertoli cell function is altered by FSH change with age. In fetal and neonatal rats, FSH is essential for Sertoli cell proliferation and the initiation of spermatogenesis (144). In utero immunoneutralization of FSH drastically reduces Sertoli cell replication, and in hypophysectomized fetal rats, exogenous FSH stimulates thymidine incorporation into the DNA of Sertoli cells (145). During this time of Sertoli cell proliferation, the number of FSH receptors in the testis is also increasing as a function of the increased cell number (146). In neonatal rats FSH also increases DNA synthesis and mitosis, but this effect diminishes prior to puberty and is not present in adults (147). The importance of this postnatal stimulation of Sertoli cells by FSH is in the initiation of spermatogenesis (148), as is evidenced by the blockade of spermatogenesis that occurs after immunoneutralization of FSH (149). Prepubertal, but not adult, unilateral castration leads to a doubling of FSH levels within 4–5 days of surgery, which, in turn, brings about a compensatory hypertrophy and hyperplasia of the Sertoli cells of the remaining testis (150, 151). Recent work using highly purified FSH in hypophysectomized adult rats shows that FSH *is* involved in the maintenance of spermatogenesis in the adult rat (152). FSH alone increases round spermatids and pachytene spermatocytes; T alone maintains elongate spermatids; and together they maintain spermatogenesis almost at intact levels (152).

In adults FSH also stimulates a number of other Sertoli cell functions, many of which may influence spermatogenesis (117), including energy metabolism, RNA and protein synthesis, receptor down-regulation, internalization of FSH-R complexes, and cAMP phosphodiesterase activity. Sertoli cells secrete over 100 different proteins bidirectionally into the seminiferous tubule lumen and into the testicular interstitial fluid (153). FSH stimulates the secretion and/or synthesis of many of these, including androgen binding protein (117), inhibin (154), insulin-like growth factor I(IGF-I) (155), plasminogen activator, transferrin, and surface glycoproteins (117).

Summary and Conclusions

In the gonads FSH is primarily responsible for slowly developing phenomena, such as differentiation of the Sertoli and granulosa cells and maturation of the gametes. Compared to an event such as ovulation, these processes require relatively constant stimulation rather than rapid fluctuations in serum levels of regulatory hormones. FSH, with its slow metabolic clearance rate and, consequently, long serum transients, provides this kind of stimulation. As a result, FSH does not need to be regulated from minute to minute. The effects of GnRH on FSH are more sluggish than its effects on LH; they appear to be primarily on synthesis of the peptide and on its glycosylation rather than on secretion. In addition, FSH levels are highly dependent upon gonadal feedback, itself a slower regulatory mechanism than GnRH. Thus, the total time domain of FSH regulation *and* action is more sluggish than that of LH, providing the basic adaptive significance to the presence of two pituitary gonadotropins in vertebrates, rather than one.

References

1. Herbert DC. Localization of antisera to LH-β and FSH-β in the rat pituitary gland. Am J Anat 1975;144:379-85.
2. Herbert DC. Immunocytochemical evidence that luteinizing hormone (LH) and follicle-stimulating hormone (FSH) are present in the same cell type in the rhesus monkey pituitary gland. Endocrinology 1976;98:1554-7.
3. Schally AV, Arimura A, Kastin AJ, et al. Gonadotropin-releasing hormone: one polypeptide regulates secretion of luteinizing hormone and follicle-stimulating hormones. Science 1971;173:1036-8.
4. Amoss M, Burgus R, Blackwell R, Vale W, Fellows R, Guillemin R. Purification, amino acid composition and N-terminus of the hypothalamic luteinizing hormone releasing factor (LRF) of ovine origin. Biochem Biophys Res Commun 1971;44:205-10.
5. Yen SCC, Rebar R, Vandenberg G, et al. Synthetic luteinizing hormone-releasing factor: a potent stimulator of gonadotropin release in man. J Clin Endocrinol Metab 1972;34:1108-11.
6. Vale W, Rivier C, Brown M, Rivier J. Pharmacology of thyrotropin-releasing factor (TRF), luteinizing hormone-releasing factor (LRF) and somatostatin. Adv Exp Med Biol 1977;87:123-56.
7. Blake CA. Stimulation of the proestrous luteinizing hormone (LH) surge after infusion of LH-releasing hormone in phenobarbital-blocked rats. Endocrinology 1976;98:451-60.
8. Blake CA. Simulation of the early phase of the proestrous follicle-stimulating hormone rise after infusion of luteinizing hormone-releasing hormone in phenobarbital-blocked rats. Endocrinology 1976;98:461-7.
9. Greeley GH Jr, Allen ME, Mahesh VB. FSH and LH response in the rat after intravenous, intracarotid or subcutaneous administration of LHRH. Proc Soc Exp Biol Med 1974;147:859-62.
10. Wise PM, Rance N, Barr GD, Barraclough CA. Further evidence that luteinizing hormone-releasing hormone also is follicle-stimulating hormone-releasing hormone. Endocrinology 1979;104:940-7.
11. Wildt L, Hausler A, Marshall G, et al. Frequency and amplitude of gonadotropin-releasing hormone stimulation and gonadotropin secretion in the rhesus monkey. Endocrinology 1981;109:376-85.
12. Luderer U, Strobl FJ, Levine JE, Schwartz NB. Differential gonadotropin responses to N-methyl-D,L-aspartate in metestrous, proestrous and ovariectomized rats. In preparation.
13. Strobl FJ, Luderer U, Schwartz NB, Levine JE. Differential gonadotropin responses to N-methyl-D,L-aspartate in intact and castrate male rats. In preparation.
14. Gay VL, Plant TM. N-methyl-D,L-aspartate elicits hypothalamic gonadotropin-releasing hormone release in prepubertal male rhesus monkeys (*Macaca mulatta*). Endocrinology 1987;120:2289-96.
15. Labrie F, Drouin J, Ferland L, et al. Mechanism of action of hypothalamic hormones in the anterior pituitary gland and specific modulation of their activity by sex steroids and thyroid hormones. Recent Prog Horm Res 1978;34:25-93.

16. Drouin J, Labrie F. Interactions between 17β-estradiol and progesterone in the control of LH and FSH release in rat anterior pituitary. Endocrinology 1981;108:52-7.
17. Fallest PC, Hiatt ES, Schwartz NB. Effects of gonadectomy on the in vitro and in vivo gonadotropin responses to gonadotropin-releasing hormone in male and female rats. Endocrinology 1989;124:1370-9.
18. Hiatt ES, Schwartz NB. Suppression of basal and GnRH-stimulated gonadotropin secretion rate in vitro by GnRH antagonist: differential effects on metestrous and proestrous pituitaries. Neuroendocrinology 1989;50:158-64.
19. Grady RR, Shin L, Charlesworth MC, et al. Differential suppression of follicle-stimulating hormone and luteinizing hormone secretion in vivo by a gonadotropin-releasing hormone antagonist. Neuroendocrinology 1985;40:246-52.
20. Kartun K, Schwartz NB. Effects of a potent antagonist to gonadotropin-releasing hormone on male rats: luteinizing hormone is suppressed more than follicle-stimulating hormone. Biol Reprod 1987;36:103-8.
21. Blake CA, Kelch RP. Administration of anti-LHRH serum to rats: effects on periovulatory secretion of LH and FSH. Endocrinology 1981;109:2175-9.
22. Chappel S, Miller C, Hyland L. Regulation of pulsatile releases of luteinizing and follicle-stimulating hormones in ovariectomized hamsters. Biol Reprod 1984;30:628-36.
23. Condon TP, Sawyer CH, Whitmayer DI. Episodic patterns of luteinizing hormone and follicle-stimulating hormone release: differential secretory dynamics and adrenergic control in ovariectomized rats. Endocrinology 1986; 118:2525-33.
24. Culler MD, Negro-Vilar A. Evidence that pulsatile follicle-stimulating hormone secretion is independent of endogenous luteinizing hormone-releasing hormone. Endocrinology 1986;118:609-12.
25. Charlesworth MC, Grady RR, Shin L, et al. Differential suppression of FSH and LH secretion by follicular fluid in the presence or absence of GnRH. Neuroendocrinology 1984;38:199-205.
26. Dahl KD, Bicsak TA, Hsueh AJW. Naturally occurring antihormones: secretion of FSH antagonists by women treated with a GnRH analog. Science 1988; 239:72-4.
27. Arslan M, Weinbauer GF, Khan SA, Nieschlag E. Testosterone and dihydrotestosterone, but not estradiol, selectively maintain pituitary and serum follicle-stimulating hormone in gonadotropin-releasing hormone antagonist treated male rats. Neuroendocrinology 1989;49:395-401.
28. Rea MA, Marshall GR, Weinbauer GF, Nieschlag E. Testosterone maintains pituitary and serum FSH and spermatogenesis in gonadotropin-releasing hormone antagonist-suppressed rats. J Endocrinol 1986;108:101-7.
29. Gallo RV. Pulsatile LH release during periods of low level LH secretion in the rat estrous cycle. Biol Reprod 1981;24:771-7.
30. Leipheimer RE, Gallo RV. Acute and long-term changes in central and pituitary mechanisms regulating pulsatile luteinizing hormone secretion after ovariectomy in the rat. Neuroendocrinology 1983;37:421-6.
31. Ellis GB, Desjardins C. Male rats secrete luteinizing hormone and testosterone episodically. Endocrinology 1982;110:1618-27.

32. Ellis GB, Desjardins C. Orchidectomy unleashes pulsatile luteinizing hormone secretion in the rat. Biol Reprod 1984;30:619-27.
33. Levine JE, Duffy MT. Simultaneous measurement of luteinizing hormone (LH)-releasing hormone, LH, and follicle-stimulating hormone release in intact and short-term castrate rats. Endocrinology 1988;122:2211-21.
34. Luderer U, Schwartz NB. 24 hour estradiol treatment is sufficient to suppress pulsatile luteinizing hormone release up to 5 days in the ovariectomized rat [Abstract]. In: Proc 71st annu meet Endocr Soc. Seattle, 1989:201.
35. Lumpkin MD, DePaolo LV, Negro-Vilar A. Pulsatile release of follicle-stimulating hormone in ovariectomized rats is inhibited by porcine follicular fluid (inhibin). Endocrinology 1984;114:201-6.
36. Urbanski HF, Pickle RL, Ramirez VD. Simultaneous measurement of gonadotropin-releasing hormone, luteinizing hormone, and follicle-stimulating hormone in the orchidectomized rat. Endocrinology 1988;123:413-9.
37. Arimura A, Debeljuk L, Schally AV. Blockade of the preovulatory surge of LH and FSH and of ovulation by anti-LH-RH serum in rats. Endocrinology 1974; 95:323-5.
38. Koch Y, Chobsieng P, Zor U, Fridkin M, Lindner HR. Suppression of gonado-tropin secretion and prevention of ovulation in the rat by antiserum to synthetic gonadotropin-releasing hormone. Biochem Biophys Res Commun 1973; 55:623-9.
39. Lopez FJ, Donoso AO, Negro-Vilar A. Endogenous excitatory amino acid neurotransmission regulates the estradiol-induced LH surge in ovariectomized rats. Endocrinology 1990;126:1771-6.
40. Schwartz NB, Rivier C, Rivier J, Vale WW. Effect of gonadotropin-releasing hormone antagonists on serum follicle-stimulating hormone and luteinizing hormone under conditions of singular follicle-stimulating hormone secretion. Biol Reprod 1985;32:391-8.
41. Schwartz NB, Talley WL. Effects of exogenous LH or FSH on endogenous FSH, progesterone, and estradiol secretion. Biol Reprod 1978;17:820-8.
42. Woodruff TK, D'Agostino J, Schwartz NB, Mayo KE. Decreased inhibin gene expression in preovulatory follicles requires primary gonadotropin surges. Endocrinology 1989;124:2193-9.
43. Gharib SD, Wierman ME, Shupnik MA, Chin WW. Molecular biology of the pituitary gonadotropins. Endocr Rev 1990;11:177-99.
44. Wierman ME, Rivier J, Wang C. Gonadotropin-releasing hormone (GnRH)-dependent regulation of gonadotropin subunit mRNA levels in the rat. Endocrinology 1989;124:272-8.
45. Chappel SC, Ulloa-Aguirre A, Coutifaris C. Biosynthesis and secretion of follicle-stimulating hormone. Endocr Rev 1983;4:179-211.
46. Weiner RI, Findell PR, Kordon C. Role of classic and peptide neuro-mediators in the neuroendocrine regulation of LH and PRL. In: Knobil E, Neill J, et al, eds. The physiology of reproduction. New York: Raven Press, 1988:1235-81.
47. Barraclough CA, Wise PM. The role of catecholamines in the regulation of pituitary luteinizing hormone and follicle-stimulating hormone secretion. Endocr Rev 1982;3:91-119.

48. Daane TA, Parlow AF. Periovulatory patterns of rat serum follicle-stimulating hormone and luteinizing hormone during the normal cycle: effects of pentobarbital. Endocrinology 1971;88:653-63.
49. Rance N, Barraclough CA. Effects of phenobarbital on hypothalamic LHRH and catecholamine turnover in proestrous rats. Proc Soc Exp Biol Med 1981; 166:425.
50. McDonald JK, Lumpkin MD, Samson WK, McCann SM. Neuropeptide Y affects secretion of luteinizing hormone and growth hormone in ovariectomized rats. Proc Natl Acad Sci USA 1985;82:561.
51. McDonald JK, Lumpkin MD, DePaolo LV. Neuropeptide-Y suppresses pulsatile secretion of luteinizing hormone in ovariectomized rats: possible site of action. Endocrinology 1989;125:186-91.
52. Kalra SP, Crowley WR. Norepinephrine-like effects of neuropeptide Y on LH release in the rat. Life Sci 1984;35:1173-6.
53. Crowley WR, Hassid A, Kalra SP. Neuropeptide Y enhances the release of luteinizing hormone (LH) induced by LH-releasing hormone. Endocrinology 1987;120:941-5.
54. Savoy-Moore RT, Schwartz NB. Differential control of FSH and LH secretion. In: Greep RO, ed. International review of physiology. Baltimore, MD: University Park Press, 1980;22(Reproductive physiology III):203-48.
55. Ying S-Y. Inhibins, activins, and follistatins: gonadal proteins modulating the secretion of follicle-stimulating hormone. Endocr Rev 1988;9:267-93.
56. De Jong FH. Inhibin. Physiol Rev 1988;68:555-607.
57. Mahesh VB. The dynamic interaction between steroids and gonadotropins in the mammalian ovulatory cycle. Neurosci Biobehav Rev 1985;9:245-60.
58. Spitzbarth TL, Horton TH, Lifka J, Schwartz NB. Pituitary gonadotropin content in gonadectomized rats: immunoassay measurements influenced by extraction solvent and testosterone replacement. J Androl 1988;9:294-305.
59. Summerville JW, Schwartz NB. Suppression of serum gonadotropin levels by testosterone and porcine follicular fluid in castrate male rats. Endocrinology 1981;109:1442-7.
60. Plant TM, Hess DL, Hotchkiss J, Knobil E. Testosterone and the control of gonadotropin secretion in the male rhesus monkey (*Macaca mulatta*). Endocrinology 1978;103:535-41.
61. Campbell CS, Schwartz NB. Time course of serum FSH suppression in ovariectomized rats injected with porcine follicular fluid (folliculostatin): effect of estradiol treatment. Biol Reprod 1979;20:1093-8.
62. Hasegawa Y, Miyamoto K, Igarashi M. Changes in serum concentrations of immunoreactive inhibin during the oestrous cycle of the rat. J Endocrinol 1989;121:91-100.
63. Ackland JF, D'Agostino J, Ringstrom SJ, Hostetler JP, Mann BG, Schwartz NB. Circulating radioimmunoassayable inhibin during periods of transient follicle-stimulating hormone rise: secondary surge and unilateral ovariectomy. Biol Reprod 1990;43:347-52.
64. Schwartz NB. Selective control of FSH secretion. In: McCann, Dhindsa, eds. Role of peptides and proteins in control of reproduction. Amsterdam: Elsevier, 1983:193-213.

65. Rivier C, Cajander S, Vaughan J, Hsueh AJW, Vale WW. Age-dependent changes in physiological action, content, and immunostaining of inhibin in male rats. Endocrinology 1988;123:120-6.

66. Medhamurthy R, Abeyawardene SA, Culler MD, Negro-Vilar A, Plant TM. Immunoneutralization of circulating inhibin in the hypophysiotropically clamped male rhesus monkey (*Macaca mulatta*) results in a selective hyperse-cretion of follicle-stimulating hormone. Endocrinology 1990;126:2116-24.

67. Culler MD, Negro-Vilar A. Destruction of testicular leydig cells reveals a role of endogenous inhibin in regulating follicle-stimulating hormone secretion in the adult male rat. Mol Cell Endocrinol 1990;70:89-98.

68. Welschen R, Dullaart J, DeJong FH. Interrelationships between circulating levels of estradiol-17β, progesterone, FSH and LH immediately after unilateral ovariectomy in the cyclic rat. Biol Reprod 1978;18:421-7.

69. Butcher R. Changes in gonadotropins and steroids associated with unilateral ovariectomy of the rat. Endocrinology 1977;101:830-40.

70. Cunningham GR, Tindall DJ, Huckins C, Means AR. Mechanisms for the testicular hypertrophy which follows hemicastration. Endocrinology 1978; 102:16-23.

71. Robertson DM, Farnworth PG, Clarke L, et al. Effects of bovine 35 kDa FSH-suppressing protein on FSH and LH in rat pituitary cells in vitro: comparison with bovine 31 kDa inhibin. J Endocrinol 1990;124:417-23.

72. Legan SJ, Coon GA, Karsch FJ. Role of estrogen as initiator of daily LH surges in the ovariectomized rat. Endocrinology 1975;96:50-6.

73. Caligaris L, Astrada JJ, Taleisnik S. Biphasic effect of progesterone on the release of gonadotropin in rats. Endocrinology 1971;89:331-7.

74. Freeman MC, Dupke KC, Croteau CM. Extinction of the estrogen-induced daily signal for LH release in the rat: a role for the proestrous surge of progesterone. Endocrinology 1976;99:223-8.

75. Hoak DC, Schwartz NB. Blockade of recruitment of ovarian follicles by sup-pression of the secondary surge of follicle-stimulating hormone with porcine follicular fluid. Proc Natl Acad Sci USA 1980;77:4953-6.

76. Knox KL, Froelich K, Spiess A, Singson P, Schwartz NB. Effect of progester-one antagonist, RU486, on preovulatory serum gonadotropin surges [Abstract]. Biol Reprod 1990;42(suppl 1):62.

77. Lee W, Mason AJ, Schwall R, Szonyi E, Mather JP. Secretion of activin by interstitial cells in the testis. Science 1988;243:396-8.

78. Vale W, Rivier J, Vaughan J, et al. Purification and characterization of an FSH releasing protein from porcine follicular fluid. Nature 1986;321:776-9.

79. Ling N, Ying S-Y, Ueno N, et al. Pituitary FSH is released by a heterodimer of the β-subunits from the two forms of inhibin. Nature 1986;321:779.

80. Baker HWG, Burger GG, de Kretser DM, et al. Studies on purification of inhibin from ovine testicular secretions using an in vitro bioassay. Int J Androl Suppl 1978;2:115.

81. Gharib SD, Wierman ME, Badger TM, Chin WW. Sex steroid hormone regula-tion of follicle-stimulating hormone subunit messenger ribonucleic acid (mRNA) levels in the rat. J Clin Invest 1987;80: 294-9.

82. Gharib SD, Bowers SM, Need LR, Chin WW. Regulation of rat LH subunit mRNAs by gonadal steroid hormones. J Clin Invest 1986;77:582.

83. Papavasiliou SS, Zmeili S, Herbon L, Duncan-Weldon J, Marshall JC, Landefeld TD. α and luteinizing hormone-β messenger ribonucleic acid (RNA) of male and female rats after castration: quantitation using an optimized RNA dot blot hybridization assay. Endocrinology 1986;119:691-8.

84. Corbani M, Counis R, Starzec A, Jutisz M. Effect of gonadectomy on pituitary levels of mRNA encoding gonadotropin subunits and secretion of luteinizing hormone. Mol Cell Endocrinol 1984;35:83-7.

85. Godine JE, Chin WW, Habener JF. Luteinizing and follicle-stimulating hormones: cell-free translations of mRNAs coding for subunit precursors. J Biol Chem 1980;255:8780-3.

86. Abbott SD, Docherty K, Roberts JL, Tepper MA, Chin WW, Clayton RN. Castration induces luteinizing hormone subunit messenger RNA levels in male rat pituitaries. J Endocrinol 1985;107:R1-4.

87. Wierman ME, Gharib SD, LaRovere JM, Badger TM, Chin WW. Selective failure of androgens to regulate follicle-stimulating hormone β messenger ribonucleic acid levels in the male rat. Mol Endocrinol 1988;2:492-8.

88. Alexander DC, Miller WL. Regulation of ovine follicle-stimulating hormone β-chain mRNA by 17β-estradiol in vivo and in vitro. J Biol Chem 1982;257:2282-6.

89. Landefeld TD, Kepa J, Karsch FJ. Regulation of a subunit synthesis by gonadal steroid feedback in the sheep anterior pituitary. J Biol Chem 1983;258:2390-3.

90. Landefeld T, Kepa J. Regulation of LH beta subunit mRNA in the sheep pituitary gland during different feedback states of estradiol. Biochem Biophys Res Commun 1984;122:1307-13.

91. Shupnik MA, Gharib SD, Chin WW. Estrogen suppresses rat gonadotropin gene transcription in vivo. Endocrinology 1988;122:1842-6.

92. Miller WL, Knight MM, Grimek HJ, Gorski J. Estrogen regulation of follicle-stimulating hormone in cell cultures of sheep pituitaries. Endocrinology 1977;100:1306-16.

93. Phillips CL, Lin L-W, Wu JC, Guzman K, Milsted A, Miller WL. 17β-estradiol and progesterone inhibit transcription of the genes encoding the subunits of ovine follicle-stimulating hormone. Mol Endocrinol 1988;2:641-9.

94. Shupnik MA, Gharib SD, Chin WW. Divergent effects of estradiol on gonadotropin gene transcription in pituitary fragments. Mol Endocrinol 1989;3:474-80.

95. Landefeld TD, Bagnell T, Levitan I. Effects of estradiol on gonadotropin subunit messenger ribonucleic acid amounts during an induced gonadotropin surge in anestrous ewes. Mol Endocrinol 1989;3:10-4.

96. Batra SK, Britt JH, Miller WL. A direct pituitary action of progesterone on basal secretion of follicle-stimulating hormone in ovine cell culture: dependence on ovaries in vivo. Endocrinology 1986;119:1929-32.

97. Attardi B, Fitzgerald T. Effects of progesterone on the estradiol-induced follicle-stimulating hormone (FSH) surge and FSH β messenger ribonucleic acid in the rat. Endocrinology 1990;126:2281-7.

98. Attardi B, Keeping HS, Winters SJ, Kotsuji F, Maurer RA, Troen P. Rapid and profound suppression of messenger ribonucleic acid encoding follicle-stimulating hormone β by inhibin from primate sertoli cells. Mol Endocrinol 1989;3:280-7.

99. Carroll RS, Corrigan AZ, Gharib SD, Vale W, Chin WW. Inhibin, activin, and follistatin: regulation of follicle-stimulating hormone messenger ribonucleic acid levels. Mol Endocrinol 1989;3:1969-76.

100. Pierce JG. Gonadotropins: chemistry and biosynthesis. In: Knobil E, Neill J, et al., eds. The physiology of reproduction. New York: Raven Press, 1988: 1335-48.

101. Denef C. Paracrine interactions in the anterior pituitary. Clin Endocrinol Metab 1986;15:1-32.

102. Childs GV, Ellison DG, Lorenzen JR, Collins TJ, Schwartz NB. Immunocyto-chemical studies of gonadotropin storage in developing castration cells. Endocrinology 1987;111:1318-28.

103. Lloyd JM, Childs GW. Differential storage and release of luteinizing hormone and follicle-releasing hormone from individual gonadotropes separated by centrifugal elutriation. Endocrinology 1988;122:1282-90.

104. Sairam MR. Gonadotropic hormones: relationship between structure and function with emphasis on antagonists. In: Li CH, ed. Hormonal proteins and peptides: gonadotropic hormones. New York: Academic Press, 1983;11:1-79.

105. Bogdanove EM, Gay VL. Studies on the disappearance of LH and FSH in the rat: a quantitative approach to adenohypophysial secretory kinetics. Endocrinology 1969;84:1118-31.

106. Bogdanove EM, Nolin JM, Campbell GT. Qualitative and quantitative gonad-pituitary feedback. Recent Prog Horm Res 1975;31:567-626.

107. Morrell AG, Gregoriadis G, Scheinberg IH, Hickman J, Ashwell G. The role of sialic acid in determining the survival of glycoproteins in the circulation. J Biol Chem 1971;246:1461-7.

108. Gay VL. Decreased metabolism and increased serum concentrations of LH and FSH following nephrectomy of the rat: absence of short-loop regulatory mechanisms. Endocrinology 1974;95:1582-8.

109. Hsueh AJW, Bicsak TA, Jia X-C, et al. Granulosa cells as hormone targets: the role of biologically active FSH in reproduction. Recent Prog Horm Res 1989; 45:209-77.

110. Vaitukaitis JL, Ross GT, Braunstein GD, Rayford PL. Gonadotropins and their subunits: basic and clinical studies. Recent Prog Horm Res 1976;32:289-331.

111. Manjunath P, Sairam MR, Sairam J. Studies on pituitary follitropin X: Biochem, receptor binding and immunological properties of deglycosylated ovine hormone. Mol Cell Endocrinol 1982;28:125-38.

112. Sairam MR, Bhargavi GN. A role for glycosylation of the α-subunit in transduction of biological signal in glycoprotein hormones. Science 1985;229:65-7.

113. Ulloa-Aguirre A, Espinoza R, Damian-Matsumura P, et al. Studies on the micro-heterogeneity of anterior pituitary follicle-stimulating hormone in the female rat. Isoelectric focusing pattern throughout the estrous cycle. Biol Reprod 1988; 38:70-8.

114. Bogdanove EM, Campbell GT, Blair ED, Mula ME, Miller AE, Grossman GH. Gonad-pituitary feedback involves qualitative change: androgens alter the type of FSH secreted by the rat pituitary. Endocrinology 1974;95:219-28.

115. Diebel ND, Yamamoto M, Bogdanove EM. Discrepancies between radioimmunoassays and bioassays for rat FSH: evidence that androgen treatment and withdrawal can alter bioassay-immunoassay ratios. Endocrinology 1973;92: 1065-78.

116. Sharma OP, Khan SA, Weinbauer GF, Arslan M, Nieschlag E. Effects of androgens on bioactivity and immunoreactivity of pituitary FSH in GnRH-antagonist-treated male rats. Acta Endocrinol (Copenh) 1990;122:168-74.

117. Bardin CW, Cheng CY, Mustow NA, Gunsalus GL. The sertoli cell. In: Knobil E, Neill J, et al., eds. The physiology of reproduction. New York: Raven Press 1988:933-74.

118. Shin J, Ji TH. Compositon of cross-linked 125-I-follitropin-receptor complexes. J Biol Chem 1985;260:12822-7.

119. Shin J, Ji TH. Photoaffinity labelling of the follitropin receptor. J Biol Chem 1985;260:14020-5.

120. Branca AA, Sluss PM, Smith RA, Reichert LE, Jr. The subunit structure of the follitropin receptor. J Biol Chem 1985;260:9988-93.

121. Smith RA, Branca AA, Reichert LE, Jr.. The subunit structure of the follitropin (FSH) receptor. J Biol Chem 1985;260:14297-303.

122. Reichert LE, Jr, Dattatreyamurty B. The follicle-stimulating hormone (FSH) receptor in testis: interaction with FSH, mechanism of signal transduction, and properties of the purified receptor. Biol Reprod 1989;40:13-26.

123. Sprengel R, Braun T, Nikolics K, Segaloff DL, Seeburg PH. The testicular receptor for follicle-stimulating hormone: structure and functional expression of cloned cDNA. Mol Endocrinol 1990;4:525-30.

124. McFarland KC, Sprengel R, Phillips KS, et al. Lutropin-choriogonadotropin receptor: an unusual member of the G-protein-coupled receptor family. Science 1989;245:494-9.

125. Rodriguez MC, Segaloff DL. The orientation of the lutropin/choriogonadotropin receptor in rat luteal cells as revealed by site-specific antibodies. Endocrinology 1990;127:674-81.

126. Grasso P, Dattatreyamurty B, Reichert LE, Jr. Reconstitution of hormone-responsive detergent-solubilized follicle-stimulating hormone receptors into liposomes. Mol Endocrinol 1988;2:420-30.

127. Zhang S-B, Dattatreyamurty B, Reichert LE, Jr. Regulation of follicle-stimulating hormone binding to receptors on bovine calf testis membranes by cholera toxin-sensitive guanine nucleotide binding protein. Mol Endocrinol 1988; 2:148-58.

128. Hunzicker-Dunn M, LaBarbera AR. Unique properties of the follicle-stimulating hormone- and cholera toxin-sensitive adenyl cyclase of immature rat granulosa cells. Endocrinology 1986;118:302-11.

129. Nishimori K, Yamoto M, Nakano R. In vitro membrane desialylation in porcine granulosa cells unmasks functional receptors for follicle-stimulating hormone. Endocrinology 1989;124:2659-65.

130. Ford KA, LaBarbera AR. Follicle-stimulating hormone (FSH) unmasks specific high affinity FSH-binding sites in cell-free membrane preparations of porcine granulosa cells. Endocrinology 1988;123:2374-81.

131. LaBarbera AR, Fisher AE. Porcine granulosa cell desensitization: prolonged FSH-responsive cAMP production in vitro. Am J Physiol 1983;244:E435-41.

132. Richards JS, Ireland JJ, Rao MC, Bernath GA, Midgley AR, Jr, Reichert LE, Jr. Ovarian follicular development in the rat: hormone receptor regulation by estradiol, follicle-stimulating hormone and luteinizing hormone. Endocrinology 1976;99:1562-70.

133. Lunenfeld B, Kaiem Z, Eshkol A. The function of the growing follicle. J Reprod Fertil 1975;45:567-74.

134. Peters H. The development of the mouse ovary from birth to maturity. Acta Endocrinol 1969;62:98-116.

135. Kim I, Shaha C, Greenwald GS. A species difference between hamster and rat in the effect of estrogens on growth of large preantral follicles. J Reprod Fertil 1984;72:179-85.

136. de Wolff-Exalto EA. Influence of gonadotrophins on early follicle cell development and early oocyte growth in the immature rat. J Reprod Fertil 1982;66: 537-42.

137. Moore PJ, Greenwald GS. Effect of hypophysectomy and gonadotropin treatment on follicular development and ovulation in the hamster. Am J Anat 1974; 139:37-48.

138. Richards JS, Hedin L. Molecular aspects of hormone action in ovarian follicular development, ovulation, and luteinization. Annu Rev Physiol 1988;50: 441-63.

139. Dorrington JH, Moon YS, Armstrong DT. Estradiol-17β biosynthesis in cultured granulosa cells from hypophysectomized immature rats. Endocrinology 1975;97:1328-31.

140. Nimrod A. Studies on the synergistic effect of androgen on the stimulation of progestin secretion in cultured rat granulosa cells: a search for the mechanism of action. Mol Cell Endocrinol 1977;8:201-11.

141. Jones PBC, Hsueh AJW. Pregnenolone biosynthesis by cultured rat granulosa cells: modulation by follicle-stimulating hormone and gonadotropin-releasing hormone. Endocrinology 1982;11:713-21.

142. Toaff ME, Strauss III JF, Hammond JM. Regulation of cytochrome $P450_{scc}$ in immature porcine granulosa cells by FSH and estradiol. Endocrinology 1983;112:1156-8.

143. Xiao S, Findlay JK, Robertson DM. The effect of bovine activin and follicle-stimulating hormone (FSH) suppressing protein/follistatin on FSH-induced differentiation of rat granulosa cells in vitro. Mol Cell Endocrinol 1990;69:1-8.

144. Means AR, Fakunding JL, Huckins C, Tindall DJ, Vital R. Follicle-stimulating hormone, the sertoli cell and spermatogenesis. Recent Prog Horm Res 1976;32:477-528.

145. Orth JM. The role of follicle-stimulating hormone in controlling sertoli cell proliferation in testes of fetal rats. Endocrinology 1984;115:1248-55.

146. Orth JM. Proliferation of sertoli cells in fetal and postnatal rats: a quantitative autoradiographic study. Anat Rec 1982;203:485-92.

147. Griswold MD, Mably ER, Fritz IB. FSH stimulation of DNA synthesis in sertoli cells in culture. Mol Cell Endocrinol 1976;4:139-49.
148. Chemes HE, Dym M, Raj HGM. The role of gonadotropins and testosterone on initiation of spermatogenesis in the immature rat. Biol Reprod 1979;21:241-9.
149. Chemes HE, Dym M, Raj HGM. Hormonal regulation of sertoli cell differentiation. Biol Reprod 1979;21:251-62.
150. Orth JM, Higginbotham CA, Salisbury RL. Hemicastration causes and testosterone prevents enhanced uptake of [3H]thymidine by sertoli cells in testes of immature rats. Biol Reprod 1984;30:263-70.
151. Waites GMH, Wenstrom JC, Crabo BG, Hamilton DW. Rapid compensatory hypertrophy of the lamb testis after neonatal hemiorchidectomy: endocrine and light microscopial morphometric analyses. Endocrinology 1983;112:2159-67.
152. Bartlett JMS, Weinbauer GF, Nieschlag E. Differential effects of FSH and testosterone on the maintenance of spermatogenesis in the adult hypophysectomized rat. J Endocrinol 1989;121:49-58.
153. Wright WW, Parvinen MM, Musto NA, et al. Identification of stage-specific proteins synthesized by rat seminiferous tubules. Biol Reprod 1983;29:257-70.
154. Sharpe RM, Swanston IA, Cooper I, Tsonis CG, McNeilly AS. Factors affecting the secretion of immunoactive inhibin into testicular interstitial fluid in rats. J Endocrinol 1988;119:315-26.
155. Closset J, Gothot A, Sente B, et al. Pituitary hormones dependent expression of insulin-like growth factors I and II in the immature hypophysectomized rat testis. Mol Cell Endocrinol 1989;3:1125-31.

Part I

Neuroendocrinology of FSH Secretion

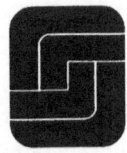

2

Modulation of Gonadotropin Secretion by Proteins of the Inhibin Family: Studies in the Female Rat

CATHERINE RIVIER AND WYLIE VALE

The secretion of FSH by anterior pituitary gonadotropes is controlled by both brain factors and those of peripheral origin. Gonadotropin releasing hormone (GnRH), a decapeptide originally characterized in mammalian hypothalamus (1, 2), stimulates FSH secretion in a variety of animal models; removal of GnRH, or blockade of its receptors, decreases basal FSH levels (reviewed in 3). However, several observations have suggested that existence of factors other than GnRH as major regulators of FSH secretion: Administration of GnRH antisera or antagonists to rats does not completely obliterate FSH release (4–10); LH can trigger a rise in FSH levels despite blockade of GnRH receptors (6) (a phenomenon that, as described below, is probably mediated through inhibin); and destruction of the dorsal anterior hypothalamus reduces LH, but not FSH, secretion by ovariectomized rats (11). At present, this GnRH-independent component of FSH release is believed to include sex steroids and gonadal proteins, such as inhibin, activin, and follistatin (reviewed in 12–114). The recent availability of recombinant human (rh) inhibin A has allowed us to reexamine the effect of this protein in a variety of animal models. Additionally, rh inhibin, combined with GnRH antagonists and inhibin antibodies, is proving to be a powerful tool with which to investigate the respective physiological role and pharmacological effects of GnRH and gonadal proteins in modulating reproductive functions.

This chapter describes and discusses studies conducted in our laboratories that were aimed at investigating the physiological role and pharmacological effects of inhibin alone or in conjunction with GnRH in mediating LH and FSH secretion by the female rat.

As briefly discussed above, GnRH represents an essential modulator of LH and FSH secretion (reviewed in 15, 16). LH is released in a pulsatile manner, and the observation of congruent GnRH and LH pulses (17, 18) had suggested that this pattern was primarily dependent on endogenous GnRH. This hypothesis is supported by the finding of markedly inhibited LH release in rats injected with GnRH antisera or antagonists (Fig. 2.1) (9, 10, 19). On the other hand, the concomitant measurement of portal GnRH levels and plasma FSH values has shown that GnRH and FSH release are not temporally associated in any consistent manner in intact rats, although a higher correlation has been found in the absence of the gonads (17, 18). In agreement with this observation, we have observed that not all rats exhibit a pulsatile pattern of FSH secretion (Fig. 2.1). Whether such pulses, when they occur, are dependent on endogenous GnRH is not firmly established. Several investigators reported that GnRH antisera, while lowering baseline FSH secretion, did not alter pulse amplitude or frequency (9, 10). On the other hand, we observed that a GnRH antagonist, injected 12 h before the assay, lowered baseline FSH secretion and also diminished pulse amplitude (Fig. 2.1) (8). It should be noted, however, that a significant degree of spontaneous FSH release occurred in the absence of GnRH drive. Thus, presently avail-

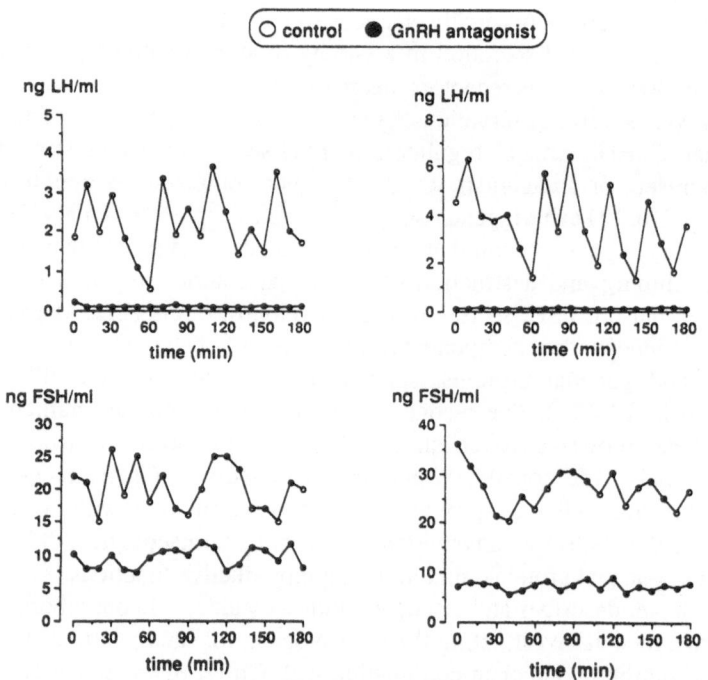

FIGURE 2.1. Effect of blockade of GnRH receptors with the GnRH antagonists [Ac-D2Nal[1], ΔCpa[2], Δ3Pal[3], Arg[5], Δ5-(p-methoxyphenyl)5-oxo-2-aminopentanoic acid[6], ΔAla[10]] GnRH (100 µg/kg, sc) on the pattern of LH and FSH secretion by ovariectomized rats. Four representative rats are shown.

able results suggest that endogenous GnRH modulates some, but not all, aspects of FSH secretion.

The physiological role played by endogenous inhibin, a 32-kD protein originally isolated and characterized from follicular fluid (20, 21) in modulating FSH secretion, is well documented. In the female rat, measurement of circulating immunoreactive inhibin and FSH values has suggested the existence of a functional relationship between the secretory rate of both compounds (22–24). Furthermore, removal of endogenous inhibin consistently increases plasma FSH, but not LH, levels (22, 25–28). Studies of the effects of immunoneutralization of endogenous inhibin have allowed a better delineation of the respective role of inhibin, GnRH, and LH in mediating FSH release. Earlier work has shown that injection of GnRH antagonists or pentobarbital blocked the primary (proestrous) rises of both LH and FSH. This treatment, however, did not markedly interfere with the secondary (estrous) FSH surge when given after the preovulatory LH rise (29–33). The observation that exogenous LH restored the estrous rise of FSH in GnRH antagonist-treated rats (32, 34) suggested that this rise was dependent on LH-induced inhibin secretion (35). We subsequently extended these studies by demonstrating that the fall in radioimmunoassayable α-inhibin levels measured during the late afternoon of proestrus was prevented by injection of a GnRH antagonist at noon on proestrus and was restored by exogenous LH (23). Because the secondary FSH surge was decreased in animals treated with the GnRH antagonist, but occurred if these animals received exogenous LH, we proposed that the estrous increase in FSH release is at least in part dependent on changes in inhibin secretion. Support for the involvement of inhibin in mediating FSH secretion, particularly during the early morning of estrus, also came from studies showing that the secondary FSH rise could be suppressed by charcoal-extracted follicular fluid (FF) (36–38), a preparation containing inhibin (4, 39, 40). However, because FF was subsequently shown to also contain activin (41, 42) and follistatin (43, 44), results obtained from these earlier studies need to be evaluated with caution.

The role played by endogenous inhibin in regulating gonadotropin secretion has been investigated with the use of antibodies raised against the N-terminal portion of the α-subunit of inhibin (45). Removal of endogenous inhibin significantly elevates baseline FSH secretion, but is reported not to alter FSH pulses (27), an observation that we confirmed (Fig. 2.2) (8). On the other hand, we have consistently failed to measure any effect of removal of endogenous inhibin on LH secretion (Fig. 2.2). Thus, our results support the role of inhibin in specifically modulating FSH, but not LH, secretion in the female rat.

Finally, studies of the pharmacological effects of inhibin are now possible due to the availability of rh inhibin A (46). We have observed that the I.V. injection of this protein A (3-, 15-, or 75-μg/kg body weight), prepared as

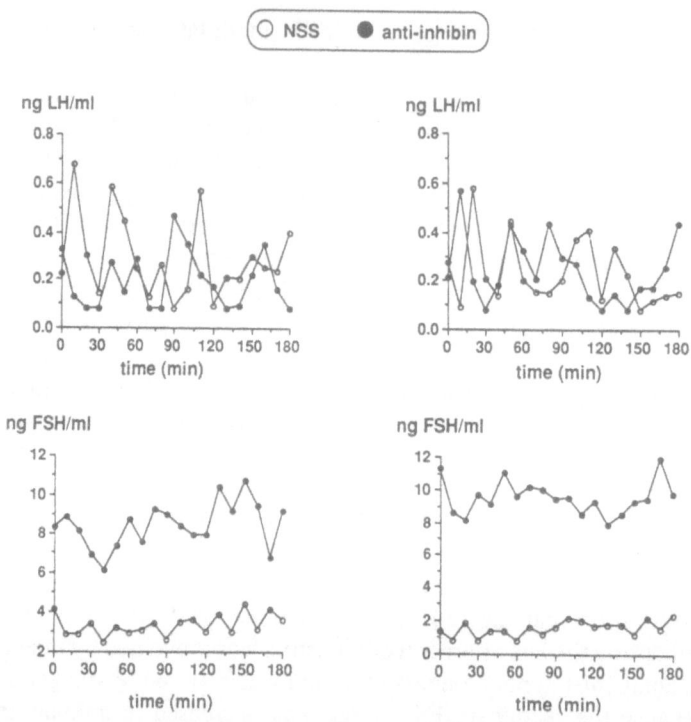

FIGURE 2.2. Effect of immunoneutralization of endogenous inhibin, using polyclonal antibodies raised against the N-terminal portion of the α-subunit of inhibin (45), on LH and FSH secretion by diestrus-2 female rats. Control animals were injected with normal sheep serum (NSS). Treatments were injected I.V. 6 h prior to the assay. Plasma radioimmunoassayable FSH levels of 4 representative rats are shown.

previously described (46), caused dose-related decreases in basal circulating radioimmunoassayable FSH values in female rats (Rivier et al., submitted to *Endocrinology*). This effect was observed in both intact (diestrus-2) and ovariectomized animals (Fig. 2.3). The inhibitory action of rh inhibin A on basal radioimmunoassayable FSH was first measurable 4 h after treatment and was maximum at 6–8 h (47), a delayed onset of action previously reported for FF (48–50).

Injection of rh inhibin A also interfered with all parameters of FSH release in gonadectomized rats (Fig. 2.4). In these experiments, LH and FSH levels were measured by RIA in the same rats following injection of the vehicle or inhibin. In contrast, inhibin did not measurably alter any parameter of LH secretion over the time course of action that we investigated (Fig. 2.4). These results suggest that at least in short-term experi-

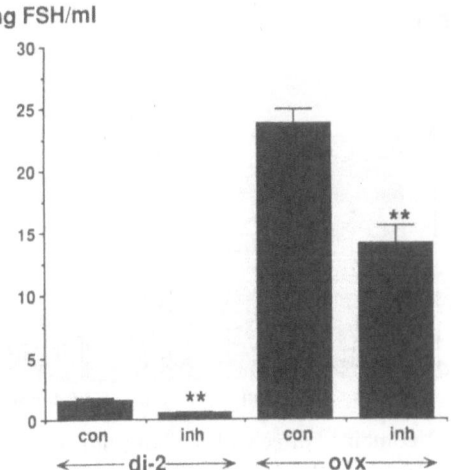

FIGURE 2.3. Effect of the I.V. injection of the vehicle (con) or rh inhibin A (inh, 25 µg/kg) on immunoreactive FSH secretion by intact diestrus-2 (di-2) or ovariectomized (ovx) rats. Blood samples were obtained 6 h after treatment. Each bar represents the means ± SEM of 5 animals (P ≤ 0.05; **P ≤ 0.01).

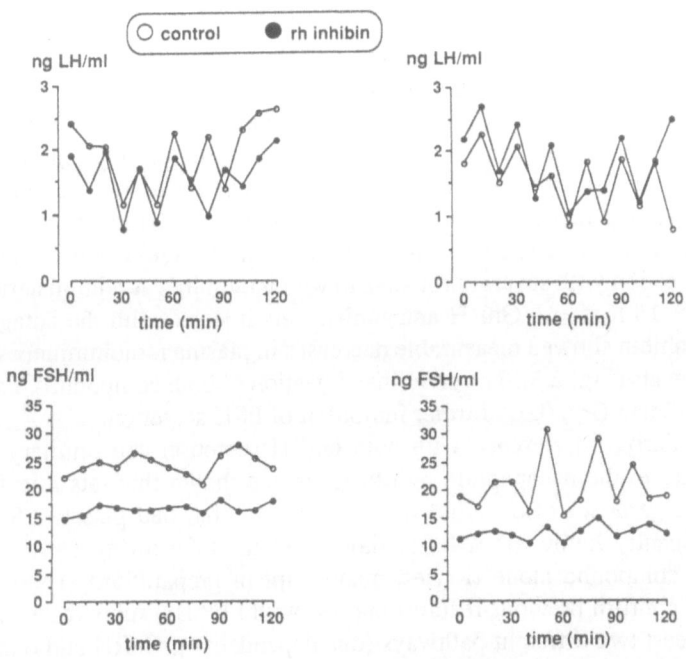

FIGURE 2.4. Effect of rh inhibin A (25 µg/kg, I.V. at 6 h) on the pattern of LH and FSH secretion by ovariectomized (ovx) female rats. Each line illustrates 1 representative animal.

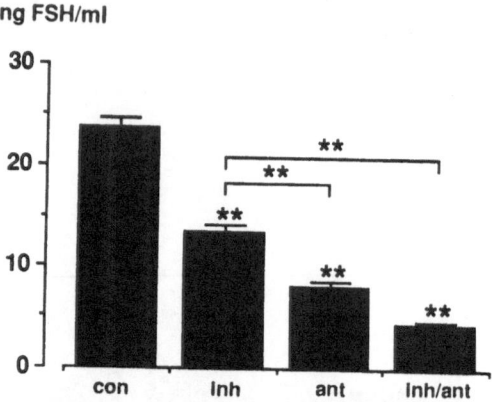

ng FSH/ml

FIGURE 2.5. Separate or combined effects of inhibin (inh) (I.V., 25 µg/kg) and the GnRH antagonist (ant) [Ac-D2Nal[1], ΔCpa[2], Δ3Pal[3], Arg[5], Δ5-(p-methoxyphenyl) 5-oxo-2-aminopentanoic acid[6], ΔAla[10]] GnRH (100 µg/kg, sc) on FSH secretion by adult ovariectomized (ovx) female rats. Blood samples were obtained 6 h after treatment. Each bar represents the means ± SEM of 5 animals (**P ≤ 0.01).

ments, inhibin specifically interferes with FSH secretion in the absence of measurable changes in LH release.

The existence of a GnRH-independent component of FSH release has been investigated in rats injected with FF and, more recently, inhibin in the presence or absence of GnRH drive. The first series of experiments has demonstrated that FF could significantly suppress FSH levels below values achieved in the absence of GnRH stimulation (4). We recently reexamined this question with several protocols in which inhibin was administered either with or 15 h after a GnRH antagonist. Rats injected with the antagonist or with inhibin showed measurable decreases in plasma radioimmunoassayable FSH levels (Fig. 2.5). The combined injection of both compounds resulted in a significant (P ≤ 0.01) further inhibition of FSH secretion.

Similarly, interference with both GnRH secretion and pituitary responsiveness to the decapeptide by estrogens has shown that rats injected with both large doses of estradiol benzoate and inhibin had plasma FSH levels significantly below (P ≤ 0.01) those measured following treatment with either compound alone (Rivier, manuscript in preparation). These results, which confirm previous results obtained with FF (51), support the existence of at least two different pathways (one dependent on GnRH and one dependent on inhibin) that modulate FSH secretion in the female rat.

One mechanism through which inhibin interferes with FSH secretion may involve a reduced FSH responsiveness to GnRH, a phenomenon observed in rats injected with purified inhibin (4, 37, 52–54) and in cultured pituitary cells exposed to the gonadal protein (55–60). Whether such changes are mediated through a decrease in FSH biosynthesis (61–63) and/ or changes in GnRH binding to the pituitary (59, 64) is unclear. We carried out several experiments designed to investigate the interaction between inhibin and GnRH in ovariectomized animals but obtained inconsistent results. Consequently, it appears that at present, the possibility that the in vivo administration of inhibin alters pituitary responsiveness to GnRH has not been fully resolved.

In conclusion, studies conducted by a variety of investigators have shown that endogenous inhibin plays a major physiological role in modulating FSH secretion in the female rat. The recent availability of rh inhibin has also allowed us to investigate the effect of this protein on gonadotropin release and to start dissecting the respective physiological roles and pharmacological effects of GnRH, sex steroids, and gonadal proteins in mediating gonadotropin secretion in the female rat. Although such studies have only very recently begun, they have demonstrated that inhibin causes a significant decrease in FSH release and may provide an important tool in evaluating the role of FSH in the process of folliculogenesis.

Acknowledgments. This work was supported by NIH grant HD-13527 and conducted in part by the Clayton Foundation for Research, California Division. C.R. and W.V. are Clayton Foundation investigators. The authors thank Drs. R. Schwall, L. Burton, A. Mason, and J. Mathers and also Genentech, Inc., for the generous gift of rh inhibin A.

References

1. Burgus R, Butcher M, Amoss M, et al. Primary structure of the ovine hypothalamic luteinizing hormone-releasing factor (LRF). Proc Natl Acad Sci USA 1972;69:278-82.
2. Matsuo H, Baba Y, Nair R, et al. Structure of the porcine LH- and FSH-releasing hormone, I. Proposed amino acid sequence. Biochem Biophys Res Commun 1971;43:1334-9.
3. McNeilly AS. The control of FSH secretion. Acta Endocrinol (Copenh) 1988;288:31-40.
4. Charlesworth C, Grady RR, Shin L, et al. Differential suppression of FSH and LH secretion by follicular fluid in the presence or absence of GnRH. Neuroendocrinology 1984;38:199-205.
5. Grady RR, Shin L, Charlesworth MC, et al. Differential suppression of follicle-stimulating hormone and luteinizing hormone secretion in vivo by a gonadotropin-releasing hormone antagonist. Neuroendocrinology 1985;40:246-52.
6. Schwartz NB, Rivier C, Rivier J, et al. Effect of gonadotropin releasing hormone

antagonists on serum follicle-stimulating hormone and luteinizing hormone under conditions of singular FSH secretion. Biol Reprod 1985;32:391-9.

7. Kartun K, Schwartz NB. Effects of a potent antagonist to gonadotropin-releasing hormone on male rats: luteinizing hormone is suppressed more than follicle-stimulating hormone. Biol Reprod 1987;36:103-8.

8. Rivier C, Meunier H, Roberts V, et al. Inhibin: role and secretion in the rat. In: Clark JH, ed. Recent progress in hormone research. Laurentian horm conf. Newport Beach, CA, August 26–30, 1989. Orlando, FL: Academic Press, 1990;46.

9. Culler MD, Negro-Vilar A. Pulsatile follicle-stimulating hormone secretion is independent of luteinizing hormone-releasing hormone (LHRH): pulsatile replacement of LHRH bioactivity in LHRH-immunoneutralized rats. Endocrinology 1987;120:2011-21.

10. Culler MD, Negro-Vilar A. Evidence that pulsatile follicle-stimulating hormone secretion is independent of endogenous luteinizing hormone-releasing hormone. Endocrinology 1986;118:609-12.

11. Lumpkin MD, McCann SM. Effect of destruction of the dorsal anterior hypothalamus on follicle-stimulating hormone secretion in the rat. Endocrinology 1984;115:2473-80.

12. Vale W, Rivier C, Hsueh A, et al. Chemical and biological characterization of the inhibin family of protein hormones. In: Clark JH, ed. Recent progress in hormone research. Proc Laurentian horm conf. San Diego: Academic Press, 1988;44:1-34.

13. Vale W, Hsueh A, Rivier C, et al. The inhibin/activin family of hormones and growth factor. In: Sporn MA, Roberts AB, eds. Peptide growth factors and their receptors. Handbook of experimental pharmacology. Heidelberg: Springer-Verlag, 1990:211-48.

14. DeKretser DM, Robertson DM. The isolation and physiology of inhibin and related proteins. Biol Reprod 1989;40:33-47.

15. Vale W, Rivier C, Brown M. Physiology and pharmacology of hypothalamic regulatory peptides. In: Morgane PJ, Panksepp J, eds. Physiology of the hypothalamus. New York: Marcel Dekker, 1980:165-251.

16. Karten MJ, Rivier JE. GnRH analog design structure-function studies toward the development of agonists and antagonists: rationale and perspective. Endocr Rev 1986;7:44-66.

17. Levine JE, Duffy T. Simultaneous measurement of luteinizing hormone (LH)-releasing hormone, LH, and follicle-stimulating hormone release in intact and short-term castrate rats. Endocrinology 1988;122:2211-21.

18. Urbanski HF, Pickle RL, Ramirez VD. Simultaneous measurement of gonadotropin-releasing hormone, luteinizing hormone, and follicle-stimulating hormone in the orchidectomized rat. Endocrinology 1988;123:413-9.

19. DePaolo LV. Differential regulation of pulsatile luteinizing hormone (LH) and follicle-stimulating hormone secretion in ovariectomized rats disclosed by treatment with a LH-releasing hormone antagonist and phenobarbital. Endocrinology 1985;117:1826-33.

20. Mason AJ, Hayflick JS, Ling N, et al. Complementary DNA sequences of ovarian follicular fluid inhibin show precursor structure and homology with transforming growth factor-β. Nature 1985;318:659-63.

21. Mayo KE, Cerelli GM, Spiess J, et al. Inhibin α-subunit cDNAs from porcine ovary and human placenta. Proc Natl Acad Sci USA 1986;83:5849-53.
22. Rivier C, Vale W. Inhibin: measurement and role in the immature female rat. Endocrinology 1987;120:1688-90.
23. Rivier C, Roberts V, Vale W. Possible role of LH and FSH in modulating inhibin secretion and expression during the estrous cycle of the rat. Endocrinology 1989; 125:876-82.
24. Hasegawa Y, Miyamoto K, Igarashi M. Changes in serum concentrations of immunoreactive inhibin during the oestrous cycle of the rat. J Endocrinol 1989; 121:91-100.
25. Rivier C, Rivier J, Vale W. Inhibin-mediated feedback control of follicle-stimulating hormone secretion in the female rat. Science 1986;234:205-8.
26. Rivier C, Vale W. Immunoneutralization of endogenous inhibin modifies hormone secretion and ovulation rate in the rat. Endocrinology 1989;125:152-7.
27. Culler MD, Negro-Vilar A. Endogenous inhibin suppresses only basal follicle-stimulating hormone secretion but suppresses all parameters of pulsatile luteinizing hormone secretion in the diestrous female rat. Endocrinology 1989; 124:2944-53.
28. Culler MD, Negro-Villar A. Passive immunoneutralization of endogenous inhibin: sex-related differences in the role of inhibin during development. Mol Cell Endocrinol 1988;58:263-73.
29. Hasegawa Y, Miyamoto K, Yazaki C, et al. Regulation of the second surge of follicle-stimulating hormone; effects of antiluteinizing hormone-releasing hormone serum and pentobarbital. Endocrinology 1981;109:130-5.
30. Blake CA, Kelch RP. Administration of antiluteinizing hormone-releasing hormone serum to rats: effects on periovulatory secretion of luteinizing hormone and follicle-stimulating hormone. Endocrinology 1981;109:2175-9.
31. Condon TP, Heber D, Stewart JM, et al. Differential gonadotropin secretion: blockade of periovulatory LH but not FSH secretion by a potent LHRH antagonist. Neuroendocrinology 1984;38:357-61.
32. Ashiru OA, Blake CA. Stimulation of endogenous follicle-stimulating hormone release during estrus by exogenous follicle-stimulating hormone of luteinizing hormone at proestrus in the phenobarbital-blocked rat. Endocrinology 1979; 105:1162-7.
33. Shander D, Anderson LD, Barraclough CA. Follicle-stimulating hormone and luteinizing hormone affect the endogenous release of pituitary follicle-stimulating hormone and the ovarian secretion of inhibin in rats. Endocrinology 1980;106:1047-53.
34. Ashiru OA, Blake CA. Variations in the effectiveness with which rat follicle-stimulating hormone can stimulate its own secretion during the rat estrous cycle. Endocrinology 1980;106:476-80.
35. Schwartz NB, Talley WL. Effects of exogenous LH of FSH on endogenous FSH, progesterone and estradiol secretion. Biol Reprod 1978;17:820-8.
36. Schwartz NB, Channing CP. Evidence for ovarian "inhibin": suppression of the secondary rise in serum follicle stimulating hormone levels in proestrous rats by injection of porcine follicular fluid. Proc Natl Acad Sci USA 1977;74:5721-4.
37. DePaolo LV, Wise PM, Anderson LD, et al. Suppression of the pituitary follicle-

stimulating hormone secretion during proestrus and estrus in rats by porcine follicular fluid: possible site of action. Endocrinology 1979;104:402-8.

38. Rush ME, Ashiru OA, Lipner H, et al. The actions of porcine follicular fluid and estradiol on periovulatory secretion of gonadotropic hormones in rats. Endocrinology 1981;108:2316-23.

39. Channing CP, Gordon WL, Liu WK, et al. Physiology and biochemistry of ovarian inhibin. Proc Soc Exp Biol Med 1985;178:339-61.

40. DeJong FH. Inhibin. Physiol Rev 1988;68:555-607.

41. Vale W, Rivier J, Vaughan J, et al. Purification and characterization of an FSH-releasing protein from porcine ovarian follicular fluid. Nature 1986;321:776-9.

42. Ling N, Ying SY, Ueno N, et al. Pituitary FSH is released by a heterodimer of the beta-subunits from the two forms of inhibin. Nature 1986;321:779-82.

43. Esch FS, Shimasaki S, Mercado M, et al. Structural characterization of follistatin: a novel follicle-stimulating hormone release inhibiting polypeptide from the gonad. Mol Cell Endocrinol 1987;1:849-54.

44. Ueno N, Ling N, Ying S-Y, et al. Isolation and partial characterization of follistatin: a single-chain M_r 35,000 monomeric protein that inhibits the release of follicle-stimulating hormone. Proc Natl Acad Sci USA 1987;84:8282-6.

45. Vaughan JM, Rivier J, Corrigan AZ, et al. Detection and purification of inhibin using antisera generated against synthetic peptide fragments. In: Conn PM, ed. Methods in enzymology. Orlando, FL: Academic Press, 1989:588-617.

46. Mason AJ, Schwall R, Renzy M, et al. Human inhibin and activin: structure and recombinant expression in mammalian cells. In: Burger HG, DeKretser DM, Findlay JK, et al., eds. Inhibin—non-steroidal regulation of follicle-stimulating hormone secretion. New York: Raven Press, 1987:77-88.

47. Rivier C, Schwall R, Mason A, et al. Effect of recombinant inhibin on LH and FSH secretion in the rat. Endocrinology 1990.

48. Grady RR, Charlesworth MC, Schwartz NB. Characterization of the FSH-suppressing activity in follicular fluid. Recent Prog Horm Res 1982;38:409-56.

49. Campbell CS, Schwartz NB. Time course of serum FSH suppression in ovariectomized rats injected with porcine follicular fluid (folliculostatin): effect of estradiol treatment. Biol Reprod 1979;20:1093-8.

50. Marder ML, Channing CP, Schwartz NB. Suppression of serum follicle stimulating hormone in intact and acutely ovariectomized rats by porcine follicular fluid. Endocrinology 1977;101:1639-42.

51. Williams AT, Lipner H. Negative feedback control of gonadotropin secretion by chronically administered estradiol and porcine follicular fluid (gonadostatin) in ovariectomized rats. Endocrinology 1981;109:1496-501.

52. Koiter TR, VanDerSchaaf-Verdonk GCJ, Kuiper H, et al. Control of follicle-stimulating hormone secretion by steroid-free bovine follicular fluid in the ovariectomized rat. J Endocrinol 1983;99:1-8.

53. DeGreef WJ, Eilers GAM, DeKonnig J, et al. Effects of ovarian inhibin on pulsatile release of gonadotrophins and secretion of LHRH in ovariectomized rats: evidence against a central action of inhibin. J Endocrinol 1987;113:449-55.

54. Lumpkin MD, DePaolo LV, Negro-Vilar A. Pulsatile release of follicle-stimulating hormone in ovariectomized rats is inhibited by porcine follicular fluid (inhibin). Endocrinology 1984;114:201-6.

55. Fukuda M, Miyamoto K, Hasegawa Y, et al. Action mechanism of inhibin in vitro—cycloheximide mimics inhibin actions on pituitary cells. Mol Cell Endocrinol 1987;51:41-50.
56. Farnworth PG, Robertson DM, DeKretser DM, et al. Effects of 31 kDa bovine inhibin on FSH and LH in rat pituitary cells in vitro antagonism of gonadotrophin-releasing hormone agonists. J Endocrinol 1988;119:233-41.
57. Campen CA, Vale W. Interaction between purified ovine inhibin and steroids on the release of gonadotropins from cultured rat pituitary cells. Endocrinology 1988;123:1320-8.
58. Robertson DM, Giacometti MS, DeKretser DM. The effects of inhibin purified from bovine follicular fluid in several in vitro pituitary cell culture systems. Mol Cell Endocrinol 1986;46:29-36.
59. Wang QF, Farnworth PG, Findlay JK, et al. Effect of purified 31K bovine inhibin on the specific binding of gonadotropin-releasing hormone to rat anterior pituitary cells in culture. Endocrinology 1988;123:2161-6.
60. Jakubowiak A, Janecki A, Steinberger A. Similar effects of inhibin and cycloheximide on gonadotropin release in superfused pituitary cell cultures. Biol Reprod 1989;41:454-63.
61. Mercer JE, Clements JA, Funder JW, et al. Rapid and specific lowering of pituitary FSHβ mRNA levels by inhibin. Mol Cell Endocrinol 1987;53:251-4.
62. Carroll RS, Corrigan AZ, Gharib SD, et al. Inhibin, activin and follistatin: regulation of follicle-stimulating hormone messenger ribonucleic acid levels. Mol Cell Endocrinol 1989;3:1969-76.
63. Attardi B, Keeping HS, Winters SJ, et al. Rapid and profound suppression of messenger ribonucleic acid encoding follicle-stimulating hormone β by inhibin from primate Sertoli cells. Mol Cell Endocrinol 1989;3:280-7.
64. Wang QF, Farnworth PB, Findlay JK, et al. Inhibitory effect of pure 31-kilodalton bovine inhibin in gonadotropin-releasing hormone (GnRH)-induced up-regulation of GnRH binding sites in cultured rat anterior pituitary cells. Endocrinology 1989;124:363-8.

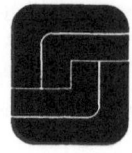

3

Control of Follicle Stimulating Hormone Secretion in the Male Rhesus Monkey (*Macaca mulatta*)

Tony M. Plant

The major drive to pituitary gonadotropin secretion is generated by the hypothalamus and is transmitted to the gonadotrophs via the hypophysial portal circulation in the form of an intermittent discharge of gonadotropin releasing hormone (GnRH). Although the morphological analysis of the network of GnRH neurons in the primate hypothalamus has received considerable attention (1), the neurobiological basis of intermittent GnRH release remains poorly understood. For the purpose of the present discussion, the neural network responsible for the generation of pulsatile GnRH secretion is viewed as a "black box" and termed the *hypothalamic GnRH pulse generator* (2, 3). In the male rhesus monkey, the secretion of follicle stimulating hormone (FSH), as well as that of luteinizing hormone (LH), appears heavily dependent upon hypothalamic input because lesions of this region of the brain that leave the vascular supply of the anterior pituitary intact reduce circulating concentrations of both gonadotropins to values that are undetectable and that fail to respond to castration (4).

The purpose of this review is to describe the systematic efforts of this laboratory over the last decade to describe the identity and site of action of the testicular hormones that regulate gonadotropin secretion in general and FSH secretion in particular in the rhesus monkey, a representative higher primate. Theoretically, testicular control of gonadotropin secretion may be achieved by the action of gonadal hormones directly at the level of the anterior pituitary to determine the responsivity of the gonadotroph to GnRH stimulation and indirectly at the level of the brain to modulate the nature of the intermittent hypophysiotropic drive to the gonadotroph.

Regulation of LH Secretion

The finding in the late 1970s that in the rhesus monkey, the maintenance of circulating testosterone (T) and estradiol (E) at preoperative levels following bilateral orchidectomy prevents the postcastration hypersecretion of both FSH and LH (5, 6) suggested that in this species, the negative feedback regulation by the testis of both gonadotropins is mediated solely by steroid hormones. This view was further supported at the time by the observation that in the male monkey, damage to the seminiferous tubules following surgically induced cryptorchidism fails to elicit a sustained increase in FSH secretion (7). Moreover, in our hands, institution of T replacement alone at the time of orchidectomy prevents circulating gonadotropins from rising above precastration control concentrations (6). This result led to the notion that testicular secretion of T alone fully accounts for the gonadal component of the negative feedback loop that governs the secretion of both LH and FSH in the male monkey. For several years this view, which is no longer tenable, as will be discussed, played a dominant role in determining the direction of this laboratory's research effort that focused on an examination of the neuroendocrine mechanisms underlying the inhibitory action of T on gonadotropin secretion.

In this context, the major action of T in the regulation of the activity of the gonadotroph in the monkey appears to reside at the level of the hypothalamus, where T (or a metabolite of this androgen) retards the frequency of the GnRH pulse generator. Evidence for this view is based on the following considerations. As in several other species, bilateral orchidectomy in the monkey results in a marked acceleration in LH pulse frequency (8). Since this mode of gonadotropin discharge is considered to be occasioned by and therefore to reflect an episodic pattern of GnRH release by the hypothalamus (see 9), it may be concluded that the testes retard the hypothalamic GnRH pulse generator. Direct evidence for this view has recently been obtained by Caraty and Locatelli (10) while examining the time course of GnRH concentrations in portal blood of entire and castrated rams. As may be seen from their elegant data (Fig. 3.1), GnRH secretion in this species is unambiguously episodic, and the frequency of its pulsatile release in orchidectomized animals is markedly higher than that in the presence of the testis.

Evidence for the hypothesis that the action of T to retard the frequency of the GnRH pulse generator plays a major role in the negative feedback regulation of LH secretion in the adult male rhesus monkey has been provided by studies employing the hypothalamic-lesioned animal, in which a normal pulsatile pattern of endocrine activity in the pituitary-testicular axis is restored with an intermittent I.V. infusion of GnRH. In this experimental model, the so-called hypophysiotropic clamp preparation, the negative feedback signal that governs

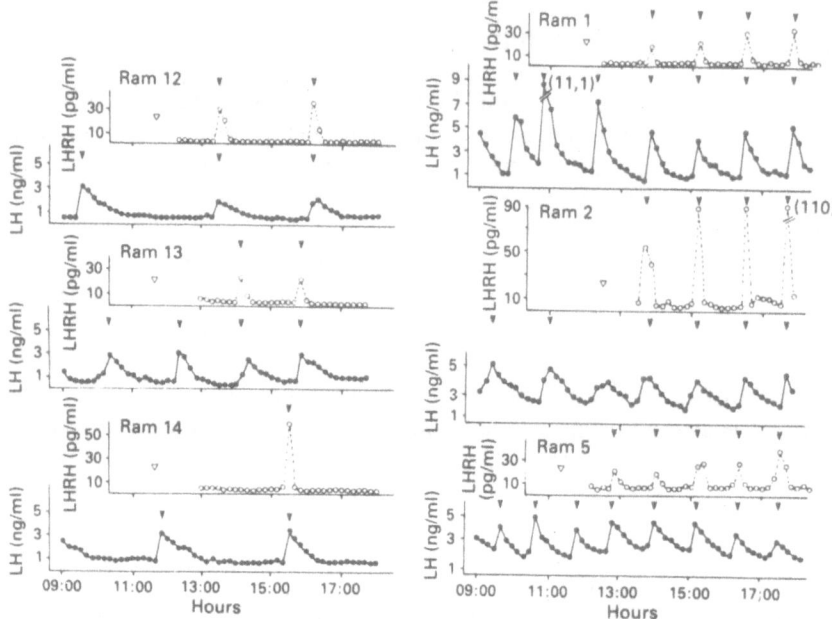

FIGURE 3.1. Time courses of GnRH (LHRH) concentrations in portal blood (open data points) and LH concentrations in the systemic circulation (solid data points) of intact (*left-hand side*) and castrated (*right-hand side*) rams. Note the acceleration in pulsatile GnRH release in the open-loop situation and the robust relationship between hypothalamic activity and intermittent LH release. Black arrows indicate algorithm-identified pulses, and white triangles indicate time at which the portal blood vessels were lesioned. Reprinted with permission from Caraty and Locatelli (10).

LH secretion may be eliminated while maintaining an unchanging pulsatile GnRH drive to the pituitary gonadotroph. When this is achieved by bilateral orchidectomy, the striking postcastration hypersecretion of LH characteristic of animals with an intact central nervous system (CNS) fails to occur (4). Instead, circulating LH concentrations remain at values indistinguishable to those observed prior to bilateral orchidectomy (Fig. 3.2). However, when the frequency of the GnRH drive to the gonadotroph in the hypophysiotropic clamp is increased to 1 pulse per hour, the frequency characteristic of the open-loop situation in animals with an intact CNS, plasma LH concentrations rise dramatically during the next 7 days (Fig. 3.2), a response reminiscent of that following castration in normal males. Taken together, the foregoing findings suggest that in the monkey, the negative feedback regulation of LH secretion by the testis is mediated primarily by the action of T to decelerate the frequency of the GnRH pulse generator and that direct actions of testicular hormones to inhibit LH release are minimal.

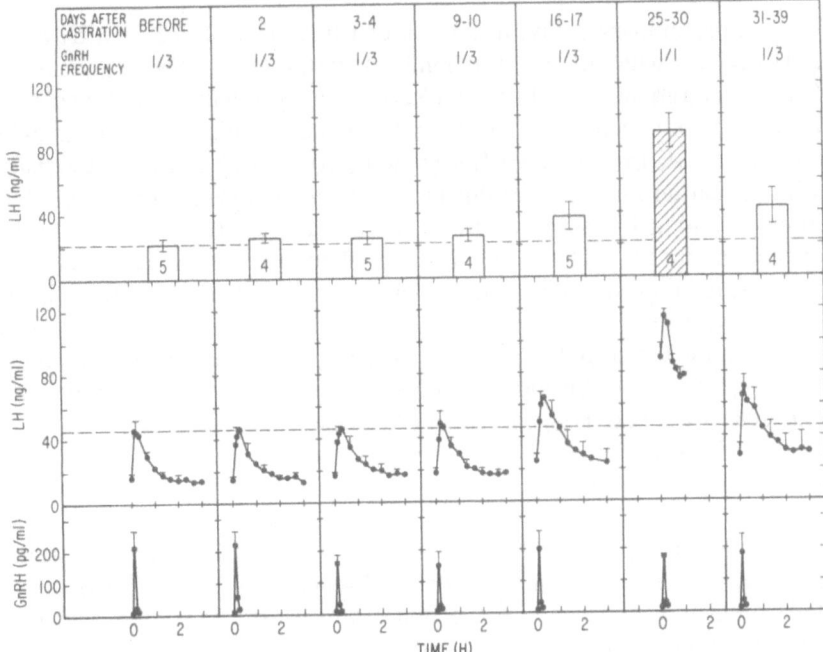

FIGURE 3.2. Mean plasma LH concentrations (*top panel*), composite plasma LH pulse profiles (*middle panel*), and composite peripheral plasma GnRH peaks in hypothalamic-lesioned GnRH-driven adult male rhesus monkeys before (*left-hand panel*) and after bilateral orchidectomy. Note that castration in the hypophysiotropic clamp fails to elicit an elevation in LH secretion. However, acceleration of the frequency of the GnRH drive (*second panel from right*) from the intact clamped frequency (1 pulse/3 h) to the open-loop frequency (1 pulse/h) results in a castration-like hypersecretion of this gonadotropin. Reprinted with permission from Plant and Dubey (4), © by The Endocrine Society.

The control systems that govern testicular regulation of LH secretion in monkey and humans appear to exhibit both similarities and differences. In the case of the former, the frequency of human pulsatile GnRH release appears to be regulated by circulating T concentrations (11, 12), and this indirect action of the steroid at the level of the brain probably plays a major role in the regulation of LH secretion in the human male, as it does in the monkey. Pituitary LH secretion in men, however, may not be fully emancipated from direct testicular feedback action. The evidence for the latter notion is based on preliminary studies of subjects with idopathic hypogonadotropic hypogonadism (IHH). As in hypothalamic-lesioned monkeys, adult patterns of endocrine activity may be elicited in the pituitary-testicular axes of men with IHH by a continuous intermittent infusion of GnRH (13).

From a preliminary study, it appears that treatment of such GnRH-driven IHH subjects with an aromatase inhibitor, testolactone, elevates circulating LH concentrations (14). In the GnRH-driven hypothalamic-lesioned monkey, on the other hand, immunoneutralization of circulating E with an ovine antiserum fails to stimulate LH secretion (15), a finding entirely consistent with the earlier result that in this model, complete opening of the feedback loop governing LH secretion by castration fails to elevate circulating LH concentrations (14). Thus, the long feedback loop governing LH secretion in humans, in contrast to that in the monkey, may involve an inhibitory action of estrogen directly at the pituitary level, in addition to the testicular deceleration of the GnRH pulse generator. Whether the former component reflects a human pituitary that is more sensitive to the inhibitory action of E or that is exposed to a greater E signal remains to be established.

The failure in the GnRH-driven hypothalamic-lesioned monkey to elicit an increase in the secretion of LH following removal of a physiological T signal by orchidectomy should not be taken as evidence that this steroid is incapable of exerting an inhibitory action directly at the level of the primate gonadotroph. Indeed, when circulating T-concentrations in GnRH-driven IHH subjects are elevated by injection of this steroid above those resulting from the endogenous hypophysiotropic signal, plasma LH concentrations decline significantly (16, 17). These findings provide unequivocal evidence that T can exert an inhibitory action on LH secretion directly at the pituitary level in humans. More recently, studies of GnRH-driven male rhesus monkeys have demonstrated that in this species also, supraphysiological levels of circulating T exert an inhibitory action on LH secretion directly at the pituitary level (Plant and Gay, unpublished observation). Additional studies of IHH patients have shown that the aromatase inhibitor, testolactone, reverses the ability of exogenous T to suppress GnRH-dependent LH secretion (14, 18), indicating that the action of the androgen may be mediated following its conversion to E. The contribution to the physiologic regulation of LH secretion of this inhibitory action of T on LH secretion, which in the monkey is demonstrable only at high levels of T, remains to be established.

Regulation of FSH Secretion

Turning now to the control of FSH secretion, it was a surprise for this laboratory to find that bilateral orchidectomy in the hypophysiotropic clamp preparation elicits a brisk and marked rise in plasma FSH concentrations (4). This elevation in FSH secretion is apparent by day 2 postcastration and continues in progressive fashion reaching a concentration an order of magnitude higher than precastration control levels 1–2 weeks later (Fig. 3.3). This result indicates that FSH secretion, in striking contrast to that of LH, is

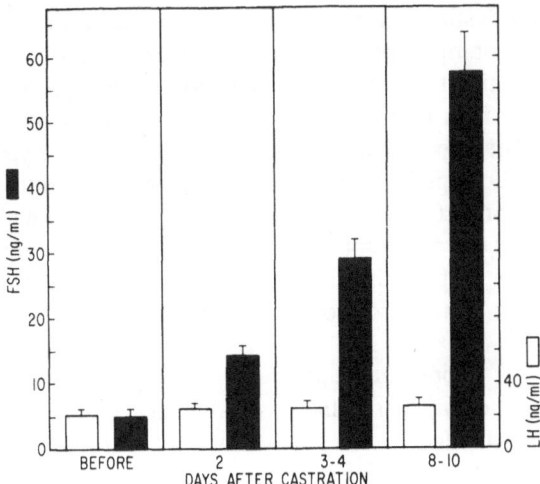

FIGURE 3.3. Mean circulating FSH (solid bars) and LH (open bars) concentrations in hypothalamic-lesioned GnRH-replaced (1 pulse/3 h) male rhesus monkeys before (*left panel*) and 2, 3–4, and 8–10 days after castration. Data were obtained from the study presented in Figure 3.2. Note the dramatic and selective rise in circulating FSH concentrations after orchidectomy in the hypophysiotropic clamp. Reprinted with permission from Plant (9), © by The Endocrine Society.

governed to a major extent by a testicular signal that exerts an inhibitory action on FSH release directly at the level of the pituitary gonadotroph. Since T-replacement instituted at the time of bilateral orchidectomy in animals with an intact CNS maintains circulating FSH at precastration control concentrations, it was reasoned that the testicular FSH inhibiting factor must be T and that this action of the steroid must be exerted directly at the level of the pituitary. This notion, however, was rejected when it became apparent that institution of T-replacement at the time of orchidectomy in the hypophysiotropic clamp fails to prevent the hypersecretion of FSH (15).

Here, the reader will recognize that the foregoing observation in the hypophysiotropic clamp seemingly contradicts the earlier finding that in monkeys with an intact CNS, T-replacement following orchidectomy maintains circulating FSH concentrations at values close to those observed prior to gonadectomy (6). This apparent paradox may be explained by positing that in both lesioned and CNS intact animals, T-replacement with steroid-containing Silastic capsules at the time of castration resulted in supraphysiologic concentrations of circulating T. This being the case, in the monkeys with an intact CNS, the decelerating action of this steroid upon the hypothalamic GnRH pulse generator would be exaggerated, and as a result, endogenous GnRH stimulation of the pituitary gonadotropes in these animals would have been compromised. In such a state of reduced hypophysiotropic drive, the concomitant loss of a testicular FSH inhibiting factor occasioned by orchidectomy fails to elicit a hypersecretion of FSH. In hypothalamic-lesioned GnRH-replaced males, on the other hand, the hypophysiotropic drive to the gonadotroph is independent of T-replacement since it is provided by the I.V. infusion of GnRH, and it is therefore maintained without interruption after combined orchidectomy and T-replacement, allowing the pituitary to respond to the loss of the FSH inhibiting factor with a postcastration hypersecretion of this gonadotropin. Evidence for this view has been obtained (19).

The failure of T to prevent the postcastration hypersecretion of FSH in the hypophysiotropic clamp raised the possibility that E secreted by the testes may play a role in the feedback regulation of FSH. This notion was addressed by examining the effect of FSH secretion of immunoneutralizing circulating E in GnRH-driven hypothalamic-lesioned males. Administration of E-antiserum in this model fails to elicit a rise in plasma FSH concentrations (15), suggesting that in this species, the testicular FSH inhibiting factor does not involve an E-component. Here, it is to be noted that in the preliminary study of GnRH-driven IHH human males referred to above (14), administration of testolactone, an aromatase inhibitor, resulted in an elevation of plasma FSH as well as that of LH, suggesting that in humans, circulating E may comprise a component of the testicular FSH inhibiting factor.

The recognition of the flaw in the earlier study of monkeys with an intact CNS, together with the failure of studies employing the hypophysiotropic clamp to provide evidence in support of a major role for testicular steroids in the suppression of FSH secretion, forced this laboratory to reexamine the possibility that the testicular control of FSH secretion in the monkey was achieved in a manner consistent with the inhibin hypothesis (20–22). In macaques, expression of the mRNAs that encode for the subunits of inhibin have recently been demonstrated in testes from pubertal and adult animals (Fig. 3.4) (23), and circulating levels of inhibin increase during the pubertal transition into adulthood (23, 24). Moreover, in adult monkeys bilateral orchidectomy results in a marked reduction in circulating concentrations of inhibin (24, 25). As a first step to determine whether inhibin may account for the testicular FSH inhibiting factor in the monkey, the effects on gonadotropin secretion of instituting combined treatment with charcoal-extracted porcine follicular fluid (pFF) and replacement with T at the time of orchidectomy were examined using the hypophysiotropic clamp (26). The results are shown in Figure 3.5. Combined T-replacement and pFF treatment maintained circulating FSH at concentrations similar to those observed prior to orchidectomy. Withdrawal of pFF treatment while maintaining T-replacement resulted in a progressive and dramatic rise in plasma FSH

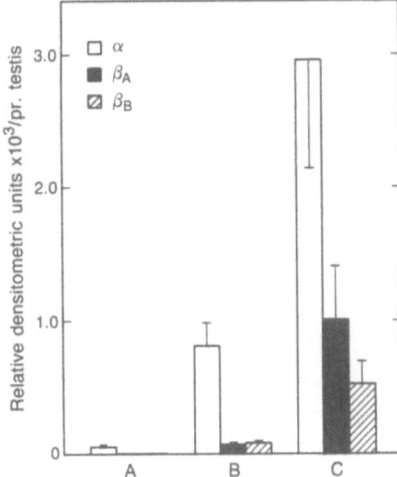

FIGURE 3.4. Steady state contents of the mRNAs encoding for the α-, β_A-, and β_B-subunits of inhibin in testes from prepubertal (A), pubertal (B), and adult (C) cynomolgus monkeys. Modified with permission from Keeping, Winters, Attardi, and Troen (23), © by The Endocrine Society.

concentrations that was reversed by the reinitiation of pFF treatment. These findings support the inhibin hypothesis and suggest that a testicular peptide, probably inhibin, plays a major role in the negative feedback regulation of FSH secretion in the male monkey.

To substantiate the foregoing view, it was first necessary to develop an alternative experimental model to the hypothalamic-lesioned GnRH-driven adult since this preparation was considered, on the basis of body weight, to be unacceptable for experiments requiring the administration of scantly available peptides and antisera. In the search for a more practical model, it was recalled that in the male rhesus monkey, the quiescence of the pituitary-testicular axis between 6 and 30 months of age is occasioned by an interruption of pulsatile hypothalamic GnRH release (27). Thus, in the context of the present problem, the 15-month-old juvenile male rhesus monkey, which weighs only 2–3 kg, is analogous to the fully adult animal bearing a hypothalamic lesion. Indeed, an adult-like pattern of hormonal activity in the pituitary-testicular axis, as reflected by circulating concentrations of LH, FSH, inhibin, and T may be prematurely induced in the prepubertal monkey by a chronic intermittent I.V. GnRH infusion (24), and subsequent bilateral orchidectomy and concomitant T-replacement elicit a selective hypersecretion of FSH qualitatively and quantitatively similar to that observed in the adult hypophysiotropic clamp (28).

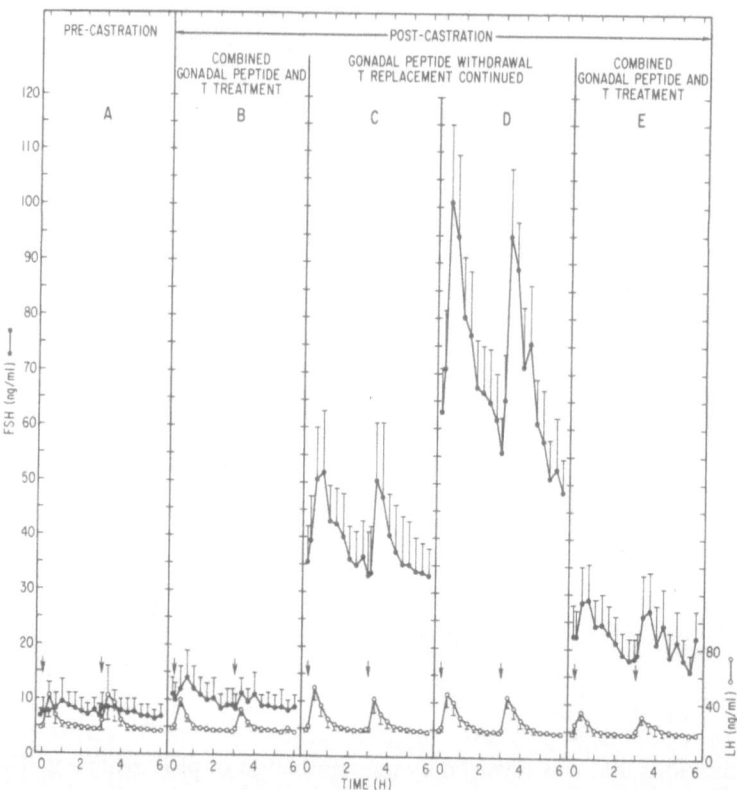

FIGURE 3.5. Changes in circulating FSH (solid circles) and LH (open circles) concentrations during 6-h windows (2 GnRH interpulse intervals) before bilateral orchidectomy (panel A) and during similar 6-h windows after bilateral orchidectomy and T-replacement with (B and E) and without (C and D) pFF treatment in GnRH-driven hypothalamic-lesioned rhesus monkeys. Arrows indicate times of GnRH infusions. The data shown in panel B were obtained 8 days postcastration. Treatment with pFF was withdrawn for 8 days on day 8 postcastration, and panels C and D show data obtained 4 and 8 days after withdrawal of pFF treatment. The treatment was then reinstituted, and panel E shows the gonadotropin profile on day 8 of reinitiated pFF treatment. Reprinted with permission from Abeyawardene and Plant (26), © by The Endocrine Society.

In collaboration with Drs. Culler and Negro-Vilar, recent studies of the juvenile hypophysiotropic clamp have shown that I.V. administration of a single bolus of inhibin antiserum raised against a synthetic fragment of the α-subunit of human inhibin elicits an increase in FSH release comparable to that observed during the first 2 days following bilateral orchidectomy in this experimental model (Fig. 3.6) (29). The change in mean plasma FSH concentrations following immunoneutralization of circulating inhibin was asso-

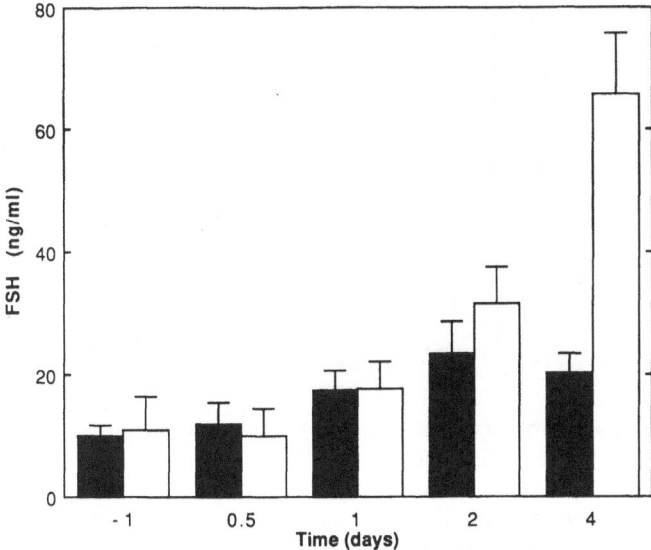

FIGURE 3.6. Mean FSH concentrations in GnRH-driven juvenile male rhesus monkeys 1 day before and 0.5, 1, 2, and 4 days after administration of inhibin antiserum (solid bar) and bilateral orchidectomy (open bar). ANOVA showed that FSH concentration on days 2 and 4 of immunoneutralization were significantly greater (P < 0.05) than those prior to injection of antiserum. Only on day 4 were mean FSH concentrations in immunized and castrated animals significantly different (P < 0.05). Reprinted with permission from Medhamurthy, Abeyawardene, Culler, Negro-Vilar, and Plant (29), © by The Endocrine Society.

ciated with a marked increase in FSH pulse amplitude (Fig 3.7). Administration of a control immune sera was without effect on FSH secretion, and the hypersecretion of FSH elicited by immunoneutralization of circulating inhibin occurred in the absence of a perturbation in the secretion of LH and T (29). Since the endocrine activity of the pituitary-testicular axis of the GnRH-driven prepubertal monkey is similar to that observed in the adult, the foregoing result provides evidence for the notion that in the sexually mature monkey, testicular inhibin is a major regulator of FSH secretion. This latter view has recently been fully substantiated by the finding that immunoneutralization of circulating inhibin in the normal adult male stimulates a dramatic hypersecretion of FSH (30).

The effects of immunoneutralizing circulating inhibin on FSH secretion have been previously studied in nonprimate species. In the adult male rat, administration of inhibin antisera similar to that employed in the study of the monkey described above fails to elicit FSH secretion (31, 32), indicating that in the rodent, inhibin's role in the postpubertal regulation of FSH secretion is

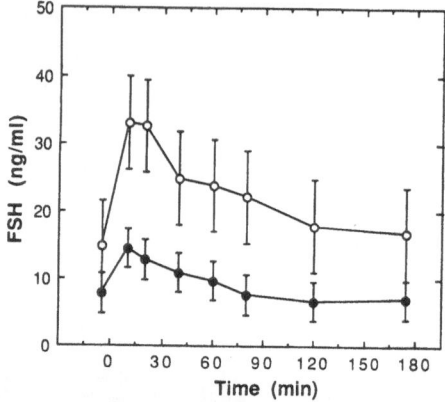

FIGURE 3.7. Pulse profiles of circulating FSH concentrations during an inter-GnRH pulse interval before (solid circles) and 2 days after (open circles) immunoneutralization of circulating inhibin. A GnRH infusion was administered at 0 min. Reprinted with permission from Medhamurthy, Abeyawardene, Culler, Negro-Vilar, and Plant (29), © by The Endocrine Society.

relatively trivial. In the ram, active immunoneutralization against the α-subunit of human inhibin results in an exaggeration of the seasonal rise of FSH secretion (33). Although the testicular regulation of FSH secretion in the adult sheep and monkey therefore appears to exhibit a common inhibin component, the FSH hypersecretion induced by immunoneutralization in the ram, in contrast to that in the adult male macaque, is associated with a concomitant elevation in circulating LH concentrations.

In view of these species differences, it becomes important to examine whether the control system underlying the testicular regulation of FSH secretion in the rhesus monkey is representative of higher primates in general. If inhibin is a major testicular regulator of FSH secretion in adult primates, it is to be expected that circulating concentrations of the testicular and pituitary hormone will be inversely related. Such a relationship between serum inhibin and FSH, however, was not observed in a recent study of men with testicular disorders associated with varying degrees of damage to the seminiferous tubules. In certain groups of azoospermic men, FSH concentrations were markedly elevated in the presence of immunoreactive inhibin levels that were indistinguishable from those in normal individuals (34). The most likely explanation for these data that contradict the inhibin hypothesis is that under pathophysiological conditions, the testes secrete inhibin peptides, such as the recently isolated α-subunit precursor protein (35, 36), that are immunologically active but biologically inactive. Support for this view has recently been provided by the report of varying degrees of α-inhibin immunoactivity in sera of hypogonadal male patients (37).

Summary

The following hypothesis is offered to account for the testicular regulation of gonadotropin secretion in the rhesus monkey. The control of LH release is governed by T-dependent changes in hypophysiotropic drive, most notably frequency, to the pituitary gonadotroph, while that of FSH is governed by changes in circulating levels of an inhibitory testicular signal, inhibin, acting directly at the pituitary. No doubt this simplistic model will require redefinition as our understanding of the hypothalamic-pituitary-testicular axis grows.

Acknowledgments. Work from the author's laboratory described in this chapter was supported by NIH grants HD-08610 and HD-16851.

References

1. Silverman A-J. The gonadotropin-releasing hormone (GnRH) neuronal systems: immunocytochemistry. In: Knobil E, Neill JD, eds. The physiology of reproduction; vol 1. New York: Raven Press, 1988:1283-1304.
2. Karsch FJ. Seasonal reproduction: a saga of reversible fertility. Physiologist 1980;23:29-38.
3. Pohl CR, Knobil E. The role of the central nervous system in the control of ovarian function in higher primates. Annu Rev Physiol 1982;44:583-93.
4. Plant TM, Dubey AK. Evidence from the rhesus monkey (*Macaca mulatta*) for the view that negative feedback control of luteinizing hormone secretion by the testis is mediated by a deceleration of hypothalamic gonadotropin-releasing hormone pulse frequency. Endocrinology 1984;115:2145-53.
5. Resko JA, Quadri SK, Spies HG. Negative feedback control of gonadotropins in male rhesus monkeys: effects of time after castration and interactions of testosterone and estradiol-17β. Endocrinology 1977;101:215-24.
6. Plant TM, Hess DL, Hotchkiss J, Knobil E. Testosterone and the control of gonadotropin secretion in the male rhesus monkey (*Macaca mulatta*). Endocrinology 1978;103:535-41.
7. Resko JA, Jackson GL, Huckins C, Stadelman H, Spies HG. Cryptorchid rhesus macaques: long term studies on changes in gonadotropins and gonadal steroids. Endocrinology 1980;107:1127-36.
8. Plant TM. Effects of orchidectomy and testosterone replacement treatment on pulsatile luteinizing hormone secretion in the adult rhesus monkey (*Macaca mulatta*). Endocrinology 1982;110:1905-13.
9. Plant TM. Gonadal regulation of hypothalamic gonadotropin-releasing hormone release in primates. Endocr Rev 1986;7:75-86.
10. Caraty A, Locatelli A. Effect of time after castration on secretion of LHRH and LH in the ram. J Reprod Fertil 1988;82:263-9.

11. Winters SJ, Troen P. A reexamination of pulsatile luteinizing hormone secretion in primary testicular failure. J Clin Endocrinol Metab 1983;57:432-5.

12. Matsumoto AM, Bremner WJ. Modulation of pulsatile gonadotropin secretion by testosterone in man. J Clin Endocrinol Metab 1984;58:609-14.

13. Santoro N, Filicori M, Crowley WF, Jr. Hypogonadotropic disorders in men and women: diagnosis and therapy with pulsatile gonadotropin-releasing hormone. Endocr Rev 1986;7:11-23.

14. Bagatell CJ, Bremner WJ. Testosterone's direct pituitary effect to inhibit gonadotropin secretion in men is mediated largely by aromatization to estradiol [Abstract]. In: Proc 72nd annu meet Endocr Soc. Atlanta, 1990;365.

15. Dubey AK, Zeleznik AJ, Plant TM. In the rhesus monkey (*Macaca mulatta*), the negative feedback regulation of follicle-stimulating hormone secretion by an action of testicular hormone directly at the level of the anterior pituitary gland cannot be accounted for by either testosterone or estradiol. Endocrinology 1987; 121:2229-37.

16. Finkelstein J, O'Dea L, Whitcomb R, Schoenfeld D, Crowley W. Testosterone infusion suppresses LH secretion at the pituitary and hypothalamic levels in the human male [Abstract]. In: Proc 70th annu meet Endocr Soc. New Orleans, 1988; 302.

17. Sheckter CB, Matsumoto AM, Bremner WJ. Testosterone administration inhibits gonadotropin secretion by an effect directly on the human pituitary. J Clin Endocrinol Metab 1989;68:397-411.

18. Finkelstein J, Whitcomb R, O'Dea L, Longcope C. Testolactone prevents the pituitary hypothalamic suppressive effects of testosterone on gonadotropin secretion in men [Abstract]. In: Proc 71st annu meet Endocr Soc. Seattle, 1989;448.

19. Abeyawardene SA, Plant TM. Reconciliation of the paradox that testosterone replacement prevents the postcastration hypersecretion of follicle-stimulating hormone in male rhesus monkeys (*Macaca mulatta*) with an intact central nervous system but not in hypothalamic-lesioned, gonadotropin-releasing hormone replaced animals. Biol Reprod 1989;40:578-84.

20. McCullagh DR. Dual endocrine activity of the testes. Science 1932;76:19-20.

21. Baker HWG, Bremner WJ, Burger HG, et al. Testicular control of follicle-stimulating hormone secretion. Recent Prog Horm Res 1976;32:429-69.

22. Franchimont P, Verstraelen-Proyard J, Hazee-Hagelstein MT, et al. Inhibin: from concept to reality. Vitam Horm 1979;37:243-302.

23. Keeping HS, Winters SJ, Attardi B, Troen P. Developmental changes in testicular inhibin and androgen-binding protein during sexual maturation in the cynomolgus monkey, *Macaca fascicularis*. Endocrinology 1990;126:2858-67.

24. Abeyawardene SA, Vale WW, Marshall GR, Plant TM. Circulating inhibin α-concentrations in infant, prepubertal and adult male rhesus monkeys (*Macaca mulatta*) and in juvenile males during premature initiation of puberty with pulsatile gonadotropin-releasing hormone treatment. Endocrinology 1989;125:250-6.

25. Fingscheidt U, Weinbauer GF, Robertson DM, deKretser DM, Nieschlag E. Radioimmunoassay of inhibin in the serum of male monkeys. J Endocrinol 1989;122:477-83.

26. Abeyawardene SA, Plant TM. Institution of combined treatment with testosterone and charcoal-extracted porcine follicular fluid immediately after orchi-

dectomy prevents the postcastration hypersecretion of follicle-stimulating hormone in the hypothalamus lesioned rhesus monkey (*Macaca mulatta*) receiving an invariant iv gonadotropin-releasing hormone infusion. Endocrinology 1989;124:1310-8

27. Plant TM. Puberty in primates. In: Knobil E, Neill JD, eds. The physiology of reproduction; vol 1. New York: Raven Press, 1988:215-37.

28. Abeyawardene SA, Plant TM. Bilateral orchidectomy and concomitant testosterone replacement in the juvenile male rhesus monkey (*Macaca mulatta*) receiving an invariant iv gonadotropin-releasing hormone (GnRH) infusion results, as in the hypothalamus lesioned GnRH-driven adult male, in a selective hypersecretion of follicle-stimulating hormone. Endocrinology 1989;125:257-9.

29. Medhamurthy R, Abeyawardene SA, Culler MD, Negro-Vilar A, Plant TM. Immunoneutralization of circulating inhibin in the hypophysiotropically clamped male rhesus monkey (*Macaca mulatta*) results in a selective hypersecretion of follicle-stimulating hormone. Endocrinology 1990;126:2116-24.

30. Medhamurthy R, Culler MD, Gay VL, Plant TM. Inhibin regulates FSH secretion in the adult male rhesus monkey, a representative higher primate [Abstract]. In: Proc 72nd annu meet Endocr Soc. Atlanta, 1990;215.

31. Culler MD, Negro-Vilar A. Passive immunoneutralization of endogenous inhibin: sex-related differences in the role of inhibin during development. Mol Cell Endocrinol 1988;58:263-73.

32. Rivier C, Cajander S, Vaughan J, Hsueh AJW, Vale W. Age-dependent changes in physiological action, content, and immunostaining of inhibin in male rats. Endocrinology 1988;123:120-6.

33. Voglmayr JK, Mizumachi M, Washington DW, Chen C-LC, Bardin CW. Immunization of rams against human recombinant inhibin α-subunit delays, augments, and extends season-related increase in blood gonadotropin levels. Biol Reprod 1990;42:81-6.

34. de Kretser DM, McLachlan RI, Robertson DM, Burger HG. Serum inhibin levels in normal men and men with testicular disorders. J Endocrinol 1989;120:517-23.

35. Sugino K, Nakamura T, Takio K, et al. Inhibin alpha-subunit monomer is present in bovine follicular fluid. Biochem Biophys Res Commun 1989;159:1323-9.

36. Robertson DM, Giacometti M, Foulds LM, et al. Isolation of inhibin α-subunit precursor proteins from bovine follicular fluid. Endocrinology 1989;125:2141-9.

37. Schneyer AL, Mason AJ, Burton LE, Zienger JR, Crowley WF, Jr. Immunoreactive inhibin α-subunit in human serum: implications for radioimmunoassay. J Clin Endocrinol Metab 1990;70:1208-12.

4

The Physiology of Puberty in Seasonally Breeding Birds

Brian K. Follett

The neuroendocrine mechanisms regulating FSH secretion in birds are very similar to those in mammals, and the 400–600 GnRH cell bodies lie in the anterior hypothalamus, passing their axons in a broad band to end on the hypophysial portal vessels. Birds possess two forms of GnRH, but it is probable that only one of these (8-Gln-GnRH) is secreted from the median eminence: Like its mammalian counterpart, the bird stimulates the release of both FSH and LH. In male birds, FSH in conjunction with androgens causes spermatogenesis, while in females it triggers oogenesis and also aids yolk uptake from the circulation. It is still unknown what role the gonadotropins play in establishing and maintaining the characteristic hierarchy of oocytes within the avian ovary that allows for daily ovulations.

The importance of FSH in avian puberty (1, 2) is illustrated in Figure 4.1, which shows the main reproductive changes in male quail that have just reached somatic maturity and have been driven to sexual maturity by exposure to a long photoperiod. FSH secretion is increased 15-fold within a week, and this causes the testes to increase from 10 to 1000 mg in 14 days. At around the time when the spermatids begin to mature, the rate of increase in testicular mass slows, and this coincides with a fall in FSH secretion. In a mature male with testes weighing 3500 mg, FSH is some 5 times greater than before puberty was triggered. The similarity of this secretory pattern with that seen in mammalian puberty is striking.

The photoperiodic control of the rate at which quail pass through puberty is quite precise, primarily because day length regulates FSH secretion in a quantitative fashion (Fig. 4.2). As photoperiod increases, so does the rate of FSH output and, hence, the rate of testicular growth.

It is worth emphasizing that the essential photoperiodic drive is independent of gonadal feedback, although the impact of such feedback is seen as the gonads mature. In castrated quail, Urbanski (3) showed that FSH levels can be set rather precisely and stably by photoperiod: Under 8L:16D, the FSH

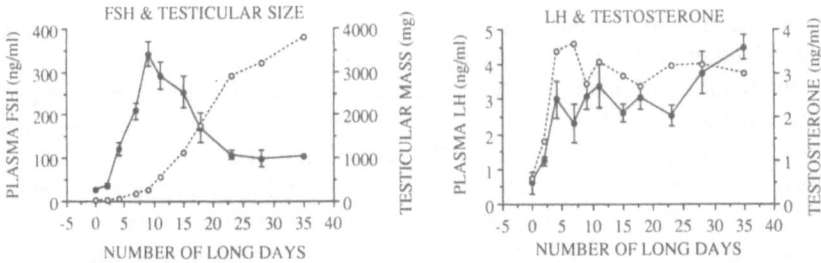

FIGURE 4.1. Endocrine changes in 1-month-old male quail passing through puberty following exposure to 20L:4D. FSH and LH (including SEM) are represented by solid symbols and lines, while testicular mass and plasma testosterone are represented by open symbols and dotted lines. Modified with permission from Follett (1) and Follett and Maung (2).

level was 250 µg/L; under 12L:12D, 670 µg/L; under 13L:11D, 1720 µg/L; and under 16L:8D, 5600 µg/L. Thus, the primary question in avian puberty appears similar to that in mammals: What *central* processes time the wave of FSH release, causing puberty to occur and sexual maturation to be attained? Before considering these physiological processes in detail, however, it is worth setting the issue of puberty in its biological context.

In birds, puberty and the age of first breeding are questions subsumed within the broader issue of life-history strategies and, as such, have attracted considerable interest from ecologists (4). The great majority of bird species first reach sexual maturity at about 12 months of age in the spring after their birth, and only a few species are physiologically capable of breeding in the year they are hatched (some quail, estrildine finches, doves, and a parrot). In most orders of birds, however, there are species that show a deferred maturity and do not breed before 2 years of age. This phenomenon is most

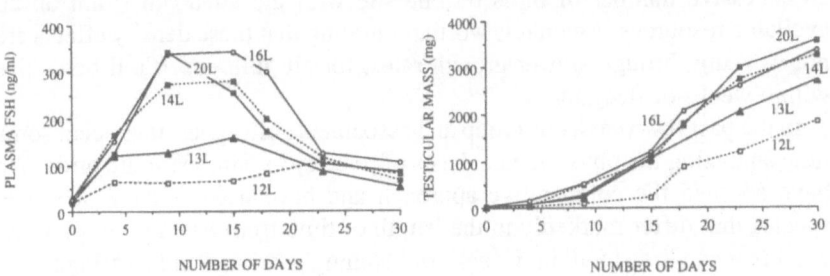

FIGURE 4.2. FSH secretion (*left*) and testicular growth (*right*) in somatically mature quail exposed to 12L:12D, 13L:11D, 14L:10D, 16L:8D, and 20L:4D. Standard errors have been omitted to improve clarity. Modified with permission from Follett and Maung (2).

apparent in seabirds (e.g., albatrosses, gulls, and penguins), but is common among other water birds (e.g., geese, storks, and waders) and some large terrestrial species, such as raptors, parrots, and ostriches. Most of these pass through puberty when 2 or 3, but some, like the large albatrosses and condors, delay until they are 9–17 years of age. This delayed puberty is closely associated with longevity of the adults and with a strategy of reproducing for many years, producing relatively few offspring each time and investing heavily in each individual. This is in contrast with most birds, which have evolved towards a shorter life span and larger clutches.

Associated with these variations in long-term reproductive strategy are three other features that impinge on avian puberty. The first is that birds are pronounced seasonal breeders so that the precise timing of puberty is confounded by the need to ensure that the gonads grow at only one season of the year. In temperate regions, seasonality is dominated by photoperiods and as will become evident, the evidence points to the fact that the delay in breeding until 1 year of age is largely the result of a photoperiodic block to earlier sexual maturation. The second feature is that body growth is extremely rapid, and most small birds have attained full body size, have fledged, and can fly at between 2 and 4 weeks of age. Even the largest species, such as albatrosses and Californian condors, have fledged at 3–5 months. Thus, the argument that the time of puberty in birds is related simply to body growth is unlikely to be sustained. The third feature, especially important ecologically, is that a bird may be old enough to pass through puberty, but is inhibited from doing so by social and other environmental factors. A good example of this comes from the work of Coulson and his colleagues (5) on the breeding biology of the herring gull (*Larus argentatus*) on the Isle of Man during a period when the population was culled from 13,000 to 3,000 breeding pairs. Over this time, the mean age of breeding dropped from 6.2 to 4.3 years. The latter age represents the normal minimum age for puberty in herring gulls, while the delay to 6 years is a result of secondary environmental factors—in this case, an excessive number of birds on one site with the attendant strain on all available resources. Again it is worth reiterating that these density effects are not working through slower growth rates, for all gulls reach full body size within weeks of fledging.

In the past few years, our group and associated colleagues have spent some time analyzing the physiological basis of puberty in photoperiodic birds. We have adopted the comparative approach and have used a range of model species that differ markedly in the length of time from hatching to puberty: quail that can breed within 6 weeks of hatching, starlings and partridges that usually breed at 1 year of age, and herring gulls and albatrosses that delay puberty for between 4 and 10 years. The persons involved have been, in alphabetical order, Creighton (6, 7), Dawson (8, 9), Goldsmith (10), Hall (11, 12), Hector (13, 14), McNaughton (15), Maung (2), Nicholls (16), and

Williams (17–19). My role is to summarize some of the broad conclusions that have been reached; most of the data quoted are for the male, but in general, many of the conclusions also apply to the female.

Birds That Breed at Less Than One Year of Age: Quail and Chickens

The quail can be viewed as having the "simplest" system. In the wild, it can breed during the summer in which it is born, and in the laboratory, it can pass through puberty at 1 month of age. To achieve this, reproductive development must begin at only a few days of age, but whether this does or does not occur depends critically upon the prevailing photoperiod. If quail are maintained under short day lengths (e.g., 8L:16D), reproductive development occurs at a negligible rate, but transfer to long days causes rapid gonadal development (Figs. 4.1 and 4.2). Photoperiodic induction in such quail is fast: FSH levels are increased by the end of the second long day, and the first detectable changes in testicular mass are measurable after 4 long days. This ability of the young quail to respond to photoperiod develops soon after hatching (20), probably towards the end of the first week when the birds weigh about 20 g (final body mass 100–125 g).

This can be seen in two ways. First, if quail are exposed to 8L:16D or 20L:4D continuously from hatching, then testicular mass (expressed as a percentage of body mass) is similar at 7 days of age but significantly different after 14 days. Also, if 7-day-old quail are moved from 8L:16D to 20L:4D, then the testes grow from 3.5 to 21.4 mg (P < 0.01) within a week; whereas, if retained under 8L:16D, they only increase in line with body mass over the same period and reach about 7 mg at 14 days of age. Before 7 days of age, it is difficult to demonstrate whether the birds are unable to respond because they cannot measure photoperiod or because the endocrine system is still too undeveloped to release hormones. However, some unpublished experiments of Nicholls point to quail being affected by the photoperiod in the first week of life. He exposed newly hatched quail to 1 week of 8L:16D or 20L:4D and then transferred all the birds to 13L:11D to test their photoresponsiveness. After 1 month testicular mass was different (8L:13L, 51.4 ± 7.6 [12] mg; and 20L:13L, 35.8 ± 3.5 [19], P < 0.05). This suggested, first, that the quail did detect day length when less than 7 days of age and, second, that short days immediately after hatching somehow changed the bird's physiological state so that subsequent longer days were more stimulatory. This was confirmed by showing that testicular growth was faster in quail given 1 week of 8L and 3 weeks of 13L than in birds exposed only to 13L:11D. The reasons behind this second effect are still unclear, but they occur also in chickens (see below) and seem a less extreme form of that seen in the many birds that delay breeding until 1 year of age. If so, this suggests that quail and chickens may be hatched in a semi-refractory state. Incidentally, this type of phenomenon also occurs in mammals (21, 22).

The domesticated chicken has many of the features found in quail, but the degree of photoperiodic control is very much less. Chickens enter puberty at about the same age, regardless of day length. An experiment quoted in Morris (23) shows the mean age to laying of the first egg as 151 days if hens were maintained from hatch under 22L:2D and as 158 days if under 6L:18D. Small as this difference is, it is highly important commercially, and much effort has been expended to shorten the time to puberty by fine-tuning the day-length treatment of growing pullets. For instance, Shanawary and Morris (24) have been able to advance puberty significantly so that 50% of a flock is in lay at 148 days of age when the birds are first exposed to a steady decrease in day length from 23L:1D to 8L:16D for 8 weeks from hatching, then to 8L:16D for 8 weeks, and finally to an abrupt increase back to extremely long days. The least effective treatment in this experiment (involving constant 8L:16D from hatch and then an abrupt increase in day length) resulted in 50% lay at 173 days of age.

Birds That Normally Breed at One Year of Age

Most birds hatch in the late spring and reach full adult body size within a few weeks; but, despite the long day lengths, they undergo no reproductive development whatsoever and remain prepubertal until the following spring. This makes ecological sense, but why do they not show an immediate reproductive response to long days as do quail? There is accumulating evidence that this inability to respond reproductively is due to the birds being hatched in a photorefractory condition very similar to that which develops in adult birds in midsummer and that ends the normal breeding season (16). That young birds were in some kind of juvenile refractory state was suggested by experiments in which white-crowned sparrows (25), ducks (26), and Chukar partridges (27) were kept continuously from hatching on long days. This greatly delayed or even prevented sexual maturation, but if the birds were exposed to 2 months of short days and then long days, they entered breeding rapidly. This response is very similar to that seen in adult refractory birds that require short days to break refractoriness and render them capable of responding to long days (16). More detailed analyses on the starling (8–10, 17–19) and the red-legged partridge (6, 7) confirm this early work and extend it to suggest that the young birds are indeed born refractory. Three types of experiment have proved significant in reaching this conclusion.

First, short days, which normally break the adult refractoriness in autumn

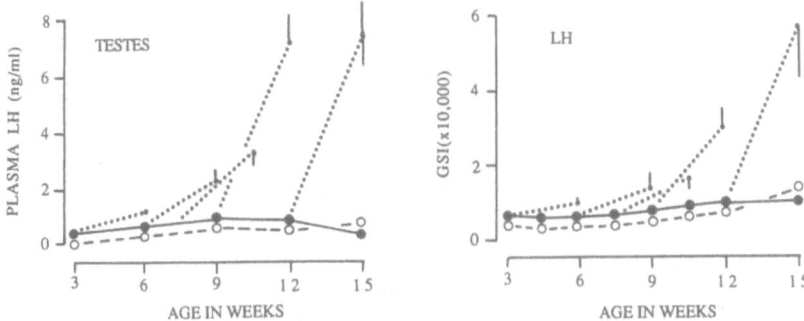

FIGURE 4.3. Plasma LH and testicular weight (expressed as the gonadosomatic index [GSI] to compensate for body growth changes from hatching [15 g] to adulthood [450 g] at 15 weeks) in partridges held from hatch on short days (solid symbols, solid lines), or long days (open symbols, dashed lines), or on short days for varying periods of time and then shifted to long days (dotted lines). Mean ± SEM. Modified with permission from Creighton (6).

(16), are equally effective in accelerating puberty in newly hatched birds. Figure 4.3 shows the results of an experiment (6) where partridges were reared from hatching on 8L:16D and groups were transferred to 20L:4D after 3, 4.5, 6, 7.5, 9, and 12 weeks. The testicular responses show clearly the basic pubertal responses in this type of bird. First, neither gonadal growth nor puberty occurs if the birds are kept on either short or long days; the former is a nonstimulatory photoperiod for gonadal growth, and the latter appears to maintain a juvenile state of refractoriness. The short days are not without action, however, for progressively they seem to dissipate the refractory condition and produce a photosensitive partridge that can respond to long days, with about 9 weeks being required for all the refractoriness to be dissipated. The gonadotropin responses to the various transfers are as expected, with the long-day-induced rises occurring only in those partridges that have dissipated some or all of their refractoriness.

The effectiveness of short days in unraveling a refractory state can be tested more directly in castrated starlings that show a *spontaneous* increase in gonadotropin secretion once the refractory state is dissipated (28). Figure 4.4 shows an experiment in which groups of starlings were reared from day 4 of life under long or short days; the nestlings were castrated when 10 days old. The data on plasma LH show a spontaneous rise at 7 weeks in the 10 starlings held on short days, but none in those maintained on long days. This response would be expected if the starlings were refractory when juveniles.

Even more persuasive evidence that puberty involves a refractoriness akin to that in adult birds at the end of the breeding season comes from the role of the thyroid glands. Removing the thyroid glands of adult refractory starlings

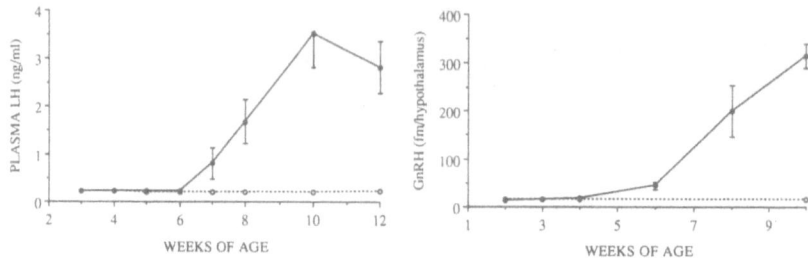

FIGURE 4.4. Effect of short days on gonadotropin secretion in castrated starlings. The left-hand graph shows plasma LH in 10 castrated starlings (solid symbols) raised on continuous short days and in 6 intact starlings (open symbols) on long days. The right-hand graph shows hypothalamic GnRH content in young female starlings raised on continuous short (solid symbols) or long (open symbols) days. Mean ± SEM. Modified with permission from Dawson and Goldsmith (9).

leads to a spontaneous disappearance of refractoriness, and so one would predict that thyroidectomy of young starlings and partridges should equally lead to gonadal growth occurring on long days without any need for prior exposure to short days (16). Figure 4.5 shows the results for the two species.

In both cases the young birds were radiothyroidectomized at a point soon after hatching, but not so early as to lead to excessive body stunting (7 days in starlings and 6 weeks in partridges). Before and subsequent to the treatment, the birds were maintained on long day lengths, as were the intact

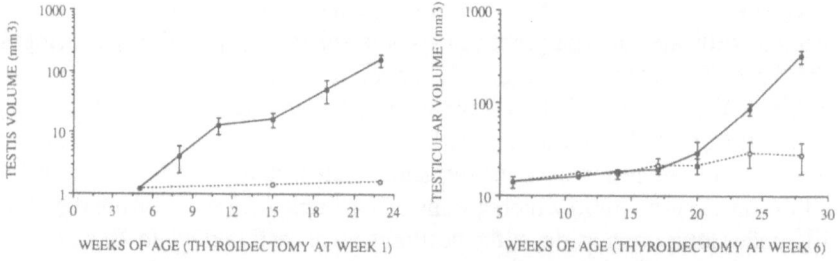

FIGURE 4.5. Spontaneous puberty of young starlings (*left*) and partridges (*right*) under long day lengths after thyroidectomy. Testicular volume (log scale) is plotted against time in birds after thyroidectomy (solid symbols) or in intact birds (open symbols). As predicted, testicular development begins some weeks after thyroid removal when the refractoriness has been dissipated. Mean ± SEM. Modified with permission from Creighton (7) and Dawson, Williams, and Nicholls (8).

controls. The results support the hypothesis: Testicular development begins spontaneously in the thyroidectomized birds some 6 weeks later, but not in the intacts, and continues rapidly until the birds are sexually mature.

A third argument that starlings are hatched in a refractory condition comes from analyzing hypothalamic GnRH. In adults, refractoriness at the end of the breeding season is so extreme that as the gonads regress, the hypothalamic GnRH content decreases 10-fold, the mean area of the GnRH perikarya decreases by 50%, and GnRH staining in the median eminence all but disappears (10, 29). Switching the adults to short day lengths leads to dissipation of the refractory state and the reappearance of GnRH in both perikarya and terminals. Thus, in the starling a virtual absence of GnRH is indicative of a refractory condition, and the content should be expected to rise as refractoriness dissipates under short days. The right panel of Figure 4.4 shows this to be true for juvenile starlings: The hypothalamic GnRH content was extremely low in juveniles reared on long days, but in those hand-reared on short days, the content rose rapidly between 6 and 8 weeks of age, which is the same time that the birds respond to long days or, if castrated, show a spontaneous rise in gonadotropin secretion. In a separate series of experiments, full-grown but prepubertal starlings on long days were moved to short days, and characteristics were analyzed immunocytochemically (10). Cell area did not alter for the first 3 weeks of short days, but then increased by one-third in the fourth week, at the same time as the GnRH staining within the perikarya doubled and stained fibers reappeared within the palisade zone of the median eminence. The starling is clearly emerging as a particularly good model for investigating plasticity in the GnRH system, perhaps because it undergoes such a highly pronounced seasonal cycle in breeding (9, 10, 29).

In summary, the long puberty in most birds that breed at 1 year of age does not derive from an age-dependent phenomenon that takes 12 months to disappear, but from a photoperiodically derived juvenile refractoriness. That refractoriness "protects" the young bird from responding to the long days into which it is born and so keeps the secretion of gonadotropins at a minimal level. The juvenile refractoriness disappears over the winter months as a result of short days, and the bird responds the following spring to long days. The refractoriness occurs within the central nervous system at or above the level of the GnRH neuron. By suitable manipulations, either of photoperiod or of thyroid function, the juvenile refractoriness can be overcome prematurely and sexually mature birds produced at 12 weeks of age.

There remain some complications to the story, however. The experiment shown in Figure 4.4 began by bringing the nestlings from the wild at 4 days of age, during which they had been exposed to long days in the nest boxes: Perhaps these 4 long days somehow induced a rapid refractoriness that was not present at birth. This possibility was tested by using nest boxes in which the day length was regulated throughout the whole period of egg laying, incubation, and rearing: The results were the same. Thus, the starlings appear to be born refractory and not to become so after hatching.

Nevertheless, there must be important processes developing during the rapid period of body growth because the starlings cannot begin to respond to short days until about 3 weeks of age. A recent experiment (15) illustrates this well. Nestling starlings were reared under short days or moved from long to short days at 2 and 3 weeks of age. The spontaneous rise in gonadotropin secretion—indicative that refractoriness had been broken—occurred at 7 weeks of age in all three groups. Thus, there must be a phase, lasting for a relatively short period but coincident with rapid body maturation, when the neural mechanisms involved in juvenile refractoriness are either still developing or cannot yet be accessed by photoperiod. Only after this time does the main photoperiodic block to puberty begin to play its powerful physiological role.

Birds That Breed at Two or More Years of Age

A long-deferred maturity is especially widespread in seabirds, which provide some spectacular examples. The large wandering and royal albatrosses, for example, do not begin breeding until 8–11 years of age. The critical factor is not size though, and a species such as the arctic tern, which migrates between the two hemispheres, rarely breeds in the Farne Islands before it is 4 years of age (30). Purely physiological studies are rare, but some endocrine data are available on the wandering albatross (13, 14), the white stork (11), and the herring gull (12, 31). One intriguing feature is illustrated in Figure 4.6 which shows testicular size in Californian gulls (*L. californicus*) sampled over a 5-year age range by Johnston (31) and in wandering albatrosses (*Diomedea*

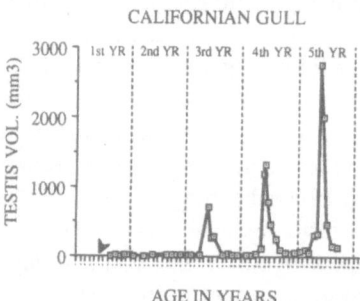
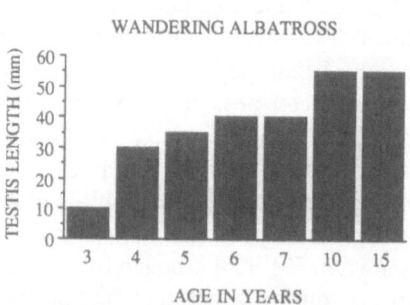

FIGURE 4.6. Testicular size in Californian gulls during the first 5 years of life (drawn from data in Johnston [31]) and wandering albatrosses of known age laparotomized in South Georgia. Modified with permission from Hector, Croxall, and Follett [13].

exulans) of known age that were laparotomized during the breeding season on Bird Island, South Georgia (13).

Testicular growth is minimal in the gull until the third year of life; then the amplitude of the testicular cycle becomes larger each year. The same appears true for the wandering albatross, although data are not available for birds up to 3 years of age since they remain at sea continuously. This pattern is consistent with the notion that the block to puberty is being progressively removed over a number of years but is anything known of the nature of the block itself?

Recently, Hall (12) has tested the hypothesis that puberty is much delayed in herring gulls (*L. argentatus*) because they are hatched in such a deeply refractory state that dissipation requires several years of exposure to winter day lengths. This is an extension, of course, of the model developed above for those birds in which the delay is for 1 year. He has exposed gulls from early in life to various photoperiodic schedules (continuous long or short days, alternating periods of 3 months of long and short days) for up to 4 years and has monitored gonadal development, hormonal changes, and molt. The results are clear-cut: None of the schedules advanced the onset of puberty by more than a few months. This leads to the conclusion that the delayed puberty in gulls is not due in the main to a refractoriness, but to some other chronological process in the brain that takes years to unwind. In many respects, the overall process looks similar to that found in primates and reindeer, but in no case do we yet understand the neural basis for the prolonged blockage to GnRH activity. Immunocytochemical studies on herring gulls indicate that all the components of the GnRH system are present from a young age; yet release must be minimal indeed for the testes remain less than 3 mm long for over 2 years.

References

1. Follett BK. Plasma follicle-stimulating hormone during photoperiodically induced sexual maturation in the male Japanese quail. J Endocrinol 1976;69:117-26.
2. Follett BK, Maung SL. Rate of testicular maturation, in relation to gonadotropin and testosterone levels, in quail exposed to various artificial photoperiods and to natural daylengths. J Endocrinol 1978;78:267-80.
3. Urbanski HF, Follett BK. Photoperiodic modulation of gonadotropin secretion in castrated Japanese quail. J Endocrinol 1982;92:73-83.
4. Lack D. Ecological adaptations for breeding in birds. London: Chapman & Hall, 1968.
5. Coulson JC, Duncan N, Thomas C. Changes in the breeding biology of the herring gull (*Larus argentatus*) induced by reduction in the size and density of the colony. J Anim Ecol 1982;51:739-56.
6. Creighton JA. Photoperiodic control of puberty in the red-legged partridge. Gen Comp Endocrinol 1988;71:17-28.

64   Brian K. Follett

7. Creighton JA. Thyroidectomy and the termination of juvenile refractoriness in the red-legged partridge (*Alectoris graeca chukar*). Gen Comp Endocrinol 1988; 72:204-8.
8. Dawson A, Williams TD, Nicholls TJ. Thyroidectomy of nestling starlings appears to cause neotenous sexual maturation. J Endocrinol 1987;112:R5-6.
9. Dawson A, Goldsmith AR. Sexual maturation in starlings raised on long or short days: changes in hypothalamic gonadotropin-releasing hormone and plasma LH concentrations. J Endocrinol 1989;123:189-96.
10. Goldsmith AR, Ivings WE, Pearce-Kelly AS, et al. Photoperiodic control of the development of the LHRH neurosecretory system of European starlings (*Sturnus vulgaris*) during puberty and the onset of photorefractoriness. J Endocrinol 1989; 122:255-68.
11. Hall MR, Gwinner E, Bloesch M. Annual cycles in moult, body mass, luteinizing hormone, prolactin and gonadal steroids during the development of sexual maturity in the white stork (*Ciconia ciconia*). J Zool (Lond) 1987;211:467-86.
12. Hall MR. Deferred sexual maturity in birds and its relationship to seasonal breeding [Abstract]. J Reprod Fertil 1990;5:27.
13. Hector JAL, Croxall JP, Follett BK. Reproductive endocrinology of the wandering albatross (*Diomedea exulans*) in relation to biennial breeding and deferred sexual maturity. Ibis 1986;128:9-22.
14. Hector JAL, Pickering SPC, Croxall JP, Follett BK. The endocrine basis of deferred sexual maturity in the wandering albatross, *Diomedea exulans* L. Funct Ecol 1990;4:59-66.
15. McNaughton F, Dawson A, Goldsmith AR. Puberty in birds: nestling starlings appear unable to respond to short days [Abstract]. J Reprod Fertil 1990;5:27.
16. Nicholls TJ, Goldsmith AR, Dawson A. Photorefractoriness in birds and comparison with mammals. Physiol Rev 1988;68:133-76.
17. Williams TD, Dawson A, Nicholls TJ, Goldsmith AR. Reproductive endocrinology of free-living nestling and juvenile starlings, *Sturnus vulgaris*; an altricial species. J Zool (Lond) 1987;212:619-28.
18. Williams TD, Dawson A, Nicholls TJ, Goldsmith AR. Short days induce premature reproductive maturation in juvenile starlings, *Sturnus vulgaris*. J Reprod Fertil 1987;80:327-33.
19. Williams TD, Dawson A, Nicholls TJ. Sexual maturation and moult in juvenile starlings *Sturnus vulgaris* in response to different daylengths. Ibis 1989;131: 135-40.
20. Maung SL. Sex steroids in bird reproduction. [Dissertation]. University College of North Wales, 1976.
21. Foster DL, Karsch FJ, Olster DL, Ryan KD, Yellon SM. Determinants of puberty in a seasonal breeder. Recent Prog Horm Res 1986;42:331-84.
22. Sisk CL. Photoperiodic regulation of gonadal growth and pulsatile luteinizing hormone secretion in male ferrets. J Biol Rhythms 1990;5:177-86.
23. Morris TR. The influence of light on ovulation in domestic birds. In: Animal reproduction, 3. Beltsville symposia in agricultural research, 1978:307-44.
24. Shanawary MM, Morris TR. Light, sexual maturity and subsequent performance [Paper]. Meet UK Branch World's Poultry Science Assn, University of Reading, 1980.

25. Farner DS, Mewaldt LR. The natural termination of the refractory period in the white-crowned sparrow. Condor 1955;57:112-7.
26. Storey CR, Nicholls TJ. Observations on the regulation of sexual quiescence in juvenile and adult male mallards (*Anas platyrhyncos*). J Zool (Lond) 1978;184: 181-6.
27. Siopes TD, Wilson WO. The effect of intensity and duration of light on photo-refractoriness and subsequent egg production of chukar partridges. Biol Reprod 1978;18:155-9.
28. Goldsmith AR, Nicholls TJ. Recovery of photosensitivity in photorefractory starlings is not prevented by testosterone treatment. Gen Comp Endocrinol 1984; 56:210-7.
29. Foster RG, Plowman G, Goldsmith AR, Follett BK. Immunocytochemical demonstration of plasticity of the luteinizing hormone-releasing hormone (LH-RH) system of photosensitive and photorefractory starlings (*Sturnus vulgaris*). J Endocrinol 1987;115:211-20.
30. Coulson JC, Horobin J. The influence of age on the breeding biology and survival of the arctic tern *Sterna paradisaea*. J Zool (Lond) 1976;178:247-60.
31. Johnston DW. The annual reproductive cycle of the California gull, I. Criteria of age and the testis cycle. Condor 1956;58:134-62.

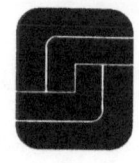

5

Hypothalamic Regulation of FSH Secretion

Jon E. Levine, Lisa A. Conaghan, Ulrike Luderer, and Frank J. Strobl

Differential regulation of LH and FSH secretion can be observed under a variety of physiological and experimental circumstances (1, 2). Situations in which FSH secretion is selectively augmented include the secondary FSH surge in female rats (3, 4), responses to unilateral (5) or bilateral ovariectomy (6), and the rise in FSH that occurs in hamsters with regressed testes following exposure to a long-day photoperiod (1). It is generally held that these selective increases in basal FSH levels result from either decreased inhibin feedback suppression (7–9), modulation of LHRH pulse frequency or amplitude (10), neurosecretion of an FSHRF distinct from the LHRH decapeptide (11), prolonged clearance rate of FSH (12), or a combination of two or more of these factors.

Evidence from experiments with rodents (13–15) also demonstrates that there can be marked differences in pulsatile release patterns of FSH and LH. It has been known for many years that LH secretion occurs in discrete, rhythmic bursts (16) and that the pulsatile neurosecretion of LHRH operates as the primary neural determinant of this episodic pattern of release (17, 18). The pattern of FSH levels in peripheral plasma, by contrast, is characterized by less frequent, irregular pulses whose amplitudes are small relative to high basal levels of the hormone (Fig. 5.1). That these relatively infrequent and irregular pulses of FSH are also stimulated by LHRH pulses has been the subject of debate (14, 19). While some have suggested that LHRH pulses stimulate pulsatile FSH secretion in rats (19), other have provided evidence that pulses of FSH are independent of LHRH control (14, 20, 21). In this chapter we review the evidence that pulse-like increments in circulating FSH levels are dependent upon pulsatile LHRH stimulation. Our strategies in studying this issue have included the examination of spontaneous LHRH and FSH release profiles (13) and the analysis of in vivo FSH responses to exogenous (22), evoked (23), and disinhibited (24) LHRH stimuli.

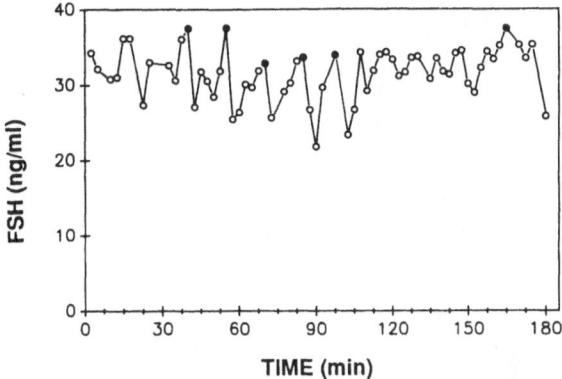

FIGURE 5.1. Peripheral FSH levels in an ovariectomized rat sampled through an indwelling jugular catheter at 2.5-min intervals. Filled circles indicate significant pulses identified by ULTRA pulse analysis as described in reference 25.

Simultaneous Measurement of LHRH and FSH Patterns

In a recent study (14), we examined the release patterns of LHRH, LH, and FSH in conscious, freely moving male rats. Hypothalamic push-pull perfusion was used to monitor pulsatile LHRH release patterns, while FSH and LH levels were determined in plasma samples obtained from indwelling atrial catheters. Animals underwent either castration or sham surgery at 24–32 h before experimentation. In the castrate group, pulsatile LHRH release occurred at a relatively high frequency, and almost all identified LHRH pulses were temporally associated with LH pulses (14). In the testes-intact group, LHRH pulses occurred less frequently, and many LHRH pulses were observed that did not appear to evoke corresponding LH pulses (silent LH pulses [see 14]). Nevertheless, the LH pulses that were observed in the intact rats were nearly all coincident with LHRH pulses. Interestingly, of the fewer irregular FSH pulses that were observed in either group, only 43.7% were temporally associated with LHRH pulses. Figures 5.2a and 5.2b depict the LHRH and FSH profiles from an intact and castrate rat, respectively, where this lack of obvious temporal association was seen. In rats sampled through jugular catheters only (14), it was likewise seen that only 23.8% of FSH pulses were temporally associated with LH pulses. Appreciable FSH temporal synchrony with LHRH or LH was also not evident when data were reexamined with respect to several different fixed latencies following LHRH or LH peaks.

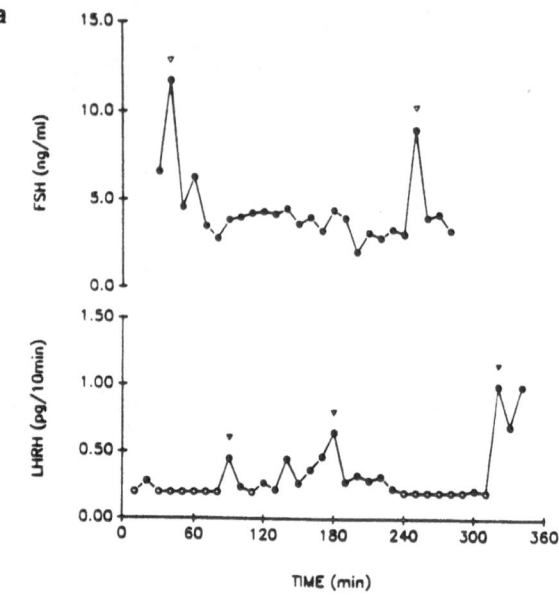

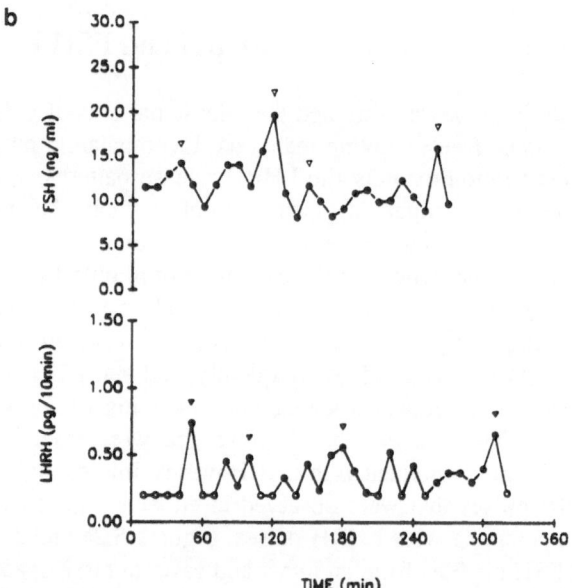

FIGURE 5.2. Simultaneous measurement of LHRH and FSH levels in a testes-intact rat (*a*) and a castrate rat (*b*). The LHRH patterns were determined in hypothalamic push-pull perfusates, and FSH levels were monitored in plasma samples obtained via jugular catheters. Inverted triangles denote significant pulses as determined by PUL-SAR analysis, as described in reference 26. Reproduced with permission from Levine and Duffy (14), © by The Endocrine Society.

The lack of a discernible relationship between LHRH and FSH pulses in male rats is in direct agreement with previous findings that LH and FSH pulses are not temporally associated in gonadectomized male (20, 21) and female rats (15) and ovariectomized hamsters (13). A study by Culler and Negro-Vilar (21) also clearly demonstrated that replacement of pulsatile LHRH bioactivity can reverse the gradual decline in basal FSH levels following LHRH immunoneutralization, but at the same time, this treatment does not directly stimulate pulsatile FSH release. In disagreement with these studies, it was recently reported that LHRH and FSH pulses were temporally associated when LHRH profiles were determined in push-pull perfusates of the anterior pituitary gland (19). The reasons for the discrepancy between our findings and those of Urbanski et al. (19) are not immediately apparent, but may ultimately be founded upon differences in pulse association criteria or sampling techniques.

In our push-pull perfusion study (14), the lack of an obvious temporal association between LHRH and FSH pulses in testes-intact rats may have been due to the presence of ovarian negative feedback mechanisms. In the castrate rats, moreover, a temporal relationship between LHRH and FSH may have been obscured by the inability of the pituitary gland to produce discrete, pulsatile FSH responses to the frequent pulsatile LHRH stimulation that is characteristic of this animal (14). Indeed, both the prolonged half-life of FSH and differential subcellular processing of the LHRH signal within FSH-secreting gonadotropes could be important factors in producing irregular FSH patterns in the peripheral circulation of the castrate. To address this possibility, we conducted experiments in which pituitaries were isolated from both hypothalamic and gonadal regulation, and the glands' relative LH and FSH secretory responses to controlled, exogenous LHRH stimuli were assessed.

Can Exogenous LHRH Pulses Produce FSH Pulses?

Although LHRH can evoke both LH and FSH release in most in vitro experiments, only large LHRH doses (which produce supraphysiological LH responses) are also capable of stimulating obvious, in vivo FSH responses (27). This apparent paradox has most often been explained on the basis of the longer half-life of FSH (12) and the resultant lengthened time for the hormone to reach equilibrium in the circulation following secretion (1). Thus, individual FSH responses to LHRH may occur in vivo, but these may simply be unresolvable under in vivo circumstances where the LHRH interpulse interval is too short to allow for production of a "clean" pulsatile FSH pattern. We recently conducted a study in which we attempted to determine if FSH pulses can be stimulated by exogenous LHRH pulses. We reasoned that

FSH pulses might be demonstrable in the absence of gonadal negative feedback and during sufficiently slow pulsatile LHRH stimulation. In the same experiments, we also analyzed the degree to which estrogen treatment can suppress LHRH-stimulated gonadotropin secretion. It was hypothesized that if the stimulatory effects of LHRH on pulsatile LH and FSH secretion are affected through similar subcellular routes, then acute suppression of one process (LHRH-stimulated LH secretion) should be accompanied by attenuation of the other (LHRH-stimulated FSH secretion).

To carry out these experiments, we developed an in vivo, isolated pituitary paradigm in which controlled exogenous LHRH stimuli can be delivered to a functioning pituitary gland that is devoid of endogenous hypothalamic control (22). Hypophysectomized rats receive pituitary transplants under the kidney capsule and are fitted with a concentric atrial catheter system that allows for pulsatile infusions of LHRH through a center catheter and blood sampling through a side port (22). Since the catheter system is protected by a jacket, tether, and swivel, the animals can recover, move freely, and receive the infusions for a virtually unlimited period of time. Ovariectomized rats prepared in this manner received pulsatile LHRH infusions for 5 days before experimental sessions. An hourly pulsatile infusion schedule was chosen, as this infusion rate approximates the likely LHRH pulse frequency rate of the gonadally intact female rat (28). On day 5, rats were bled at 10-min intervals for 4 h. Pulsatile LHRH infusions were continued during sampling sessions. After the first hour of sampling, rats received s.c. injections of either oil vehicle or estradiol benzoate (2 µg). Figures 5.3 and 5.4 depict representative LH and FSH data obtained from oil-treated (Figs. 5.3 and 5.4, top panels) and estrogen-treated (Figs. 5.3 and 5.4, bottom panels) rats. While the LHRH infusions (50 ng/min/5 min) consistently evoked physiologically proportioned LH pulses in all animals, the same pulsatile LHRH stimulation was ineffective in eliciting FSH pulses. Using a standard pulse analysis criterion (22), it was found that 77.5% of the LHRH pulses elicited significant LH pulses, but only 7.5% of the same LHRH stimuli were followed by significant FSH pulses Thus, the same LHRH stimuli that provided an adequate stimulus for secretion of LH pulses were totally ineffective in stimulating FSH pulses.

Our failure to observe significant FSH pulses from grafted tissue was accompanied by an additional important finding: The injection of 2 µg of estradiol benzoate profoundly inhibits LHRH-stimulated LH secretion, while it is without effect on FSH secretion. See Figures 5.3 (bottom), 5.4 (bottom), and 5.5. This observation provides additional evidence that the mechanism by which LHRH stimulates pulsatile LH secretion differs from that which mediates the effects of LHRH on FSH secretion.

Although LHRH infusions were ineffective in stimulating FSH pulses, it was of interest to note that basal levels of FSH were raised by continued

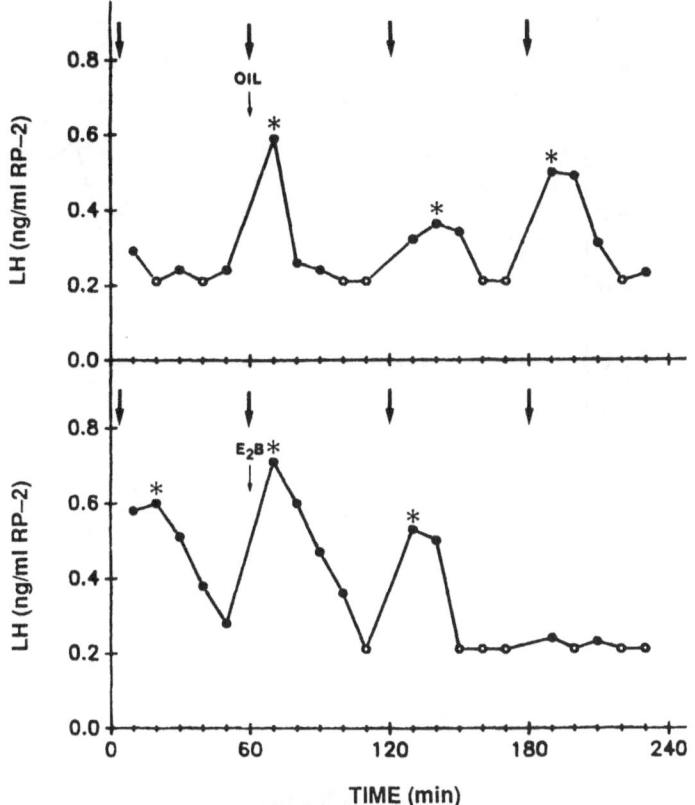

FIGURE 5.3. Peripheral LH levels in hypophysectomized, ovariectomized rats bearing pituitary transplants and receiving pulsatile LHRH infusions. The top panel depicts results obtained from an animal treated with oil vehicle, and the bottom panel shows the results of an experiment in which an animal received 2-μg estradiol benzoate, s.c. Darker arrows at the top of each panel indicate the times of pulsatile LHRH infusions during sampling sessions. Asterisks denote significant pulses of LH. Reprinted with permission from Strobl and Levine (22), © by The Endocrine Society.

exposure of the transplanted pituitaries to pulsatile LHRH stimulation (22). Using LHRH immunoneutralization and pulsatile LHRH agonist administration, Culler and Negro-Vilar (21) similarly found that basal FSH levels can be altered by blockade or restoration of pulsatile LHRH stimulation independently of the spontaneous occurrence of pulse-like increments in peripheral FSH levels. Taken together, these findings are consistent with the hypothesis that basal FSH secretion is at least partially dependent on pulsatile LHRH release, while the irregular, pulse-like fluctuations of FSH in plasma that we

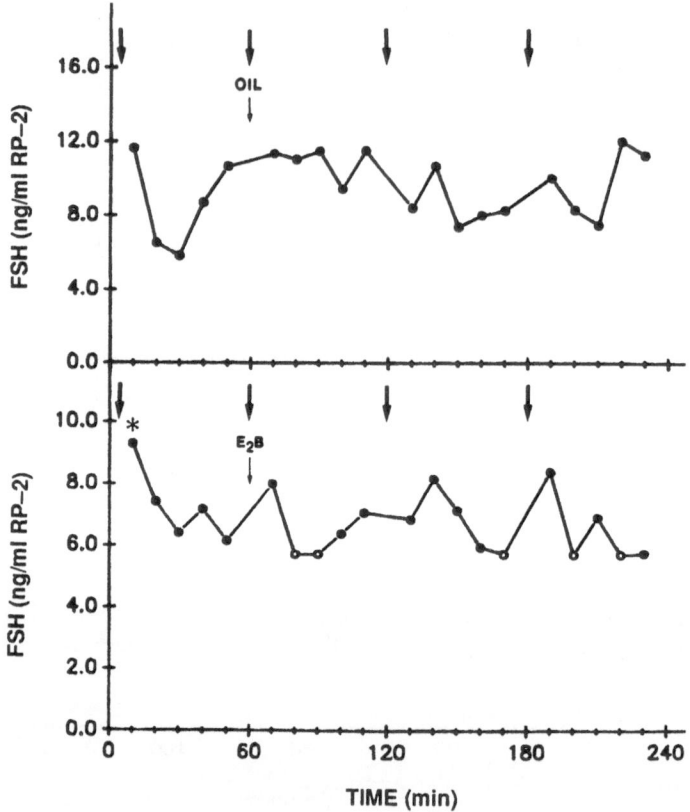

FIGURE 5.4. Peripheral FSH levels in rats whose LH levels are depicted in Figure 5.3.

(14) and others (21) have documented using standard pulse analysis criteria would appear to arise via an LHRH-independent mechanism. Further support for this hypothesis was gained in recent experiments using the LHRH secretagogue, N-methyl-D,L-aspartate (NMA), as described below (23).

Can Evoked LHRH Pulses Stimulate FSH Pulses?

Peripheral administration of the aspartate analog, NMA, evokes an acute increase in the secretion of LH in rats (29), sheep (30), and monkeys (31). The mechanism by which NMA induces LH secretion involves an acute increase in LHRH neurosecretion, inasmuch as this action can be blocked by prior administration of LHRH antagonist (31). The significance of NMA-activated LHRH neurosecretion is not clear; it may simply reflect an ability

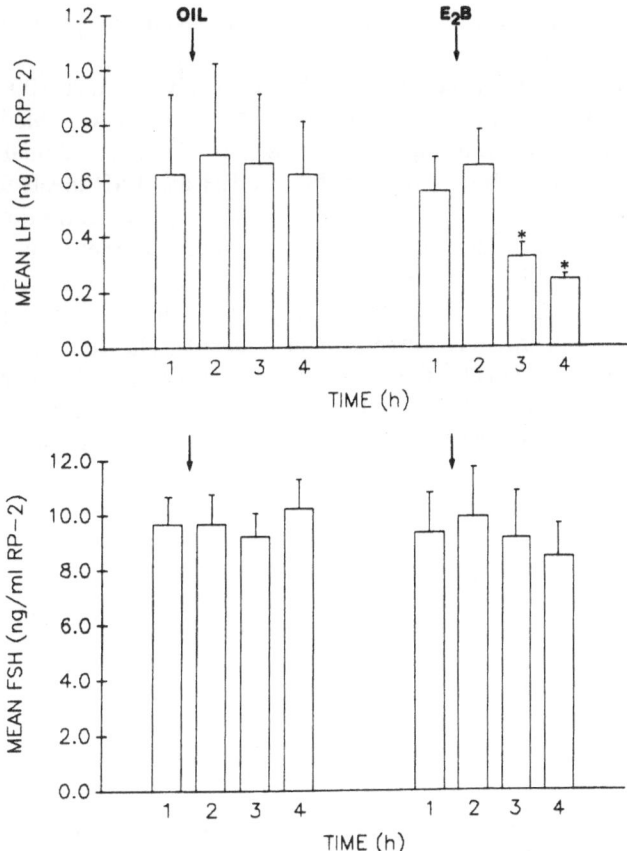

FIGURE 5.5. Mean LH (*top panel*) and FSH (*bottom panel*) levels in hypophysectomized, pituitary-grafted rats treated with oil vehicle or estradiol benzoate (2 μg, s.c.) at the times indicated. Estrogen treatment significantly suppressed LH, but not FSH secretion. Reprinted with permission from Strobl and Levine (22), © by The Endocrine Society.

of the drug to excite virtually any neuronal system through ubiquitously distributed NMA receptors. Alternatively, NMA may activate receptors that normally play a direct physiological role in the regulation of LHRH pulses (32), LH surges (33), or puberty (34).

In a recent study, we utilized NMA as an LHRH secretagogue to investigate the relative dependency of LH and FSH secretion on the acute secretion of LHRH. The study was based on the premise that if pulsatile LHRH secretion normally functions to stimulate both LH and FSH pulses, then the pharmacological provocation of an endogenous LHRH discharge should, in turn, evoke coincident LH and FSH responses. Furthermore, both gonadotropin responses should be susceptible to blockade by pretreatment with LHRH antagonist.

Castrated and sham-castrated male rats received either 100-µg LHRH antagonist or oil vehicle at 2100 h and on the next day were bled at 10-min intervals through atrial catheters between 0900–1200. Animals received 5-mg NMA after 1 h of sampling. Plasma LH and FSH levels were determined by RIA. As shown in Figures 5.6 and 5.7, NMA injections induced transient, pulse-like increases in LH secretion that were entirely blocked by pretreatment with LHRH antagonist. The profile of the LH secretory responses to NMA were similar or slightly more robust than endogenous LH pulses observed previously in intact male rats (14). The same injections were entirely ineffective in eliciting increases in FSH secretion. In agreement with the foregoing results in hypophysectomized, pituitary-grafted rats, these results demonstrate that the amount of endogenously secreted LHRH required to induce a pulse of LH is inadequate to stimulate a coincident pulse of FSH secretion. These findings are therefore incompatible with the pro-

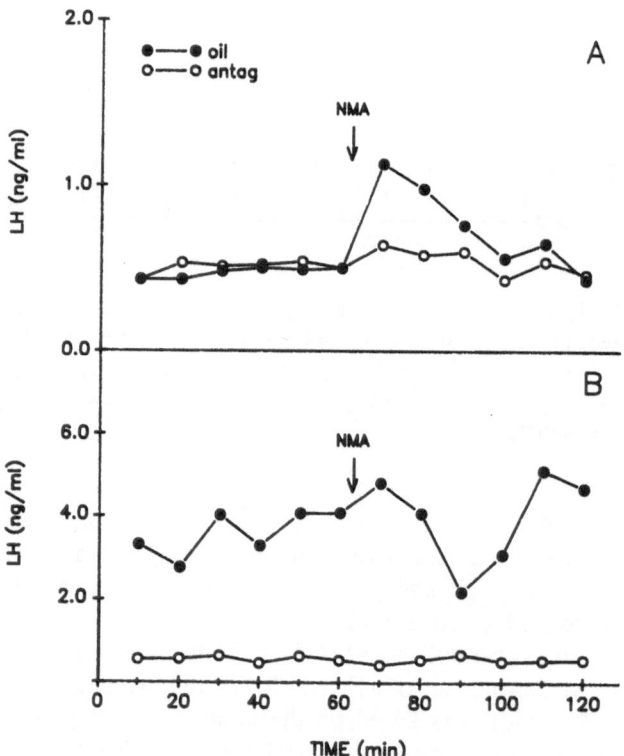

FIGURE 5.6. The LH levels in (A) intact and (B) castrate male rats after pretreatment with oil vehicle (closed circles) or LHRH antagonist (open circles). Rats in each group received 5-mg NMA, I.V., at the times indicated.

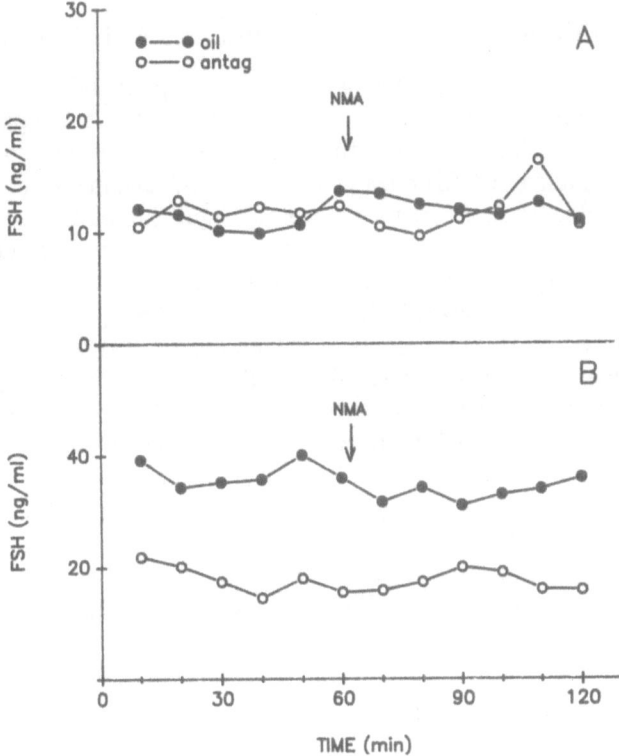

FIGURE 5.7. The FSH levels in rats whose LH data are depicted in Figure 5.6.

posal that pulse-like increments in circulating FSH levels are directly stimulated by LHRH pulses.

As reported previously (1), treatment with LHRH antagonist also reduced circulating FSH levels by approximately 60%. This finding reinforces the idea that basal secretion of FSH is at least partially dependent upon the neurosecretion of LHRH (1, 21). That the LHRH support of basal FSH secretion differs qualitatively from LHRH stimulation of LH pulses is suggested by the differing time courses of the antagonism of LH and FSH secretion; while the effect of the antagonist on pulsatile LH secretion is virtually immediate, its effects on basal FSH secretion requires up to 12 h to be manifest. These differential effects on LH and FSH cannot be explained on the basis of the slower clearance of FSH from the circulation (1). It would appear, therefore, that LHRH support of FSH secretion is mediated by subcellular processes that operate over significantly longer times than the relatively short intervals over which pulse-like increments occur. As suggested in a succeeding section, these observations may reflect a predominant effect of LHRH on FSH biosynthetic processes (35), as opposed to FSH release mechanisms.

Can Disinhibited LHRH Pulses Stimulate FSH Pulses?

The neurons that produce the endogenous opioid peptide (EOP) are known to tonically inhibit the secretion of LH via the intrahypothalamic suppression of LHRH release, since administration of the opiate receptor antagonist, naloxone, stimulates LHRH release in vitro (36, 37) and in vivo (24, 38). We recently conducted experiments that were designed, in part, to determine if the transient removal of EOP inhibitory tone also results in an acute increase in FSH secretion (24). We again reasoned that larger endogenous LHRH pulses should produce larger FSH pulses, if indeed FSH pulses are normally stimulated by LHRH. In this study, however, our strategy was to relieve the LHRH release apparatus from physiological inhibition and thereby produce LHRH pulses of increased, yet physiological amplitude. As shown in Figure 5.8, we first used push-pull perfusion of the hypothalamus to document that naloxone treatment (2.5 mg/kg, s.c.) produces an acute increase in the amplitude of LHRH release in ovarian-intact rats and in animals ovariectomized at 4 days or 8 days prior to experiments. Naloxone was equally effective in producing acute increases in LH secretion in intact and ovariectomized animals (Fig. 5.9). By contrast, FSH secretion was not significantly affected

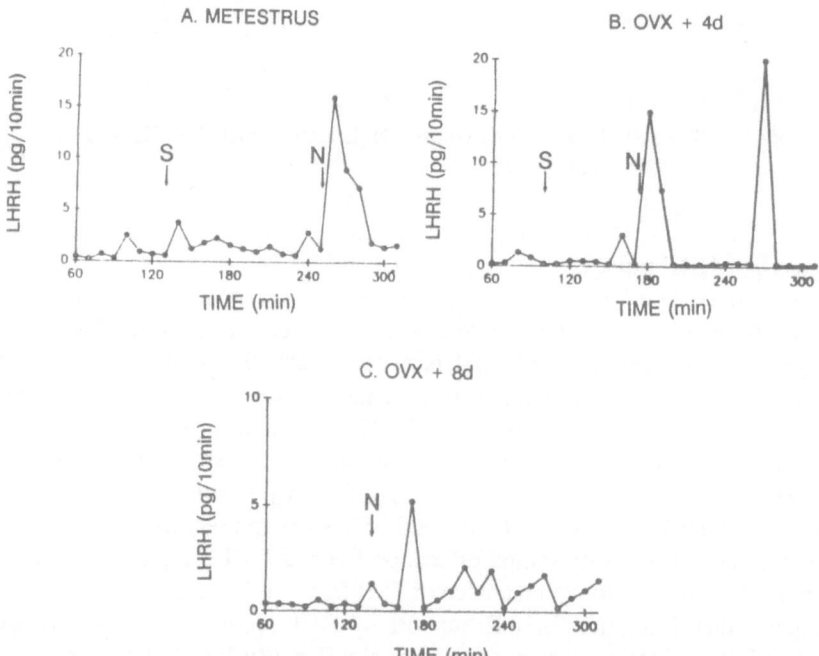

FIGURE 5.8. Effects of naloxone on in vivo LHRH release. Naloxone (2.5 mg/kg, s.c.) evoked transient increases in LHRH pulse amplitude in ovary-intact (A) and ovariectomized (B and C) rats, while saline injections were without effect. Reprinted with permission from Karahalios and Levine (24), © by S. Karger AG, Basel.

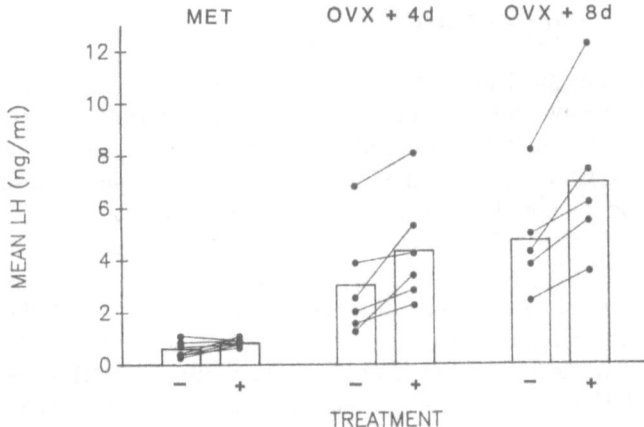

FIGURE 5.9. Effects of naloxone on mean LH secretion in ovarian-intact and 4-day or 8-day ovariectomized rats. Pairs of points represent mean LH levels in individual animals for the hour preceding (−) and the hour following (+) naloxone injection. Histograms indicate grand mean levels for each condition, before and after naloxone administration. Statistical analysis revealed a significant effect of the opiate antagonist in each group. Reprinted with permission from Karahalios and Levine (24), © by S. Karger AG, Basel.

by naloxone administration (Fig. 5.10) in any group. Since both LHRH and LH release, but not FSH release, were potentiated by treatment with naloxone, it can be concluded that disinhibited LHRH pulses are inadequate stimuli for the acute secretion of FSH.

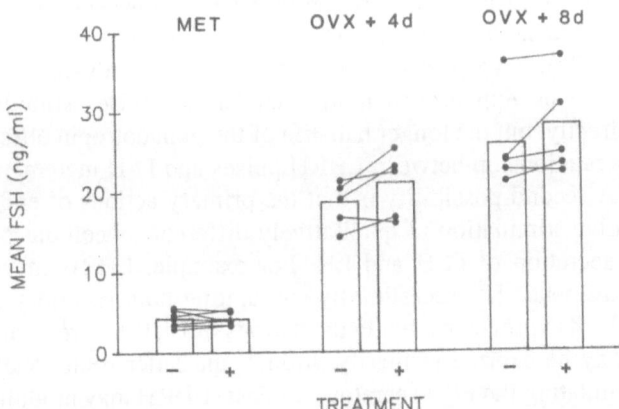

FIGURE 5.10. Lack of effect of naloxone on mean FSH levels in ovarian-intact and 4-day or 8-day ovariectomized rats. Depicted are FSH levels from rats whose LH data are described in Figure 5.9. See legend to Figure 5.9 for explanation of symbols. Naloxone treatment produced no significant effect upon FSH levels in any of the three treatment groups. Reprinted with permission from Karahalios and Levine (24), © S. Karger AG, Basel.

Summary and Conclusions

Using four independent experimental strategies, we have found no evidence to support the hypothesis that pulses of LHRH are capable of directly stimulating pulse-like increments in FSH in the rat. Spontaneous pulsatile LHRH release profiles were determined in castrate and testes-intact male rats and found to be temporally associated with LH pulses but not with FSH levels. Exogenous LHRH pulses were similarly found to be effective in stimulating LH, but not FSH pulses, from ectopic pituitary glands. Endogenous LHRH pulses produced by activation of NMA receptors or opiate receptor antagonism were also found to be adequate stimuli for the secretion of LH, while being inadequate for affecting any change in circulating FSH patterns. Thus, since LHRH pulses are not temporally associated with FSH pulses and because physiologically proportioned LHRH pulses are incapable of acutely stimulating FSH pulses, we must conclude that pulse-like FSH increments in the peripheral circulation are not driven by endogenous pulsatile LHRH stimulation.

What role then, if any, does LHRH neurosecretion play in supporting FSH secretion? Clearly, the primary FSH surge in proestrous rats represents one physiological circumstance in which a large increase in LHRH release and/or responsiveness to LHRH leads to an acute increase in the secretion of FSH (39). Basal FSH secretion also appears to be dependent upon LHRH support since LHRH antagonist treatments ultimately lower FSH levels (40) and because prolonged pulsatile LHRH stimulation can sustain higher circulating levels of FSH in hypophysectomized, pituitary-grafted rats (22).

The support of basal FSH secretion by LHRH, however, appears to be temporally dissociable from the acute stimulation of LH pulses by the decapeptide (22). Two possible explanations can be advanced for these observations. One explanation holds that LHRH pulses stimulate FSH secretion directly, but the longer half-life of the gonadotropin obscures any momentary relationship between LHRH pulses and FSH increments in the periphery. A second possibility is that the primary actions of endogenous LHRH involve stimulation of qualitatively different subcellular processes leading to secretion of FSH and LH. For example, LHRH in vivo may ultimately influence LH secretion by stimulating both secretory (14) and synthetic (35, 41) processes, while the actions of LHRH in regulating FSH secretion may be exerted primarily through the latter route. Rather than directly stimulating the FSH secretory process, LHRH may modulate some subcellular process leading to the accumulation of FSH in the releasable hormone pool. The most likely mechanism for this would be transcriptional regulation, as it has been recently shown that pulsatile infusions of LHRH increase FSHβ mRNA in rats (35, 41) and sheep (42) and that chronic LHRH antagonist and antiserum administration prevent the postcastration rise in FSHβ mRNA levels and suppress FSHβ mRNA levels in intact male rats (43).

The origins of relatively rapid, pulse-like increments in circulating FSH levels remains unresolved. Our observations, taken together with the finding that FSH fluctuations still occur after LHRH immunoneutralization (20, 21), make it extremely unlikely that they are dependent upon acute stimulation by LHRH. While it remains a possibility that a FSHRF (11) distinct from the LHRH decapeptide stimulates this irregular, episodic pattern of secretion (14, 20, 21), such a substance has yet to be identified. Moreover, the erratic occurrence of pulse-like FSH fluctuations and the irregular profiles of individual pulses do not suggest an underlying neurosecretory drive.

An alternative hypothesis holds that the rat pituitary gland intrinsically releases FSH in an irregular, discontinuous manner and that this "noisy" secretion provides enough variability in the pattern of circulating FSH levels to occasionally exceed standard pulse criteria. Such an irregular pattern could conceivably arise from paracrine (intrapituitary) regulation of FSH secretion, a possibility that receives some support from the observation that "minipulses" of other pituitary hormones from isolated tissue have been reported (44, 45). Such a mechanism could be mediated by selective regulation of secretion from FSH-containing granules, which have been shown to be morphologically distinct from LH-containing granules (46).

Yet another explanation for pulse-like increments in FSH secretion must also be considered: Despite the best intentions of the most careful of investigators, sampling procedures themselves may introduce a significant source of noise in the measurement of FSH patterns in peripheral blood. We are currently testing this possibility by comparing the degree to which FSH levels fluctuate in normal animals versus hypophysectomized rats receiving constant infusions of exogenous FSH. Assuming that these experiments will confirm that FSH pulses are not artifactual in origin, we are hopeful that their biological basis can be identified in subsequent studies.

Acknowledgments. We wish to thank NIADDK, Dr. Gordon Niswender, and Dr. Leo Reichert, Jr., for supplying the gonadotropin RIA materials and Drs. William Ellinwood and Martin J. Kelly for supplying the EL-14 LHRH antiserum. This work was supported by NIH R01 HD-20677 (J.E.L.), NIH T32 HD-07068 (J.E.L. and N.B. Schwartz), NIH P01 HD-21921 (J.E.L. and N.B. Schwartz), and NIH K04 HD-00879 (J.E.L., R.C.D.A.).

References

1. Schwartz NB, Milette JJ, Cohen IR. Animal models which demonstrate divergence in secretion or storage of FSH and LH. In: Burger HG, de Kretser DM,

Findlay JK, Igarashi M, eds. Serono symposium on inhibin-non-steroidal regulation of follicle stimulating hormone secretion. New York: Raven Press, 1987:239-52.

2. Chappel SC, Ulloa-Aguirre A, Coutifaris C. Biosynthesis and secretion of follicle-stimulating hormone. Endocr Rev 1983;4:179-211.

3. Butcher RL, Collins WE, Fugo NW. Plasma concentrations of LH, FSH, prolactin, progesterone and estradiol 17β throughout the 4-day estrous cycle of the rat. Endocrinology 1974;94:1704-8.

4. Nequin LG, Alvarez JA, Schwartz NB. Measurement of serum steroid and gonadotropin levels and uterine and ovarian variables throughout the 4-day and 5-day estrous cycles in the rat. Biol Reprod 1979;20:659-70.

5. Butcher R. Changes in gonadotropins and steroids associated with unilateral ovariectomy of the rat. Endocrinology 1977;101:830-40.

6. Spitzbarth TL, Horton TH, Llfka J, Schwartz NB. Pituitary gonadotropin content in gonadectomized rats: immunoassay measurements influenced by extraction solvent and testosterone replacement. J Androl 1988;9:294-305.

7. Savoy-Moore RT, Schwartz NB. Differential control of FSH and LH secretion. In: Greep RO, ed. International review of physiology. Baltimore, MD: University Park Press, 1980;22(Reproductive physiology III):203-48.

8. Ying S-Y. Inhibins, activins, and follistatins: gonadal proteins modulating the secretion of follicle-stimulating hormone. Endocr Rev 1988;9:267-93.

9. De Jong FH. Inhibin. Physiol Rev 1988;68:555-607.

10. Wildt L, Hausler A, Marshall G, et al. Frequency and amplitude of gonadotropin-releasing hormone stimulation and gonadotropin secretion in the rhesus monkey. Endocrinology 1981;109:376-85.

11. Mizunuma H, Samson WK, Lumpkin MD, Moltz JH, Fawcett CP, McCann SM. Purification of a bioactive FSH-releasing factor. Brain Res Bull 1984;10:623-9.

12. Bogdanove EM, Gay VL. Studies on the disappearance of LH and FSH in the rat: a quantitative approach to adenohypophysial secretory kinetics. Endocrinology 1969;84:1118-31.

13. Chappel S. Miller C, Hyland L. Regulation of pulsatile releases of luteinizing hormone and follicle-stimulating hormones in ovariectomized hamsters. Biol Reprod 1984;30:628-36.

14. Levine JE, Duffy MT. Simultaneous measurement of luteinizing hormone (LH)-releasing hormone, LH, and follicle-stimulating hormone release in intact and short-term castrate rats. Endocrinology 1988;122:2211-21.

15. Lumpkin MD, Depaolo LV, Negro-Vilar A. Pulsatile release of follicle-stimulating hormone in ovariectomized rats is inhibited by porcine follicular fluid (inhibin). Endocrinology 1984;114:201-6.

16. Gay VL, Sheth NA. Evidence for periodic release of LH in castrated male and female rats. Endocrinology 1972;90:158-62.

17. Levine JE, Pau K-YF, Ramirez VD, Jackson GL. Simultaneous measurement of luteinizing hormone-releasing hormone (LHRH) and luteinizing hormone release in unanesthetized, ovariectomized sheep. Endocrinology 1982;111:1449-55.

18. Clarke IJ, Cummins JT. The temporal relationship between gonadotropin releasing hormone (GnRH) and luteinizing hormone (LH) secretion in ovariectomized ewes. Endocrinology 1982;111:1737-9.

19. Urbanski HF, Pickle RL. Ramirez VD. Simultanous measurement of gonado-tropin-releasing hormone, luteinizing hormone, and follicle-stimulating hormone in the orchidectomized rat. Endocrinology 1988;123:413-9.

20. Culler MD, Negro-Vilar A. Evidence that pulsatile follicle-stimulating hormone secretion is independent of endogenous luteinizing hormone-releasing hormone. Endocrinology 1986;118:609-12.

21. Culler MD, Negro-Vilar A. Pulsatile follicle-stimulating hormone secretion is independent of luteinizing hormone-releasing hormone (LHRH): pulsatile re-placement of LHRH bioactivity in LHRH-immunoneutralized rats. Endocrinol-ogy 1987;120:2011-21.

22. Strobl FJ, Levine JE. Estrogen inhibits LH, but not FSH secretion in hypo-physectomized pituitary-grafted rats receiving pulsatile LH-releasing hormone infusions. Endocrinology 1988;123:622-30.

23. Strobl FJ, Luderer U, Schwartz NB, Levine JE. Differential gonadotropin re-sponses to N-methyl-D,L-aspartate in intact and castrate male rats [Abstract 495.17]. Soc Neurosci 20th annu meet. St. Louis, MO: Society for Neuroscience, 1990:1202.

24. Karahalios DG, Levine JE. Naloxone stimulation of in vivo LHRH release is not diminished following ovariectomy. Neuroendocrinology 1988;47:504-10.

25. Van Cauter E. Estimating false-positive and false-negative errors in analyses of hormonal pulsatility. Am J Physiol 1988;254:E786-94.

26. Merriam GR, Wachter KW. Algorithms for the study of episodic hormone secretion. Am J Physiol 1982;243:E310-8.

27. Fallest PC, Hiatt ES, Schwartz NB. Effects of gonadectomy on the in vitro and in vivo gonadotropin responses to gonadotropin-releasing hormone in male and female rats. Endocrinology 1989;124:1370-9.

28. Gallo RV. Pulsatile LH release during periods of low-level LH secretion in the rat estrous cycle. Biol Reprod 1981;24:771-7.

29. Price MT, Olney W, Cicero TJ. Acute elevations of serum luteinizing hormone induced by kainic acid, N-methyl-aspartic acid or homocysteic acid. Neuroendo-crinology 1978;26:352-8.

30. Estienne MJ, Schillo KK, Hileman SM, Green MA, Hayes SH. Effect of N-methyl-D,L-aspartate on luteinizing hormone secretion in ovariectomized ewes in the absence and presence of estradiol. Biol Reprod 1990;42:126-30.

31. Wilson RC, Knobil E. Acute effects of N-methyl-D,L-aspartate on the release of pituitary gonadotropins and prolactin in the adult female rhesus monkey. Brain Res 1982;248:177-9.

31. Gay VL, Plant TM. N-methyl-D,L-aspartate elicits hypothalamic gonadotropin-releasing hormone release in prepubertal male rhesus monkeys (*Macaca mulatta*). Endocrinology 1987;120:2289-96.

32. Arslan M, Pohl CR, Plant TM. D,L-2-amino-5-phosphonopentanoic acid, a spe-cific N-methyl-D-aspartic acid receptor antagonist, suppresses pulsatile LH re-lease in the rat. Neuroendocrinology 1988;47:465-8.

33. Lopez FJ, Donoso AO, Negro Vilar A. Endogenous excitatory amino acid neuro-transmission regulates the estradiol-induced LH surge in ovariectomized rats. Endocrinology 1990;126:1771-6.

34. Urbanski HJ, Ojeda SR. A role for N-methyl-D-aspartate (NMDA) receptors in

the control of LH secretion and initiation of female puberty. Endocrinology 1990;126:1774-6.

35. Dalkin AC, Haisenleder DJ, Ortolano GA, Ellis TR, Marshall JC. The frequency of gonadotropin-releasing hormone stimulation differentially regulates gonadotropin subunit messenger ribonucleic acid expression. Endocrinology 1989;125: 917-24.

36. Leadem CA, Crowley WR, Simpkins JW, Kalra SP. Effects of naloxone on catecholamine and LHRH release from the perfused hypothalamus of the steroid-primed rat. Neuroendocrinology 1985;497-500.

37. Wilkes MM, Yen SSC. Augmentation by naloxone of efflux of LRF from superfused medial basal hypothalamus. Life Sci 1982;28:2355-9.

38. Orstead KM, Spies HG. Inhibition of GnRH release by endogenous opioid peptides in female rabbits. Neuroendocrinology 1987;46:14-23.

39. Arimura A, Debeljuk L, Schally AV. Blockade of the preovulatory surge of LH and FSH and of ovulation by anti-LHRH serum in rats. Endocrinology 1974;95: 323-5.

40. Grady RR, Shin L, et al. Differential suppression of follicle-stimulating hormone and luteinizing hormone secretion in vivo by a gonadotropin-releasing hormone antagonist. Neuroendocrinology 1985;40:246-52.

41. Gharib SD, Wierman ME, Shupnik MA, Chin WW. Molecular biology of the pituitary gonadotropins. Endocr Rev 1190;11:177-99.

42. Leung K, Kaynard AH, Negrini BP, Kim KE, Maurer RA, Landefeld TD. Differential regulation of gonadotropin subunit messenger ribonucleic acids by gonadotropin-releasing hormone pulse frequency in ewes. Mol Cell Endocrinol 1987;1:724-8.

43. Rodin DA, Lalloz MRA, Clayton RN. Gonadotropin-releasing hormone regulates follicle-stimulating hormone β-subunit gene expression in the male rat. Endocrinology 1989;125:1282-9.

44. Gambacciani M, Liu JH, et al. Intrinsic pulsatility of LH release from the human pituitary in vitro. Neuroendocrinology 1987;45:402-6.

45. Shin SH, Reifel CW. Adenohypophysis has an inherent property for pulsatile prolactin secretion. Neuroendocrinology 1981;32:139-44.

46. Inoue K, Kurosumi K. Ultrastructural immunocytochemical localization of LH and FSH in the pituitary of the untreated male rat. Cell Tissue Res 1984;235: 77-83.

6

Photoperiodic Control of Reproduction in Male Hamsters: Role of FSH in Early Stages of Photostimulation

Fred W. Turek and Neena B. Schwartz

Photoperiodism

Reproductive activity for most birds and mammals inhabiting the temperate zones of the world is confined to a period of the year such that the birth of the young occurs when the probability of survival for both adults and offspring is maximum. While various environmental signals are used to synchronize the mating season to the appropriate season of the year (1), a primary factor that is the overriding one in many species for regulating various stages of the reproductive cycle is the annual change in day length (2, 3). For many species with a short gestation period (e.g., hamsters, voles, ferrets, and most temperate zone birds), reproductive activity takes place in association with the lengthening or long days of spring and summer; while for species with a long-duration gestation period (e.g., horses, sheep, and deer), mating activity occurs in association with the shortening or short days of fall and winter.

In many animals, a period of sensitivity to the light cycle is followed by a period of insensitivity (for reviews see 3, 4). For example, in many species of birds, gonadal regression follows photic-induced gonadal development even though the animals are maintained on photostimulatory long days. In order to become responsive to long days again, the birds must first be exposed to short days for a species-specific period of time. Similarly, gonadal regression that occurs in golden hamsters in response to exposure to short days is followed by gonadal recrudescence after a prolonged exposure to short days. In order to become responsive again to the inhibitory effects of short days, hamsters must be exposed to long days for about 11 weeks (5). The physiological state in which an animal is temporarily incapable of responding to a particular light cycle that had previously altered neuroendocrine-gonadal activity is referred to as the *refractory* condition.

Thus, depending on the species, the photoperiod may regulate one or more phases of the seasonal reproductive cycle. Furthermore, while changes in day length may be absolutely necessary to induce specific or all stages of the reproductive cycle in some species, in other species the changing day length acts to entrain, or synchronize, an endogenous, imprecise, *circannual* timing system (i.e., a clock) to the 365-day cycle in the physical environment (6, 7). After first providing a brief discussion of the major physiological events that mediate the effects of light on the neuroendocrine-gonadal axis, this review will focus on the important role that the follicle stimulating hormone (FSH) appears to play during the early stages of photostimulated testicular activity.

Photoperiodic Response: Cascade of Events

Over the past two decades, many of the underlying neural and endocrine events that mediate the effects of the seasonal change in day length on reproduction have been elucidated. While experiments on many different species have contributed to our understanding of the physiology of the photoperiodic response, studies in the male of two hamster species (i.e., the golden or Syrian hamster, *Mesocricetus auratus,* and the Djungarian or Siberian hamster, *Phodopus sungorus*) that have been carried out in many different laboratories provide a particularly detailed picture of how the seasonal change in day length regulates reproduction in mammals. Since the cascade of neural and endocrine events that make up the photoperiodic response is probably quite similar across diverse mammalian species, a review of the events in these two well-studied hamster species is meant to provide an overall view of most of what we know and do not know about the physiological mechanisms that underlie the effects of light on the mammalian neuroendocrine-gonadal axis. Briefly described below is the pathway by which information about day length enters the organism and eventually reaches the testes in male hamsters.

Photoreception

In hamsters, as in all other mammalian species, the first step in the cascade of events that mediates the effects of light on the neuroendocrine-gonadal axis involves the reception of light by photoreceptors located in the eye (3, 8). While this may seem like an obvious and trivial finding, it is not. In all nonmammalian vertebrate classes, extraocular photoreceptors located deep in the brain represent a primary if not sole route by which photic signals about the annual change in day length are first "perceived" by the organism (3, 9). Although light reception, as the first step in the photoperiodic response, involves the eyes in mammals, it appears that the mammalian photoreceptors, like those for lower vertebrates, are also separate from the photoreceptors that relay light information to the visual system. The photoreceptive system involved in photoperiodic time measurement in the Djungarian hamster is clearly much less sensitive (by several orders of magnitude) than that involved in vision, and recent studies in this species indicate that blue cones may be the dominant photoreceptor mediating the effects of light on both circadian and seasonal rhythms (10, 11).

While recent studies have begun to characterize the photoreceptors that mediate the effects of light on neuroendocrine-gonadal function in mammals, essentially nothing is known about the interretinal neural events or the ganglion cells that are the next step in this pathway. The finding that only a small number of ganglion cells appear to project to the circadian clock located in the suprachiasmatic nucleus (12, 13), an area of the hypothalamus involved in photoperiodic time measurement (see below), raises the distinct possibility that within the retina a unique neural system that is independent from the visual response system is involved in transmission of the light information used by the brain to evaluate the length of the day. Such a vision-independent system in the retina is perhaps expected since the neural pathway from the retina to the brain for the transmission of information about day length is clearly independent of the transmission of visual information to the brain.

Circadian Clock: Suprachiasmatic Nucleus

Moore and Lenn (14) established a number of years ago that there were direct projections from the retina to the bilaterally paired suprachiasmatic nuclei (SCN) of the hypothalamus. Beginning with the seminal work of Moore and Eichler (15) and Stephan and Zucker (16), literally hundreds of studies have been carried out that have conclusively demonstrated that a circadian clock(s) exists within the SCN, and that this clock serves as a "pacemaker," regulating most if not all circadian rhythms in rodents and, probably, in all mammalian species. The importance of these findings in the context of the present paper is that it has been well established in hamsters that the circadian clock in the SCN plays a key role in measuring the length of the day (for reviews see 2, 17–19). Indeed, destruction of the SCN renders hamsters (and the few other mammalian species that have been examined) incapable of responding appropriately to changes in daylength (3, 17, 20). Despite the close proximity of the SCN to the hypothalamic neurons that regulate pituitary gonadotropin release, the transmission of information from the day length-measuring system to these neurons is not a direct one.

Pineal Gland and Melatonin

While the results of a number of studies carried out over the past two decades were defining the role of the circadian clock in measuring the seasonal change in day length in mammals, other independent studies carried out over the same time period established a central role for the pineal gland in the photoperiodic response (for reviews see 2, 19, 21–23). Indeed, while there is still the occasional reference to the pineal gland being a vestigial organ in mammals, there is no question that the pineal gland mediates the effects of day length on neuroendocrine-gonadal activity. In both the golden and Djungarian hamster, pinealectomy prevents short-day-induced gonadal regression (21–23). While the effects of pinealectomy on the photoperiodic response may vary depending on the species, there are conclusive data in all mammalian species that have been examined in detail to indicate that the pineal gland is always somehow involved in the photoperiodic response.

A number of investigators have contributed substantially to our understanding of how the SCN/circadian clock and the pineal gland work together to mediate the effects of day length on the hypothalamic-pituitary-gonadal axis. The key link is the pineal hormone, melatonin. One of the circadian rhythms regulated by the SCN is the synthesis and release of melatonin, and the complete pathway by which circadian neural signals from the SCN reach the pineal gland and control the timing of melatonin release appears to have been established (for reviews see 24, 25).

In all mammalian species, serum levels of melatonin are high during the nighttime and low during the daytime (19, 22, 26, 27). The important link to the reproductive system was made by Goldman and his colleagues working with the Djungarian hamster (as well as Karsch and his colleagues in sheep) who established that the duration of peak melatonin levels in the circulation determined whether a long-day or a short-day reproductive response was observed (2, 22, 26, 27). In the Djungarian hamster, the long-duration serum melatonin peak associated with long nights (and thus short days) results in an inhibition of the reproductive system, while the short-duration serum melatonin peak associated with short nights (and thus long days) is stimulatory to neuroendocrine-gonadal activity. While there is some data to suggest that the melatonin duration hypothesis may not represent the entire story of how the melatonin signal affects the seasonal reproductive response (28, 29), there is no question that the duration of high nighttime melatonin levels plays a key role in transmitting information about day length to the reproductive system.

Although the importance of melatonin in the photoperiodic response is no longer in question, essentially nothing is known about (1) where melatonin acts in the brain to influence hypothalamic-pituitary function, or (2) how the melatonin duration signal is decoded to provide information that eventually leads to the inhibition or stimulation of neuroendocrine-gonadal activity.

Recent advances in melatonin binding assays have focused attention on a number of brain regions that may be the target sites for melatonin's action on the reproductive system. Particularly intriguing is the finding that high concentrations of melatonin binding sites are found in the pars tuberalis (30–32), a portion of the pituitary gland that has not previously been linked to the photoperiodic response and whose role in the control of pituitary gonadotropin release is not known. Equally intriguing is the finding that radiolabeled melatonin binds in high amounts in the SCN itself (33, 34). Since there is limited data to implicate a role for melatonin in the control of circadian signals generated within the SCN of mammals (35), the function of melatonin's presumed action in the SCN remains unknown. Perhaps melatonin's effects on reproduction in seasonally breeding animals involve an action on the same circadian clock that regulates its own rhythm of release. While it is uncertain where or how melatonin acts to influence hypothalamic-pituitary function, its effects on this axis are dramatic.

Hypothalamic-Pituitary-Gonadal Axis

Short-day-induced testicular regression in hamsters is associated with a clear decrease in serum testosterone levels (and associated testosterone-induced behaviors) and in the complete inhibition of spermatogenesis (36, 37). This decrease in testicular function is undoubtedly due to the decrease in serum levels of LH, FSH, and prolactin that are observed during exposure to an inhibitory light cycle. A number of experiments carried out in the golden hamster, as well as in other species, have established that two processes are involved in photic-induced changes in pituitary gonadotropin release (3, 38). One process appears to depend on steroid hormone feedback since exposure to short days renders castrated male hamsters extremely sensitive to the negative-feedback effects of steroid hormones on pituitary LH and FSH release. A second process does not appear to depend on steroid hormone feedback since the photoperiod can alter pituitary gonadotropin release in the absence of the testes. The relationship between the steroid-dependent and steroid-independent processes is not clear, nor have the cellular and molecular mechanisms that must underlie these two processes been identified.

Contrary to what might be expected, hypothalamic GnRH levels are either increased or show no change when hamsters are exposed to short days, despite the decrease in serum gonadotropin levels (39). Such findings have been interpreted to indicate that exposure to short days inhibits hypothalamic GnRH release without an associated decrease in content. Nevertheless, it remains to be determined empirically what changes in hypothalamic GnRH release are associated with photostimulation or photoinhibition of pituitary gonadotropin release. Recent in vitro studies indicate that the photoperiod does not induce any intrinsic changes in hypothalamic function (40) and suggest that the photoperiodic control of hypothalamic activity occurs at a level above the GnRH neurons.

Thus, following the transfer from an inhibitory to a stimulatory light cycle, photoperiodic information travels along a pathway that involves an unknown photoreceptive system in the eye, a neural input to a circadian clock located in the SCN, neural circadian signals from the SCN that control the release of pineal melatonin, and a melatonin duration signal that somehow alters hypothalamic-pituitary function, which ultimately leads to an inhibition or stimulation of pituitary gonadotropin release. Changes in pituitary gonadotropin release, of course, lead to changes in gametogenesis and steroidogenesis in the gonads. The final step in the response of the brain to changes in day length has an interesting feature in itself: There is a differential effect of photoperiod on pituitary LH and FSH release during the early stages of photostimulation. The remainder of this review focuses on this differential response, with an emphasis on the importance of pituitary FSH release during the first few days of light activation of the neuroendocrine-gonadal axis.

Critical Role of FSH During Early Stages of Photostimulated Testicular Growth

Both serum FSH levels and testes weight increase more rapidly than serum LH levels when juvenile male Djungarian hamsters are transferred from short to long days (41). In one study significant changes in serum FSH levels were observed within 3 days and significant testicular growth within 5 days of photostimulation, while significant increases in serum LH levels in the same animals did not occur until 21 days' exposure to long days (41). A critical role for FSH during the early stages of testicular growth is demonstrated by the finding that administration of FSH to animals maintained on a short nonstimulatory photoperiod led to increased testis weight within 7 days, while no significant increase in testis weight was observed in animals exposed to short days and given LH. Furthermore, in animals exposed to a long stimulatory day length for 7 days, but whose FSH levels were suppressed due to treatment with porcine follicular fluid (pFF) known to contain inhibin, testis weight was decreased compared to untreated animals or control animals treated with porcine serum during exposure to long days (Fig. 6.1) (42). Further, the suppressive effects of pFF injections on testis growth were not observed in animals exposed to a long photoperiod and treated simultaneously with FSH. Taken together, these results suggest that FSH and not LH plays a central role during the early phase of testis growth in response to photostimulation.

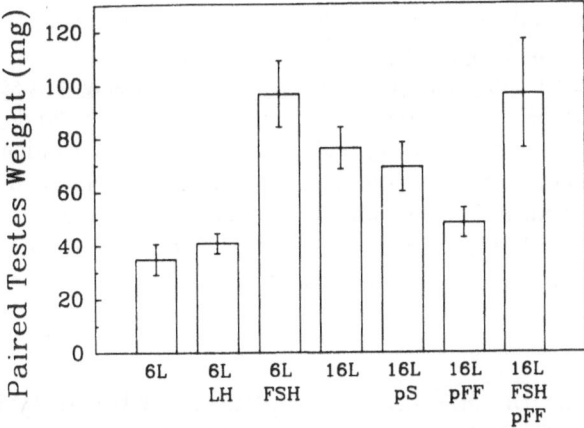

FIGURE 6.1. Mean (±SEM) paired testes weight (mg) of young male Djungarian hamsters exposed to 6L:18D (6L), exposed to 6L:18 and implanted with a minipump containing ovine LH (6L LH), exposed to 6L:18D and implanted with a minipump containing ovine FSH (6L FSH), exposed to 16L:8D (16L), exposed to 16L:8D and injected twice a day with pig serum (16L pS), exposed to 16L:8D and injected twice a day with porcine follicular fluid (16L pFF), or exposed to 16L:8D and implanted with a minipump containing ovine FSH and injected twice a day with porcine follicular fluid (16L FSH pFF) for 7 days. All animals were exposed to 6L:18D for 3 weeks to induce gonadal regression before the 7 days of treatment. Reprinted with permission from Milette, Schwartz, and Turek (42), © by The Endocrine Society.

In another study on Djungarian hamsters, Niklowitz et al. (43) demonstrated that treatment with FSH caused regrowth of the testes and restoration of tubular lumen and diameter and restored complete spermatogenesis in animals maintained on photoinhibitory short days. In contrast, treatment with LH had little effect on spermatogenesis despite increased intratesticular and peripheral testosterone levels. These authors concluded that normal levels of intratesticular testosterone are not sufficient to restore spermatogenesis in the Djungarian hamster and that FSH is required for quantitatively normal spermatogenesis. Taken together with the results from the studies of Simpson et al. (41) and Milette et al. (42), it appears that FSH plays a more central role than LH in the regulation of the early stages of spermatogenesis following photostimulation in the hamster.

After prolonged photostimulation, serum FSH levels decline (41), and this decline may be due to an increased production of inhibin as the testes mature. Inhibin is thought to act primarily at the level of the pituitary to decrease synthesis of FSH by the gonadotrope (44). Thus, the rapid testicular growth observed in young male Djungarian hamsters during the early phase of photostimulation may occur when the immature testis is not yet producing sufficient inhibin to suppress pituitary FSH release.

FSH appears to play a critical role during the early stages of spontaneous testicular recrudescence following prolonged exposure to short days (i.e., the refractory period, see above) in both the golden and Djungarian hamsters. Spontaneous testicular growth in the golden hamster is preceded by a sharp increase in serum FSH levels long before any clear increase in serum LH levels is observed (45), while in the Djungarian hamster, during this recrudescence period pituitary FSH increases weeks before any increase in LH or prolactin (43).

Mechanisms for Differential Regulation of Pituitary LH and FSH Release in Photostimulated Hamsters

The observation that serum FSH levels increase while serum LH levels remain low during the early stages of photostimulated testicular growth demonstrates that the release of these two hormones is under differential control at this time. While the physiological basis for this differential control of LH and FSH release remains unknown, some obvious possibilities can be ruled out. For example, exposure to short days does not appear to have any direct effect in inducing an altered responsiveness of the pituitary gland to GnRH-stimulated LH and FSH release. Single injections of synthetic GnRH into castrated hamsters previously exposed to short or long days for 60 days induces a similar dose-dependent rise in serum LH and FSH levels (46). Similarly, the differential effects of photostimulation on pituitary LH and FSH release do not appear to be dependent on a differential effect of testosterone on pituitary gonadotropin release. When castrated testosterone-treated hamsters are transferred from short to long days, the time course for the escape from the short-day-induced supersensitivity to the negative-feedback effects of testosterone is similar for both pituitary LH and FSH release (47). Likewise, the time course for the escape from the short-day-induced supersensitivity to the negative-feedback effects of testosterone, which occurs in castrated testosterone-treated hamsters during prolonged exposure to short days (i.e., during the onset of photorefractoriness), is similar for both pituitary LH and FSH release (48).

While the differential effects on pituitary gonadotropin release observed during the early stages of photostimulation do not appear to depend on the differential effects of testosterone on pituitary gonadotropin release, this response does appear to be gonad dependent. This conclusion is based on the observation that serum LH and FSH levels rise in parallel when castrated golden hamsters are transferred from short to long days (49). Thus, in the absence of the gonads, there does not appear to be a differential effect of photoperiod on pituitary gonadotropin release. One possibility raised by this finding is that a nonsteroidal gonadal factor (e.g., inhibin) is involved in the differential control of pituitary LH and FSH release during the early stages of photostimulation.

While the rise in FSH in the absence of a concomitant increase in serum LH levels could be due to a separate hypothalamic releasing factor for FSH (50, 51), the existence of such an FSHRF remains controversial. A particularly intriguing possibility for why photostimulation leads to an initial rise in serum FSH levels in the absence of an increase in serum LH is that the pattern of hypothalamic GnRH release during the early stages of photostimulation may favor the release of pituitary FSH over LH. There is now substantial evidence from studies in both animals and humans that the pattern of GnRH stimulation plays a role in the differential synthesis and secretion of FSH and LH, with low-amplitude, slow-frequency pulses of GnRH favoring FSH release and high-amplitude, high-frequency GnRH pulses favoring pituitary LH release (52). A photoperiodic animal in which pituitary gonadotropin release is at a minimum due to exposure to a nonstimulatory light cycle may prove to be an interesting model with which to examine the importance of different patterns of GnRH stimulation (e.g., in frequency and/or amplitude) in the differential release of LH or FSH by the pituitary gland.

References

1. Bronson F. Seasonal regulation of reproduction in mammals. In: Knobil E, Neill J, eds. The physiology of reproduction, vol 2. New York: Raven Press, 1988:1831-71.
2. Nelson RJ, Badura LL, Goldman BD. Mechanisms of seasonal cycles of behavior. Annu Rev Psychol 1990;41:81-108.
3. Turek FW, Campbell CS. Photoperiodic regulation of neuroendocrine-gonadal activity. Biol Reprod 1979;20:32-50.
4. Watson-Whitmyre M, Stetson M. Reproductive refractoriness in hamsters: environmental and endocrine etiologies. In: Stetson M, ed. Processing of environmental information in vertebrates. New York: Springer-Verlag, 1988:219-49.
5. Stetson M. Termination of photorefractoriness in golden hamsters—photoperiodic requirements. J Exp Zool 1977;202:81-8.
6. Gwinner E. Circannual rhythms. Berlin, Heidelberg, New York: Springer-Verlag, 1989.
7. Karsch FJ, Robinson JE, Woodfill CJI, Brown MB. Circannual cycles of luteinizing hormone and prolactin secretion in ewes during prolonged exposure to a fixed photoperiod: evidence for an endogenous reproductive rhythm. Biol Reprod 1989; 41:1034-46.
8. Legan SJ, Karsch FJ. Importance of retinal photoreceptors to the photoperiodic control of seasonal breeding in the ewe. Biol Reprod 1983;29:316-25.
9. Underwood H, Groos G. Vertebrate circadian rhythms: retinal and extraretinal photoreception. Experientia 1982;38:1013-21.

10. Milette JJ, Hotz MM, Takahashi JS, Turek FW. Characterization of the wavelength of light necessary for initiation of neuroendocrine-gonadal activity in male Djungarian hamsters [Abstract]. Biol Reprod 1987;36:110.

11. Hotz MM, Milette JJ, Takahashi JS, Turek FW. Spectral sensitivity of the circadian clock's response to light in Djungarian hamsters [Abstract]. Soc Res Biol Rhythms 1990;2:49.

12. Pickard G. Morphological characteristics of retinal ganglion cells projecting to the suprachiasmatic nucleus: a horseradish peroxidase study. Brain Res 1980; 183:458-65.

13. Pickard G, Friauf E. Morphological features of lucifer yellow (LY) filled retinal ganglion cells innervating the suprachiasmatic nucleus (SCN) [Abstract]. Neurosci Soc 1990;16:602.

14. Moore RY, Lenn NJ. A retinohypothalamic projection in the rat. J Comp Neurol 1972;146:1-15.

15. Moore RY, Eichler VB. Loss of a circadian adrenal corticosterone rhythm following suprachiasmatic lesions in the rat. Brain Res 1972;42:201-6.

16. Stephan FK, Zucker I. Circadian rhythms in drinking behavior and locomotor activity of rats are eliminated by hypothalamic lesions. Proc Natl Acad Sci USA 1972;69:1583-6.

17. Morin LP, Fitzgerald KM, Rusak B, Zucker I. Circadian organization and neural mediation of hamster reproductive rhythms. Psychoneuroendocrinology 1977; 2:73-98.

18. Turek F, Van Cauter E. Rhythms in reproduction. In: Knobil E, Neill J, eds. The physiology of reproduction, vol 2. New York: Raven Press, 1988:1789-1830.

19. Underwood H, Goldman BD. Vertebrate circadian and photoperiodic systems: role of the pineal gland and melatonin. J Biol Rhythms 1987;2:279-315.

20. Stetson M, Watson-Whitmyre M. Nucleus suprachiasmaticus: the biological clock in the hamster. Science 1976;191:197-9.

21. Hoffmann K. The role of the pineal gland in the photoperiodic control of seasonal cycles in hamsters. In: Follett BK, Follett DE, eds. Biological clocks in seasonal reproductive cycles. Bristol: Wright, 1981:237-50.

22. Bartness TJ, Goldman BD. Mammalian pineal melatonin: a clock for all seasons. Experientia 1989;45:939-44.

23. Reiter RJ. Circannual reproductive rhythms in mammals related to photoperiod and pineal function: a review. Chronobiologia 1974;1:365-95.

24. Smale L, Cassone VM, Moore RY, Morin LP. Paraventricular nucleus projections mediating pineal melatonin and gonadal responses to photoperiod in the hamster. Brain Res Bull 1989;22:263-9.

25. Youngstrom TG, Weiss ML, Nunez AA. A retinal projection to the paraventricular nuclei of the hypothalamus in the Syrian hamster (*Mesocricetus auratus*). Brain Res Bull 1987;19:747-50.

26. Wayne NL, Malpaux B, Karsch RJ. How does melatonin code for day length in the ewe: duration of nocturnal melatonin release or coincidence of melatonin with a light-entrained sensitive period? Biol Reprod 1988;39:66-75.

27. Bittman EL, Dempsey RJ, Karsh FJ. Nightly duration of pineal melatonin secretion determines the reproductive response to inhibitory day length in the ewe. Biol Reprod 1984;30:585-93.

28. Reiter RJ. The melatonin message: duration versus coincidence hypotheses. Life Sci 1987;40:2119-31.

29. Stetson M, Sarafidis E, Rollag M. Sensitivity of adult male Djungarian hamsters (*Phodopus sungorus*) to melatonin injections throughout the day: effects on the reproductive system and the pineal. Biol Reprod 1986;35:618-23.

30. de Reviers M-M, Ravault J-P, Tillet Y, Pelletier J. Melatonin binding sites in the sheep pars tuberalis. Neurosci Lett 1989;100:89-93.

31. Morgan PJ, Williams LM, Davidson G, Lawson W, Howell E. Melatonin receptors on ovine pars tuberalis: characterization and autoradiographic localization. J Neuroendocrinol 1989;1:1-4.

32. Weaver DR, Carlson LL, Reppert SM. Melatonin receptors and signal transduction in melatonin-sensitive and melatonin-insensitive populations of white-footed mice (*Peromyscus leucopus*). Brain Res 1990;506:353-7.

33. Vanecek J, Pavlík A, Illnerová H. Hypothalamic melatonin receptor sites revealed by autoradiography. Brain Res 1987;435:359-62.

34. Williams LM. Melatonin-binding sites in the rat brain and pituitary mapped by in-vitro autoradiograph. J Mol Endocrinol 1989;3:71-5.

35. Cassone VM. Effects of melatonin on vertebrate circadian systems. TINS 1990; 13:457-70.

36. Sinha Hikim AP, Amador AG, Bartke A, Russell LD. Structure/function relationships in active and inactive hamster Leydig cells: a correlative morphometric and endocrine study. Endocrinology 1989;125:1844-56.

37. Sinha Hikim AP, Amador AG, Klemcke HG, Bartke A, Russell LD. Correlative morphology and endocrinology of Sertoli cells in hamster testes in active and inactive states of spermatogenesis. Brain Res Bull 1989;125:1829-43.

38. Turek FW, Ellis GB. Steroid-dependent and steroid-independent aspects of the photoperiodic control of seasonal reproductive cycles in male hamsters. In: Follett BK, Follett DE, eds. Biological clocks in seasonal reproductive cycles. Bristol: Wright, 1981:251-60.

39. Pickard GE, Silverman AJ. Effects of photoperiod on hypothalamic luteinizing hormone releasing hormone in the male hamster. J Endocrinol 1979;83:421-28.

40. Jetton AE, Schwartz NB, Turek FW. Effects of photoperiod and melatonin on in vitro hypothalamic gonadotropin releasing hormone (GnRH) release in Djungarian hamsters [Abstract]. Neurosci Soc 1990;16:285.

41. Simpson SM, Follett BK, Ellis DH. Modulation by photoperiod of gonadotropin secretion in intact and castrated Djungarian hamsters. J Reprod Fertil 1982;66:243.

42. Milette JJ, Schwartz NB, Turek FW. The importance of follicle-stimulating hormone in the initiation of testicular growth in photostimulated Djungarian hamsters. Endocrinology 1988;122:1060-6.

43. Niklowitz P, Khan S, Bergmann M, Hoffman K, Nieschlag E. Differential effects of follicle-stimulating hormone and luteinizing hormone on Leydig cell function and restoration of spermatogenesis in hypophysectomized and photoinhibited Djungarian hamsters (*Phodopus sungorus*). Biol Reprod 1989;41:871-80.

44. Scott RS, Burger HG. Mechanism of action of inhibin. Biol Reprod 1981;24:541.

45. Turek FW, Elliot JA, Alvis JD, Menaker M. Effect of prolonged exposure to nonstimulatory photoperiods on the activity of the neuroendocrine-testicular axis of golden hamsters. Biol Reprod 1975;13:475-81.

46. Turek FW, Alvis JD, Menaker M. Pituitary responsiveness to LRF in castrated male hamsters exposed to different photoperiodic conditions. Neuroendocrinology 1977;24:140-6.
47. Ellis GB, Turek FW. Time course of the photoperiod-induced change in sensitivity of the hypothalamic-pituitary axis to testosterone feedback in castrated male hamsters. Endocrinology 1979;104:625-30.
48. Ellis GB, Losee S, Turek FW. Prolonged exposure of castrated male hamsters to a nonstimulatory photoperiod: spontaneous change in sensitivity of the hypothalamic-pituitary axis to testosterone feedback. Endocrinology 1979;104:631-5.
49. Ellis G, Turek FW. Photoperiodic regulation of serum luteinizing hormone and follicle-stimulating hormone in castrated and castrated-adrenalectomized male hamsters. Endocrinology 1980;106:1338-44.
50. Mizunuma H, Samson WK, Lumpkin MD, Moltz JH, Fawcett CP, McCann SM. Purification of a bioactive FSH-releasing factor (FSHRF). Brain Res Bull 1983;10:623.
51. Vale W, Rivier J, Vaughan J, et al. Purification and characterization of an FSH releasing protein from ovarian follicular fluid. Nature 1986;321:776.
52. Marshall JC, Dalkin AC, Goodman GT, Haisenleder, Kelch RP, Paul SJ. GnRH pulse patterns in the regulation of FSH secretion [Abstract]. Symposium on Regulation and Actions of Follicle Stimulating Hormone, Serono Symposia, USA. Evanston, 1990. (See Chapter 13, this volume.)

7

Light Regulates c-*fos* Gene Expression in the Hamster SCN: Implications for Circadian and Seasonal Control of Reproduction

JON M. KORNHAUSER, DWIGHT E. NELSON, KELLY E. MAYO, AND JOSEPH S. TAKAHASHI

The naturally occurring daily cycle of light and darkness in the environment exerts important control upon the function of the reproductive system in mammals, providing external timing cues that influence reproductive physiology in two distinct ways. First, the light-dark cycle serves to synchronize the circadian timekeeping system, and this circadian pacemaker regulates daily periodic events of the neuroendocrine axis. Second, many mammals breed on a seasonal basis, and the length of the day is the most important environmental factor regulating these dramatic seasonal changes in reproduction. The circadian pacemaking system mediates effects of this type by measuring changes in the photoperiod corresponding to seasonal alterations in day length (1). The suprachiasmatic nucleus (SCN) of the hypothalamus is the site of the predominant circadian pacemaker regulating behavioral and physiological processes in mammals, including the reproductive axis, (2–4). Timing signals from this pacemaker coordinate circadian components of reproductive rhythms; for example, the time of occurrence of the preovulatory surges in luteinizing hormone (LH) and follicle stimulating hormone (FSH) and of ovulation during proestrus (1, 5). The SCN also mediates the effects of alterations in photoperiod on seasonal changes in reproductive function. Thus, the circadian pacemaker in the SCN utilizes photic information for synchronization of endogenous rhythms to the environmental 24-h light cycle and for measurement of changes in day length for photoperiodic regulation of reproduction.

Light synchronizes, or entrains, this circadian pacemaker to the ambient daily light cycle by shifting the phase of the oscillation generated by the

SCN. The cellular and molecular mechanisms by which this entrainment occurs (and, indeed, the nature of the pacemaking mechanism itself) are not understood. In golden hamsters, even light pulses of quite short duration can produce a significant phase shift (a steady state change in phase) of the circadian rhythm of locomotor activity (6). Therefore, transduction of a brief light signal leads to long-term changes in pacemaker function. Several other long-term cellular processes, such as the regulation of cell growth and the cell cycle (7–11) and of learning and memory (12, 13), are characterized by changes in transcription and/or translation in response to appropriate extra-cellular signals. In these systems, cellular immediate-early genes have been shown to couple transient stimuli to coordinated changes in gene expression (7, 8). A number of these immediate-early genes, which respond rapidly to extracellular signals, have been identified. Many of the protein products of these genes are transcription factors that can interact with DNA to regulate the transcription of specific target genes (14). The product of one such gene, c-*fos* (15), can form heterodimers with the c-*jun* (16) gene product (another immediate-early gene) or with related members of the Jun family to form the AP-1 transcription factor (11). This AP-1 protein complex recognizes a specific DNA sequence and binds to it with high affinity to regulate transcription (17). In culture, c-*fos* is induced in neuronal cells by a number of stimuli, including exposure to serum (8) and nerve growth factor or other growth factors (18, 19), or by depolarization either by cholinergic neurotransmitters or by high extracellular K^+ (20, 21). Expression of c-*fos* is stimulated in the rat hippocampus by pentylenetetrazol-induced seizure activity (22), in the paraventricular nucleus by water deprivation (23), and in spinal cord neurons following peripheral stimulation (24).

We have found that light exposure leads to rapid increases in levels of c-*fos* mRNA in the SCN of the golden hamster (25), and it has also been shown that Fos-like immunoreactivity in the SCN of both hamster (26) and rat (27–29) is stimulated by light. To begin to address the question of whether Fos mediates transcriptional events involved in phase shifting of the circadian pacemaker, we have further characterized the photic induction of c-*fos* mRNA utilizing in situ hybridization techniques. Using defined light stimuli for which the effects on the hamster's circadian rhythm of activity have been measured, we have compared the photic induction of c-*fos* mRNA and the behavioral phase shifts produced by light. Specifically, we examined whether the photic induction of c-*fos* was quantitatively correlated with phase shifting of locomotor activity in two respects. First, we asked if induction of c-*fos* mRNA by light, like the phase-shifting effect of light, depends upon the circadian time at which the light occurs. Second, we compared the photic threshold of c-*fos* mRNA induction and the threshold for phase-shifting circadian rhythms.

Photic Induction of c-*fos* mRNA in the Suprachiasmatic Nucleus

Presentation of a pulse of light to a hamster during the night at circadian time (CT) 19 causes a dramatic induction of c-*fos* mRNA in the SCN (Fig. 7.1). (CT12 is defined as the time of onset of running-wheel activity in nocturnal species, such as the hamster, corresponding to the time of lights off on a light-dark cycle.) The increase in c-*fos* mRNA levels illustrated here was induced by a 5-min light pulse, after which the animal was returned to darkness for 25 min before sacrifice. This dark-field photomicrograph shows that hybridization to a complementary RNA probe for c-*fos* is localized mainly in the ventrolateral portion of each SCN and extends dorsally from the SCN toward the paraventricular nuclei. This pattern matches that of retinohypothalamic tract projections to the SCN described by Johnson et al. (30), as determined by anterograde labeling using cholera toxin-horseradish peroxidase. No other effect of light on c-*fos* mRNA was observed in any other areas of the brain, including such retinorecipient regions as the lateral geniculate nucleus or intergeniculate leaflet (data not shown). To verify this light-stimulated induction of c-*fos* mRNA detected by in situ hybridization, we also performed RNA blot analysis of total RNA isolated from microdissections of brain tissue containing the SCN. A single transcript of approximately 2.2 kb in size is detected in the RNA from light-pulsed but not dark control animals (25). This corresponds to the reported size of c-*fos* mRNA in mouse (31) and rat (18, 19).

Upon stimulation, c-*fos* gene expression generally responds very rapidly and transiently. Transcription of the c-*fos* gene is rapidly increased by second-messenger-mediated regulatory factors, and this transcriptional activation does not require new protein synthesis. The brief duration of the elevation of c-*fos* mRNA levels is accounted for by two mechanisms: The Fos protein negatively autoregulates the transcription of the c-*fos* gene, and c-*fos* messenger RNA is rapidly degraded. Similar to what has been observed in other types of cells, c-*fos* mRNA induction by light in the SCN exhibits a transient time course (Fig. 7.2A). When light is presented at CT19 and continues until the time of sampling, c-*fos* mRNA levels are maximal after about 30 min and then decline (Fig. 7.2A). The induction of c-*fos* mRNA after a 5-min light pulse (at CT19) followed by a return to darkness for varying lengths of time until sampling shows a similar time course (Fig. 7.2B). Two hours following the light pulse, c-*fos* mRNA levels return nearly to basal levels. These measurements of c-*fos* mRNA levels were made utilizing in situ hybridization and quantification of autoradiographic silver-grain densities in the SCN.

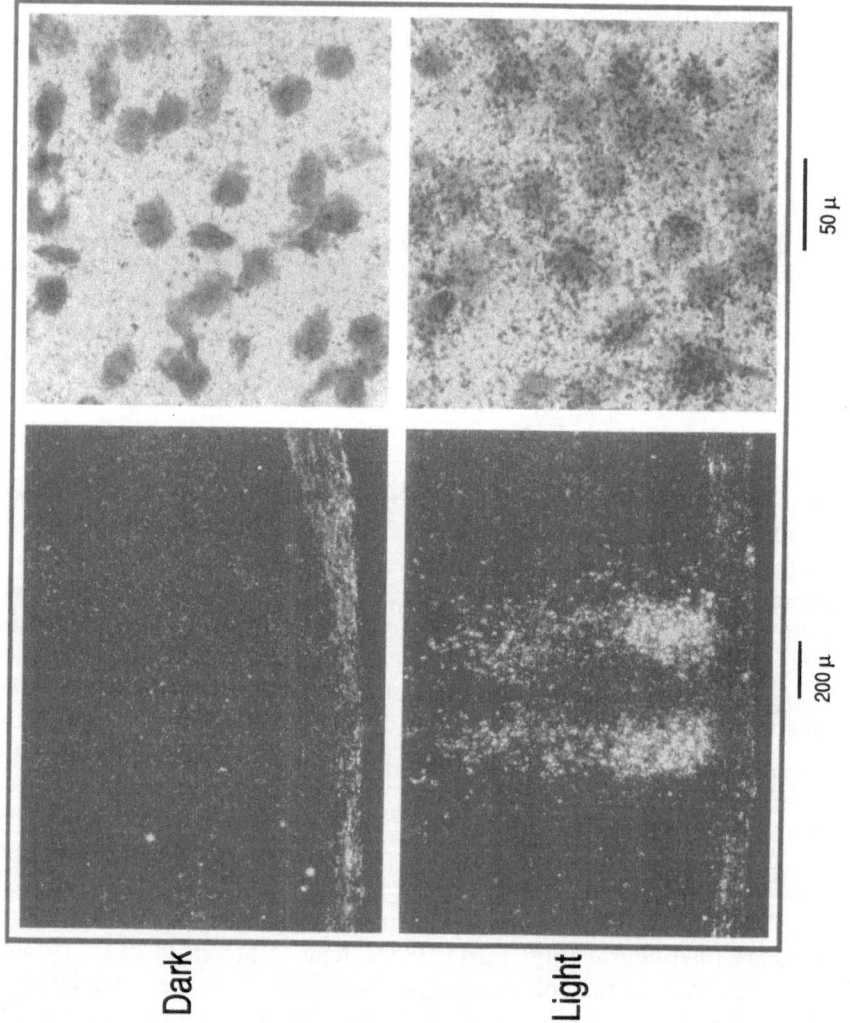

Circadian Gating of c-*fos* Induction by Light

Light has distinct effects on the hamster's circadian system at different CTs (32). During the early part of the subjective night, light causes phase delays or a shifting of the animal's rhythm to a later phase. Light during the latter part of the night leads to phase advances. In contrast, light does not affect the phase of the activity rhythm when presented during the subjective day (Fig. 7.3A). (Experiments of this type are conducted in constant darkness; *subjective day* refers to the period of the hamster's internally generated daily rhythm when the animal is inactive.) We investigated whether the induction of c-*fos* mRNA by light might also depend upon the CT when the light is presented. As already shown, light at CT19 greatly increases c-*fos* mRNA levels in the SCN. Photic stimulation at CT14, which causes a phase delay in the circadian rhythm, and at CT21, which induces a phase advance, also elevate c-*fos* mRNA levels (Fig. 7.3B). Remarkably, light pulses during the subjective day at CT3, CT6 (not shown), and CT9, which produce no behavioral phase shifts, do not cause a detectable increase in c-*fos* mRNA in the SCN (Fig. 7.3B). Hamsters receiving no light, examined at all 5 CTs displayed no specific c-*fos* hybridization in the area of the SCN. The expression of c-*fos*, then, is not simply regulated by light, but is controlled at another level by circadian phase. The ability of light to induce expression of this immediate-early gene, like its ability to phase-shift the pacemaker, is gated in some way by the state of the circadian pacemaker.

◀ FIGURE 7.1. Light-induced c-*fos* mRNA in the SCN. At CT19, hamsters were exposed to either 5 min of light (503 nm) or to the same handling without light. Animals were then returned to darkness for 25 min, and brains were removed and sectioned for in situ hybridization to an ^{35}S-labeled c-*fos* complementary RNA probe (25). Dark-field photographs of a dark control animal (*upper left*) and a light-pulsed animal (*lower left*) are shown. The paired SCN are located at the base of the anterior hypothalamus; the strong hybridization observed in the brain of the light-exposed hamster is localized to the ventrolateral portion of each SCN. The third ventricle vertically divides the 2 nuclei, and the optic chiasm extends horizontally below them in the photographs. The hybridization observed in the optic chiasm represents nonspecific labeling and is observed with either a sense or an antisense RNA probe. The photographs on the right are bright-field images of the same two sections at higher magnification, showing autoradiographic silver grains that indicate cellular hybridization. Reprinted with permission from Kornhauser, Nelson, Mayo, and Takahashi (25), © by Cell Press.

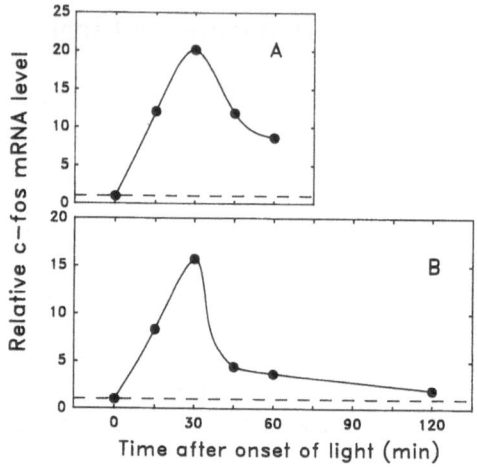

FIGURE 7.2. Time course of the photic induction of c-*fos* mRNA in the SCN. *A*: After various durations of light exposure (15–60 min) at CT19, in situ detection of c-*fos* mRNA in the SCN was performed. The hybridization was quantified, and the ratio of this signal to that in dark control animals is plotted. Quantification of hybridization was performed essentially as described (25) with the following exception: The "signal" in each section was defined by taking a measurement from a 75 × 75-μm area within the SCN and subtracting a background measurement from an area of equal size lateral to the SCN. This background-subtraction method was used rather than defining the signal as the ratio of the SCN to the lateral measurement. *B*: Five-minute light pulses were delivered at CT19, after which the hamsters were returned to darkness for varying durations until sampling. Quantified SCN c-*fos* mRNA levels were determined by in situ detection, as in *A*. Adapted with permission from Kornhauser, Nelson, Mayo, and Takahashi (25), © by Cell Press.

Photic Threshold for c-*fos* mRNA Induction

The response of the hamster's circadian system to varying levels of illumination has been characterized (6, 32). The magnitude of the phase shift in locomotor activity exhibits a monotonic, saturable dependence on the irradiance of the light stimulus (of a given wavelength and duration). Figure 7.4 illustrates the amount of behavioral phase shift produced by 5-min light pulses (503-nm wavelength) of varying irradiance occurring at CT19 (open circles). To compare the sensitivity to light of the c-*fos* mRNA induction and of this photic response of the circadian system, we performed in situ hybridization following 5-min light stimuli of different illumination levels and quantified the photic increase in specific c-*fos* hybridization within the SCN

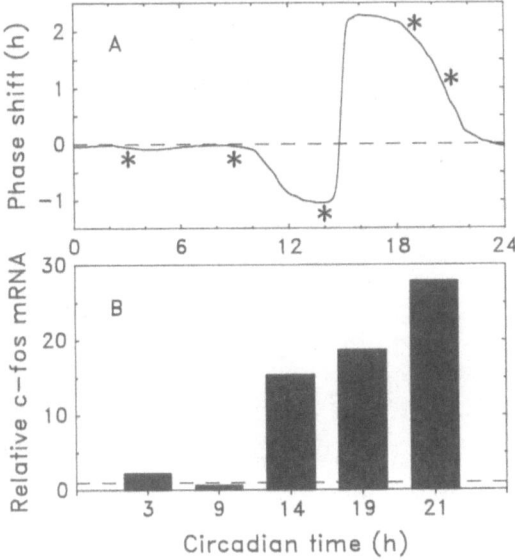

FIGURE 7.3. Dependence of photic induction of phase shifting and c-*fos* mRNA on circadian phase. *A*: A phase response curve for the golden hamster showing the dependence of the magnitude and direction of the behavioral phase shift on the phase of the rhythm at which the light stimulus occurs. From Takahashi, DeCoursey, Bauman, and Menaker (32). Asterisks indicate circadian phases when photic c-*fos* induction was measured (shown in *B*). *B*: Hamsters were placed in constant darkness for 7 days before the experiment and then received a 5-min light pulse at CT3, CT9, CT14, CT19, or CT21. Animals were returned to darkness for 25 min and in situ hybridization was performed. Quantified c-*fos* mRNA levels in the SCN (as described in Fig. 7.2) are shown as a function of the circadian time at which the light pulse was given. Values represent the mean signal in the SCN of light-pulsed hamsters relative to the signal in animals receiving no light. Adapted with permission from Kornhauser, Nelson, Mayo, and Takahashi (25), © by Cell Press.

(Fig. 7.4, closed circles). The threshold for a detectable increase in expression of the c-*fos* gene is virtually identical to the threshold for light-induced phase shifts, suggesting that this alteration in gene expression could be related to mechanisms involved in phase-shifting the pacemaker.

It is interesting that the inhibition of pineal melatonin synthesis by light, a photic response that is also mediated by a pathway involving the SCN, is significantly more sensitive to light than either circadian entrainment or the c-*fos* induction response (Nelson and Takahashi, unpublished data). This indicates that dim-light stimuli which can activate SCN neurons and produce

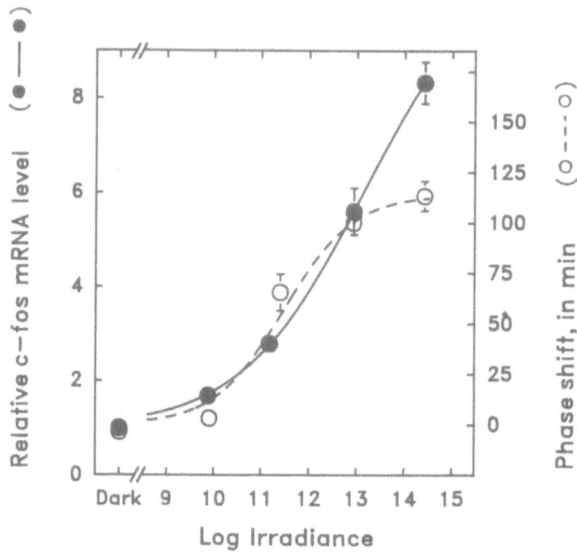

FIGURE 7.4. Dependence of c-*fos* mRNA induction and of phase shifting of locomotor activity on irradiance of light stimuli. Hamsters were entrained to a 14L:10D cycle and then placed in constant darkness for 7 days prior to the experiment. Light pulses of 5-min duration and varying irradiance were presented at CT19. Animals were then either returned to darkness for 25 min and quantitative in situ hybridization performed or returned to darkness and their locomotor activity recorded to estimate steady state phase shifts of the onset of activity. Measurements of c-*fos* mRNA levels in the SCN are indicated by the closed circles; group data for behavioral phase shifts are shown by the open circles. Quantification of in situ hybridization was performed exactly as described. Reprinted with permission from Kornhauser, Nelson, Mayo, and Takahashi (25), © by Cell Press.

physiological responses, are not necessarily adequate to evoke either this transcriptional modulation of c-*fos* or phase shifts, reinforcing the idea that these two events may share common elements or mechanisms. The phase-shifting response to light and the induction of c-*fos* mRNA differ only in that more intense light stimuli produce increasing levels of c-*fos* expression in the irradiance range where the magnitude of the phase-shifting response has saturated. Since Fos participates in transcriptional regulation at AP-1 sites through its interactions with Jun proteins, which may either be in limiting concentrations or regulated differentially by light, this result is still consistent with a hypothesized role for Fos/AP-1 in the regulation of genes intrinsic to the mechanism of phase-shifting the circadian pacemaker.

Significance of c-*fos* to Circadian Pacemaker Mechanisms

Stimulation of the hamster's visual system by light leads to a rapid and dramatic increase in SCN expression of the c-*fos* gene; the anatomical specificity of this response is striking: The c-*fos* mRNA induction is confined to structures in and near the SCN known to participate in photic entrainment of circadian rhythms. This well-defined distribution indicates that c-*fos* may be quite useful as a cellular marker of light-activated cells in the region of the pacemaker nuclei of the brain, facilitating studies involving behavioral, surgical, or pharmacological manipulations of circadian responses to light.

We have also demonstrated that in addition to this spatial specificity, this effect of light on gene expression in the SCN is correlated with two other characteristics of circadian entrainment by light. First, the photic induction of c-*fos* mRNA exhibits a distinct temporal specificity, being restricted to CTs when light causes phase shifts of the hamster's circadian rhythm of locomotor activity. Second, the threshold illumination that measurably increases c-*fos* gene expression and the threshold irradiance that is required to produce phase shifts of the circadian clock are very similar. This close correspondence between parameters of light stimuli that are appropriate to entrain behavioral circadian rhythms and those that can alter expression of c-*fos* suggests that regulation of transcription by AP-1 may mediate the effects of light on the circadian clock. If this proves to be the case, then the identification of target genes affected by AP-1 might prospectively lead to the characterization of molecular components of the pacemaker mechanism itself.

It is reasonable to hypothesize that transcriptional and translational events may participate in the generation and the entrainment of circadian rhythms. A critical period for protein synthesis in circadian rhythmicity in the golden hamster has been demonstrated (33–35), as it has for other systems in which long-term modifications in gene expression occur as a consequence of appropriate extracellular stimuli (36–38). Specific gene products play critical roles in the control and generation of circadian rhythms, as demonstrated by the identification of single-gene mutations in quite diverse organisms (39), including *Neurospora* (40), *Drosophila* (41, 42), and the golden hamster (43), all of which produce disruptions of the period of circadian rhythms. In the golden hamster, light pulses of only 3-sec duration or less produce significant phase shifts in the locomotor activity rhythm (6). Thus, if modification of gene expression is indeed involved in this response, one might expect that rapidly responding genes encoding transcriptional regulatory molecules, such as c-*fos*, would likely participate in mediation of the transcriptional events elicited by light. A particularly intriguing aspect of this relationship between c-*fos* gene expression and the circadian clock is that the circadian pacemaker and the visual photic input converge to influence the expression of c-*fos* such that the phase of the pacemaker gates the induction of c-*fos* transcription by light. Further investigation into this apparent mutual interdependence between c-*fos* expression and the circadian pacemaker may help to define the molecular mechanisms regulating rhythms and to elucidate the means by which the animal can utilize photic information, reflecting both daily and seasonal variations, to regulate and coordinate processes of reproductive physiology.

Acknowledgments. We thank Dr. Lester Lau for his gift of the c-*fos* cDNA clone and Dr. Daniel Linzer for helpful discussions. This research was supported by grants from the NIH, NSF, and McKnight Foundation to K.E.M. and NIMH, NIH, and NSF to J.S.T.

References

1. Turek FW, Van Cauter E. Rhythms in reproduction. In: Knobil E, Neill J, et al., eds. The physiology of reproduction. New York: Raven Press, 1988;1789-830.
2. Moore RY. Organization and function of a central nervous system circadian oscillator: the suprachiasmatic hypothalamic nucleus. Fed Proc 1983;42:2783-9.
3. Rusak B, Zucker I. Neural regulation of circadian rhythms. Physiol Rev 1979;59:449-526.
4. Meijer JH, Rietveld WJ. Neurophysiology of the suprachiasmatic circadian pacemaker in rodents. Physiol Rev 1989;69:671-707.
5. Stetson MH, Anderson PJ. Circadian pacemaker times gonadotropin release in free-running female hamsters. Am J Physiol 1980;238:R23-7.
6. Nelson DE, Takahashi JS. Sensitivity of the visual pathway for entrainment of a circadian pacemaker: temporal integration of photic inputs. J Physiol (Lond) (in press).
7. Müller R, Bravo R, Burckhardt J, Curran T. Induction of c-*fos* gene and protein by growth factors precedes activation of c-*myc*. Nature 1984;312:716-20.
8. Greenberg ME, Ziff EB. Stimulation of 3T3 cells induces transcription of the c-*fos* protooncogene. Nature 1984;311:433-7.
9. Lau LF, Nathans D. Expression of a set of growth-related immediate early genes in BALB/c 3T3 cells: coordinate regulation with c-*fos* or c-*myc*. Proc Natl Acad Sci USA 1987;84:1182-6.
10. Sassone-Corsi P, Lamph WW, Verma IM. Regulation of proto-oncogene *fos*: a paradigm for early response genes. Cold Spring Harbor Symp Quant Biol 1988; 53:749-60.
11. Curran T, Franza BR. Fos and Jun: the AP-1 connection. Cell 1988;55:395-7.
12. Goelet P, Castellucci VF, Schacher S, Kandel ER. The long and short of long-term memory—a molecular framework. Nature 1986;322:419-22.
13. Cole AJ, Saffen DW, Baraban JM, Worley PF. Rapid increase of an immediate early gene messenger RNA in hippocampal neurons by synaptic NMDA receptor activation. Nature 1989;340:474-6.

14. Mitchell PJ, Tjian R. Transcriptional regulation in mammalian cells by sequence-specific DNA binding proteins. Science 1989;245:371-8.

15. Van Beveren C, van Straaten F, Curran T, Müller R, Verma IM. Analysis of FBJ-MuSV provirus and c-*fos* (mouse) gene reveals that viral and cellular *fos* gene products have different carboxy termini. Cell 1983;32:1241-55.

16. Rauscher FJ III, Cohen DR, Curran T, et al. Fos-associated protein p39 is the product of the *jun* proto-oncogene. Science 1988;240:1010-6.

17. Curran T, Rauscher FJ, Cohen DR, Franza BR. Beyond the second messenger: oncogenes and transcription factors. Cold Spring Harbor Symp Quant Biol 1988; 53:769-77.

18. Kruijer W, Schubert D, Verma IM. Induction of the proto-oncogene *fos* by nerve growth factor. Proc Natl Acad Sci USA 1985;82:7330-4.

19. Milbrandt J. Nerve growth factor rapidly induces c-*fos* mRNA in PC12 rat pheochromocytoma cells. Proc Natl Acad Sci USA 1986;83:4789-93.

20. Greenberg M, Ziff EB, Greene LA. Stimulation of neuronal acetylcholine receptors induces rapid gene transcription. Science 1986;234:80-3.

21. Greenberg ME, Greene LA, Ziff EB. Nerve growth factor and epidermal growth factor induce rapid transient changes in proto-oncogene transcription in PC12 cells. J Biol Chem 1985;260:14101-10.

22. Morgan JI, Cohen DR, Hempstead JL, Curran T. Mapping patterns of c-*fos* expression in the central nervous system after seizure. Science 1987;237:192-7.

23. Sagar SM, Sharp FR, Curran T. Expression of c-*fos* protein in brain: metabolic mapping at the cellular level. Science 1988;240:1328-31.

24. Hunt SP, Pini A, Evan G. Induction of c-*fos*-like protein in spinal cord neurons following sensory stimulation. Nature 1987;328:632-4.

25. Kornhauser JM, Nelson DE, Mayo KE, Takahashi JS. Photic and circadian regulation of c-*fos* gene expression in the hamster suprachiasmatic nucleus. Neuron 1990; 5:127-34.

26. Rusak B, Robertson HA, Wisden W, Hunt SP. Light pulses that shift rhythms induce gene expression in the suprachiasmatic nucleus. Science 1990;248:1237-40.

27. Rea M. Light increases Fos-related protein immunoreactivity in the rat suprachiasmatic nuclei. Brain Res Bull 1989;23:577-81.

28. Aronin N, Sagar SM, Sharp FR, Schwartz WJ. Light regulates expression of a Fos-related protein in rat suprachiasmatic nuclei. Proc Natl Acad Sci USA 1990; 87:5959-62.

29. Earnest DJ, Iadarola M, Yeh HH, Olschowka JA. Photic regulation of c-*fos* expression in neural components governing the entrainment of circadian rhythms. Exp neurol 1990;109:353-61.

30. Johnson RF, Morin LP, Moore RY. Retinohypothalamic projections in the hamster and rat demonstrated using cholera toxin. Brain Res 1988;462:301-12.

31. Müller R, Slamon DJ, Tremblay JM, Cline MJ, Verma IM. Differential expression of cellular oncogenes during pre- and postnatal development of the mouse. Nature 1982;299:640-4.

32. Takahashi JS, DeCoursey PJ, Bauman L, Menaker M. Spectral sensitivity of a novel photoreceptive system mediating entrainment of mammalian circadian rhythms. Nature 1984;308:186-8.

33. Takahashi JS, Turek FW. Anisomycin, an inhibitor of protein synthesis, perturbs the phase of a mammalian circadian pacemaker. Brain Res 1987;405:199-203.

34. Inouye ST, Takahashi JS, Wollnik F, Turek FW. Inhibitor of protein synthesis phase shifts a circadian pacemaker in mammalian SCN. Am J Physiol 1988;255: R1055-8.

35. Wollnik F, Turek FW, Majewski P, Takahashi JS. Phase shifting the circadian clock with cycloheximide: response of hamsters with an intact or a split rhythm of locomotor activity. Brain Res 1989;496:82-8.

36. Pardee AB. G_1 events and regulation of cell proliferation. Science 1989;246: 603-8.

37. Montarolo PG, Goelet P, Castellucci VF, Morgan J, Kandel ER, Schacher S. A critical period for macromolecular synthesis in long-term heterosynaptic facilitation in Aplysia. Science 1986;234:1249-54.

38. Davis HP, Squire LR. Protein synthesis and memory: a review. Psychol Bull 1984;96:518-59.

39. Rosbash M, Hall JC. The molecular biology of circadian rhythms. Neuron 1989; 3:387-98.

40. Dunlap JC. Closely watched clocks: molecular analysis of circadian rhythms in *Neurospora* and *Drosophila*. Trends Genet 1990;6:159-65.

41. Konopka RJ. Genetics of biological rhythms in *Drosophila*. Annu Rev Genet 1987;21:227-36.

42. Young MW, Bargiello TA, Baylies MK, Saez L, Spray DC. Molecular biology of the *Drosophila* clock. In: Jacklet JW, ed. Neuronal and cellular oscillators. New York: Marcel Dekker, 1989:529-42.

43. Ralph MR, Menaker M. A mutation of the circadian system in golden hamsters. Science 1988;241:1225-7.

Part II

Synthesis and Secretion of FSH: Molecular Regulation

Part II

Samples and Selection of
Marketable Residues

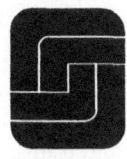

8

Estradiol Inhibition of Expression of the Human Glycoprotein Hormone α-Subunit Gene Through an ERE-Independent Mechanism

Ruth A. Keri, Bogi Andersen, Giulia C. Kennedy,
Debora L. Hamernik, and John H. Nilson

The α-subunit comprises one-half of all glycoprotein hormones. Expression of the α-subunit gene occurs in a variety of cell types (gonadotrophs, thyrotrophs, and syncytiotrophoblasts) and is regulated by a multitude of hormones, including gonadotropin releasing hormone (GnRH), thyrotropin releasing hormone (TRH), estradiol, thyroxine, and others. Thus, this gene serves as a useful model to study various mechanisms underlying hormonal regulation and cell-specific expression. In this report we focus on the approaches we have used to characterize the cis-acting elements required for placenta- and pituitary-specific expression and hormonal responsiveness of the α-subunit gene.

Two Distinct Cis-Acting Elements Required for Placenta-Specific Expression of the Human α-Subunit Gene

Based on transient transfection studies in human choricarcinoma cell lines, at least two cis-acting elements in the 5' flanking region of the α-subunit gene are absolutely required for placenta expression. The first of these elements resides between −180 and −146 and is referred to as the upstream regulatory element or URE (1–3). This element binds to two distinct proteins that are unique to choricarcinoma cells (4). Alone, however, the URE has no effect on transcriptional activity of the α-subunit gene (1, 2). The URE must act in conjunction with an adjacent element that lies between −146 and −110. This region contains 2 tandem 18-bp repeats known as the cAMP response elements, or CRE. While the URE is contingent upon the CRE for transcriptional activation, the CRE can act independently to confer cAMP responsiveness to both the α-subunit gene and heterologous promoters (1, 2, 5). The

CRE bind a ubiquitous, 43-kD protein called CREB (6–8). Each CRE contains an 8-bp palindrome, TGACGTCA, that is critical for binding of CREB and transcriptional activation by cAMP (9). Together, the URE and CRE act to confer placenta-specific expression to the α-subunit gene; thus, they are jointly referred to as the placenta-specific enhancer.

In addition to mediating cAMP responsiveness, the CRE can also confer responsiveness to phorbol esters (10). The addition of both cAMP and PMA results in a synergistic increase in transcription of the α-subunit gene (6, 10). Thus, the CRE can mediate the effects of both the A- and C-kinase pathways, as well as contribute to the cell-specific expression of the α-subunit gene.

While much is known about the cis-acting elements required for placenta-specific expression of the α-subunit gene, the elements necessary for pituitary expression remain undefined. This lag in our understanding of pituitary expression is partially due to the lack of pituitary cell lines that express the α-subunit gene. Thus, as an alternative approach to study pituitary expression, we have used transgenic mice.

Tissue-Specific Expression of Human and Bovine α-Subunit Chimeric Genes in Pituitaries of Transgenic Mice

To begin to determine whether the elements responsible for pituitary expression of the α-subunit gene are similar to those that are required for placenta expression, we produced two strains of transgenic mice. These mice harbor chimeric genes containing the 5' flanking regions and promoters from the human (HαCAT) or bovine (BαCAT) α-subunit genes linked to the bacterial reporter gene encoding chloramphenicol acetyl transferase, or CAT (Fig. 8.1) (11). An obvious difference between the two flanking regions is their length; HαCAT contains 1500 bp of 5' flanking region, while BαCAT contains 315 bp. Another difference between the two regions is the lack of a functional CRE in the bovine construct (11). As mentioned above, the presence of a functional CRE is critical for placenta-specific expression of the α-subunit gene. Thus, using these two constructs, we sought to determine whether a functional CRE was necessary for expression of the α-subunit gene in the pituitary and also to begin to localize any other element(s) necessary for pituitary-specific expression.

Transgenic founder mice containing either the HαCAT or BαCAT chimera were bred with naive animals, and tissues from adult progeny were examined for expression of CAT (Fig. 8.2). Of 8 tissues examined from both strains of mice, only pituitary and brain tissues contained detectable levels of CAT (11). Expression in brain tissue was not entirely surprising, given reports of luteinizing hormone (LH) (12) and thyroid stimulating hormone (TSH) (13) immunoreactivity in the brain. Thus, these results indicate that sufficient 5' flanking sequence is present in both constructs to direct pituitary-specific expression of CAT.

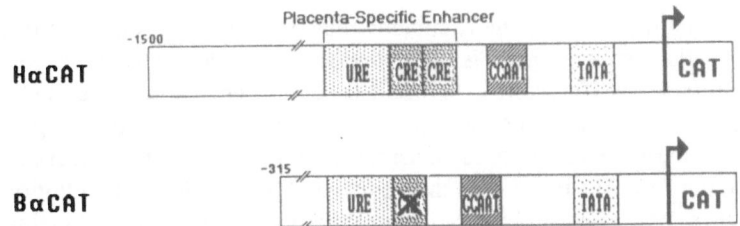

FIGURE 8.1. Constructs used to establish transgenic mice. HαCAT and BαCAT were constructed by fusing either the human or bovine 5' flanking regions and promoters, respectively, to the bacterial chloramphenicol acetyl transferase gene. The human gene construct contains 1500 bp of proximal 5' flanking sequence, whereas 315 bp of 5' flanking region was used for the bovine chimera. In addition, HαCAT contains 2 tandem, functional CRE, while BαCAT contains a single, nonfunctional CRE homolog (11).

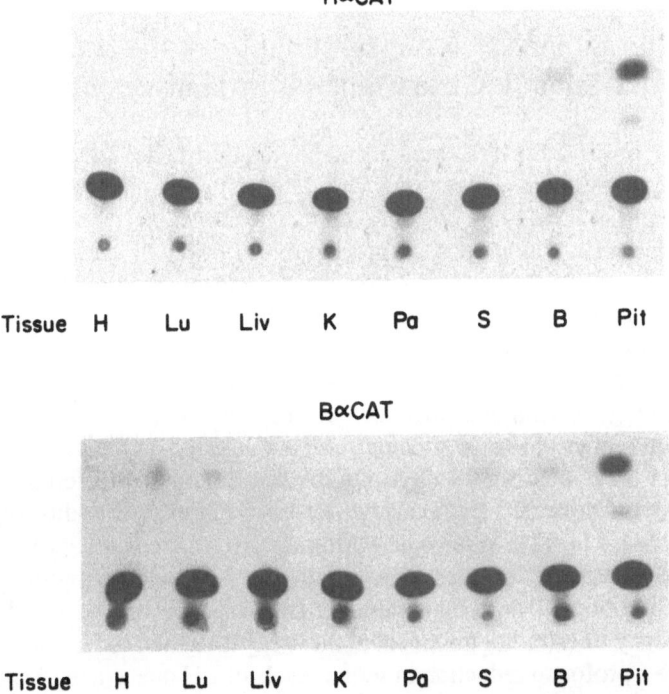

FIGURE 8.2. Tissue-specific expression of HαCAT and BαCAT chimeras in transgenic mice. Adult transgenic mice harboring either HαCAT (*top*) or BαCAT (*bottom*) were euthanized, and the following tissues were examined for expression of the CAT enzyme: heart (H), lung (Lu), liver (Liv), kidney (K), pancreas (Pa), spleen (S), brain (B), and pituitary (Pit). Cell lysates were prepared, and CAT assays were performed as previously described in reference 11. Similar results were obtained from either 2 or 3 independent lines of mice harboring either HαCAT or BαCAT, respectively. Reprinted with permission from Bokar et al. (11).

All mammals express the α-subunit gene in the pituitary. Given this strict conservation of function, it is likely that the same element(s) is responsible for pituitary-specific expression of all α-subunit genes. Because the bovine and human α-subunit genes are nearly 85% homologous out to 315 bp (11), it is likely that the element(s) responsible for pituitary-specific expression lies within the first 315 bp of both the human and bovine genes. In addition, the bovine α-subunit gene chimera lacks a functional CRE, thus indicating that this element is not required for pituitary-specific expression of the bovine gene and, presumably, the human gene. Moreover, because the URE binding protein appears to be unique to the placenta (2), it is likely that a completely different set of elements is required for pituitary-specific expression. Studies that use progressive deletions of the 5' flanking region of the α-subunit gene to further map the elements required for pituitary-specific expression are currently in progress.

Estradiol Suppression of Transcription of the Human and Bovine α-Subunit Gene Chimeras in Transgenic Mice

Once we observed that the human and bovine transgenes were expressed in a tissue-specific manner, we sought to determine whether these genes were under similar hormonal control as are their endogenous counterparts. Estradiol can either stimulate or suppress transcription of the α-subunit gene depending on dose, duration of treatment, and physiological status of the animal (14). In all species tested to date, chronic administration of estradiol causes suppression of α-subunit gene transcription (14).

To assess whether the 5' flanking regions of the human and bovine α-subunit gene chimeras mediate the response to estradiol, adult female transgenic mice were ovariectomized and treated chronically with 17β-estradiol or vehicle for 14 days. On the last day, pituitary, brain, and liver tissues were collected and analyzed for CAT activity. Estradiol suppressed CAT activity by 82% in mice harboring the HαCAT construct (Fig. 8.3 top). Similarly, BαCAT expression was reduced 72% with estradiol treatment (Fig. 8.3 bottom). The concentration of LH in serum was measured to assess the efficacy of estradiol treatment in these experiments, as estradiol is known to cause a profound reduction in serum levels of LH due to a marked suppression of both the endogenous α- and LHβ subunit genes. In both the HαCAT and BαCAT experiments, estradiol treatment almost completely suppressed secretion of LH. From these results, we can conclude that sufficient flanking sequence is present in both transgenes to confer responsiveness to estradiol. Again, based on the high degree of homology between the human and bovine genes, we suggest that the element(s) responsible for this effect would be downstream of –315 bp.

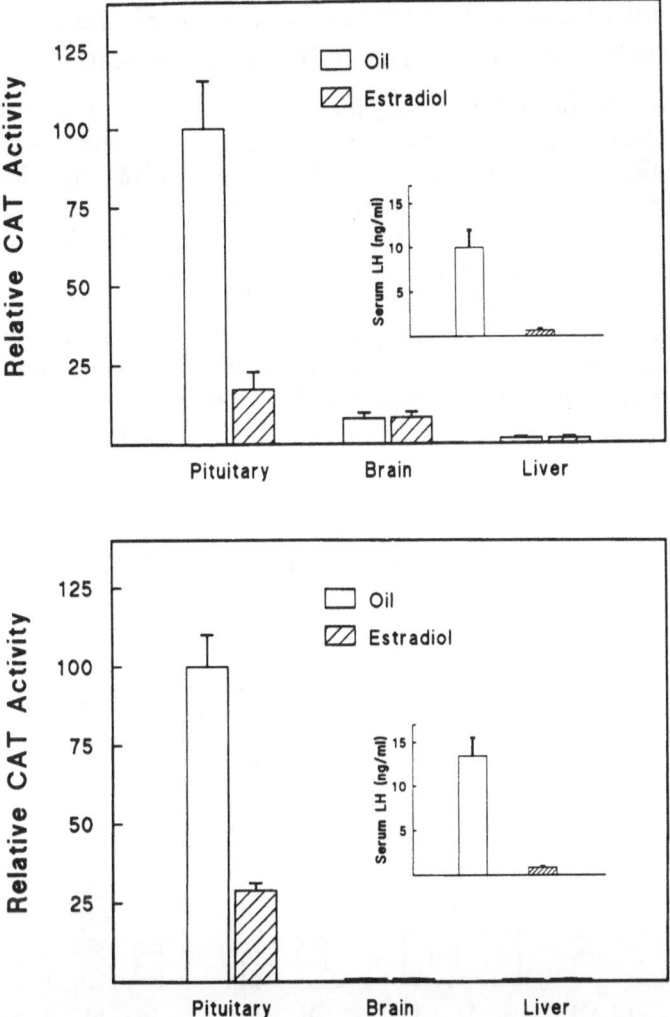

FIGURE 8.3. Estradiol regulation of both HαCAT and BαCAT chimeras in transgenic mice. Adult female transgenic mice harboring either HαCAT (*top*) or BαCAT (*bottom*) were ovariectomized and treated for 14 days with a single daily injection of either 300-ng estradiol in safflower oil or oil alone. On the last day the mice were euthanized, and CAT activity in the pituitary, brain, and liver was assessed. Serum samples were collected the last 3 days of the experiment and examined for LH and estradiol content. LH values are shown as insets. Serum levels of estradiol in estradiol-replaced mice averaged 130 pg/mL. Reported values are means and SEM from 16 (HαCAT) or 21 (BαCAT) mice per group. The data shown for each construct are the compilation of two separate experiments performed on different days. Reprinted with permission from Keri et al. (26).

Estradiol Inhibition of Transcription of the Human α-Subunit Gene Through an Indirect Mechanism

Pulsatile secretion of GnRH is required for maintenance of α-subunit mRNA levels (15). In addition, chronic treatment with estradiol causes reduction of GnRH mRNA levels (16, 17) and inhibits its secretion (18). Thus, it has been suggested that estradiol regulates transcription of the α-subunit gene indirectly by regulating GnRH. Conversely, pituitary effects of estradiol on α-subunit gene expression have also been reported (19–21).

To determine if estradiol could regulate α-subunit gene expression in a GnRH-independent manner, we performed a transient transfection experiment using human choriocarcinoma cells (JAR). These cells were cotransfected with an expression vector encoding the human estrogen receptor (HEO) (22) and 1 of 3 additional vectors: HαCAT, the same construct that was used in the transgenic mice; pSV2CAT, a CAT vector containing the SV40 enhancer and promoter that does not contain an estrogen response element (ERE); and ERESV1CAT, which contains the *Xenopus* vitellogenin ERE (23) 5' to the SV40 promoter linked to CAT (Fig. 8.4). Following

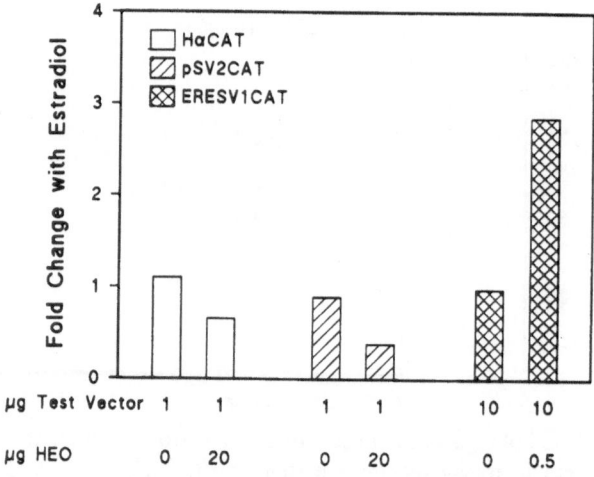

FIGURE 8.4. Failure of estradiol to regulate HαCAT in a transient transfection system. Various amounts of reporter plasmids were cotransfected with 0, 0.5, or 20 μg of HEO, a human estrogen receptor expression vector. HαCAT is described in Figure 8.1. pSV2CAT contains the SV40 promoter and enhancer linked upstream to the CAT gene. ERESV1CAT contains the vitellogenin ERE upstream of the SV40 promoter linked to CAT. Following transfection, each plate was subcultured, with half of the cells receiving estradiol and the other half receiving control media. Values reported as CAT activity are representative determinations from a single experiment and are expressed as % conversion/μg protein/h. Reprinted with permission from Keri et al. (26).

cotransfection, cells were treated with control media or media containing 10^{-7}M 17β-estradiol. As expected, expression of ERESV1CAT was induced following addition of estradiol. This induction indicated that a response to estradiol would be observed if an ERE were present within any of the vectors tested. Although a slight suppression of transcription was observed with HαCAT, the same degree of inhibition was observed with 2 non-ERE-containing vectors, pSV2CAT and RSVCAT (data not shown). Thus, the modest degree of suppression observed with these 3 vectors was a generalized vector-independent inhibition of transcription. Similar results were also observed in transiently transfected MCF-7 cells derived from a human breast carcinoma (data not shown).

Although the HαCAT chimera could be regulated by estradiol in transgenic mice, this same effect was not observed in either transient transfection system. This may have been due to the use of cell lines that were not of pituitary origin. To circumvent this possibility, we opted to determine if the human α-subunit gene contained a high affinity binding site for the estrogen receptor. Estrogen receptor regulates transcription through direct binding to DNA; thus, if a high-affinity site were detected, we could conclude that the human α-subunit gene contained an ERE.

To determine if the human α-subunit gene 5' flanking region contained a high-affinity binding site for the estrogen receptor, filter binding studies were performed as described previously (24). To ascertain whether this approach would detect a DNA-receptor interaction, ERESV1CAT was first analyzed. ERESV1CAT was digested with *Bgl*I followed by incubation with purified calf-uterus estrogen receptor. This mixture was then filtered over nitrocellulose, which only retains DNA-protein complexes. Retained DNA was then eluted from the filter and analyzed by agarose gel electrophoresis. As shown in Figure 8.5, a fragment that contained the vitellogenin ERE (band II) was selectively retained on the filter when compared with vector alone (band I). In contrast, none of the fragments obtained from the HαCAT digestion were selectively retained on the filter, indicating that this region of the human α-subunit gene did not contain an ERE.

Similar results were obtained with multiple enzymatic digestions of HαCAT DNA, ensuring that a site was not disrupted by restriction analysis (data not shown). To determine if an ERE existed within a region of the human α-subunit gene other than the 5' flanking region, a genomic clone of this gene was analyzed for interaction with estrogen receptor. This clone contained 7 kb of 5' flanking sequence and 10 kb of the gene proper. However, this clone yielded results similar to those of HαCAT; that is, none of the fragments exhibited a high-affinity interaction with the estrogen receptor (Fig. 8.5). From the transfection analyses and filter-binding assays, we conclude that the human α-subunit gene is regulated by estradiol, but through a mechanism that does not involve a canonical ERE.

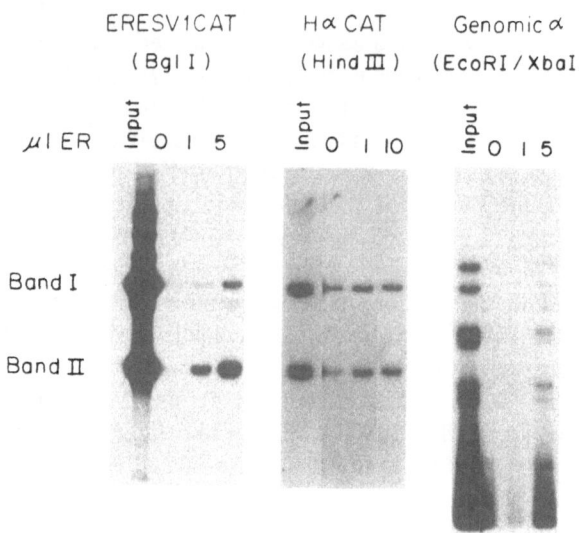

FIGURE 8.5. Failure of estrogen receptor to bind the human α-subunit gene with high affinity. HαCAT and ERESV1CAT are described in the legends to Figures 8.1 and 8.4, respectively. A genomic human α-subunit clone has been described previously in reference 25. It contains 7 kbp of 5' flanking region and 10 kbp of the gene proper. Input DNA was restricted with the indicated enzymes. The resulting fragments were incubated with increasing amounts of estrogen receptor purified from calf uterus and then filtered over nitrocellulose. Retained fragments were eluted and analyzed by agarose gel electrophoresis. Some degree of retention was observed for all fragments due to their large size. However, fragments containing a high-affinity binding site for the estrogen receptor could be identified by their preferential retention compared with the other fragment(s) in the reaction mixture. Reprinted with permission from Keri et al. (26).

GnRH Regulation of the Human and Bovine α-Subunit Gene Chimeras

Although HαCAT was responsive to estradiol in transgenic mice, this same suppression could not be repeated by transfection analysis, and this region lacked a high-affinity binding site for the estrogen receptor. It is possible that the suppression of α-subunit gene transcription occurred through a suppression of GnRH synthesis and/or secretion. Since GnRH is required for maintenance of α-subunit mRNA levels (15), inhibition of GnRH would indirectly lead to inhibition of α-subunit mRNA accumulation.

To determine if a GnRH response element existed within the 5' flanking region of the human α-subunit gene promoter, HαCAT transgenic mice were ovariectomized and treated with estradiol for 7 days to suppress transcription from the HαCAT chimera. Following this treatment period, the mice were treated for an additional 7 days with estradiol ± GnRH. As expected, estradiol treatment resulted in an 80% reduction of CAT expression. However, addition of GnRH resulted in a complete recovery of CAT activity, indicating that GnRH can completely reverse the suppressive effect of estradiol (data not shown). Similar results were obtained using BαCAT transgenic mice (data not shown). Thus, a GnRH-responsive region can be localized to within 315 bp of the 5' flanking region of the bovine α-subunit gene.

Whether the sole effect of estradiol is to cause suppression of GnRH remains to be determined. It is possible that estradiol may exert some effect on α-subunit gene transcription directly at the pituitary, but through an indirect mechanism. As these experiments were performed in vivo, we cannot eliminate the possibility that estradiol inhibition does have a pituitary component. To assess whether estradiol also acts at the pituitary, it will be necessary to use primary cultures of pituitary cells maintained in the presence of GnRH. Precise localization of the element(s) required for GnRH and estradiol responsiveness should lead to a greater understanding of the roles that these two hormones play in regulating transcription of the α-subunit gene.

Summary

The cis-acting elements required for placenta-specific expression of the human α-subunit gene are downstream of −180 bp. In addition, both the human and bovine proximal 5' flanking regions contain the elements responsible for pituitary-specific expression and responsiveness to estradiol and GnRH. Thus, a small region (315 bp) of 5' flanking region from both the human and bovine α-subunit genes contains an array of tightly packed cis-acting elements that are responsible for conferring both tissue-specific expression and hormonal responsiveness.

While a functional cAMP response element is required for placenta expression of the human α-subunit gene, pituitary expression and responsiveness to both estradiol and GnRH are probably CRE-independent processes because the proximal 5' flanking region of the bovine α-subunit gene lacks a functional CRE yet is expressed pituitary specifically and responds to both hormones. Consequently, pituitary-specific expression of the α-subunit gene and regulation by estradiol and GnRH is likely to involve a set of cis-acting elements that is distinct from that required for placenta-specific expression.

Acknowledgments. This work was supported by grants from the Ohio Edison Biotechnology Fund and the National Institutes of Health DK-28559 (J.H.N.) and by a Public Health Service Cancer Research Center Grant, P30 CA-43703.

This work was also supported by a Public Health Service pharmacological sciences training grant GM-07382 (R.A.K.), a Fogarty International Fellowship WO-4162 (B.A.), and National Research Service Awards DK-08132 (G.C.K.) and HD-07138 (D.L.H.).

References

1. Silver BJ, Bokar JA, Virgin JB, Vallen EA, Milsted A, Nilson, JH. Cyclic AMP regulation of the human glycoprotein hormone α-subunit is mediated by an 18-bp element. Proc Natl Acad Sci 1987;84:2198-202.
2. Delegeane AM, Ferland LH, Mellon PL. Tissue-specific enhancer of the human glycoprotein hormone α-subunit gene: dependent on cyclic AMP-inducible elements. Mol Cell Biol 1987;7:3994-4002.
3. Jameson JL, Jaffe RC, Deutsch PJ, Albanese C, Habener JF. The gonadotropin α-gene contains multiple protein binding domains that interact to modulate basal and cAMP-responsive transcription. J Biol Chem 1988;263:9879-86.
4. Jameson JL, Powers AC, Gallagher GD, Habener JF. Enhancer and promoter element interactions dictate cyclic adenosine monophosphate mediated and cell-specific expression of the glycoprotein hormone α-subunit gene. Mol Endocrinol 1989;3:763-72.
5. Deutsch PJ, Jameson JL, Habener JF. Cyclic AMP responsiveness of human gonadotropin α-gene transcription is directed by a repeated 18-bp enhancer. J Biol Chem 1987;262:12169-74.
6. Hoeffler JP, Deutsch PJ, Lin J, Habener JF. Distinct adenosine 3',5'-monophosphate and phorbol ester-responsive signal transduction pathways converge at the level of transcriptional activation by the interactions of DNA-binding proteins. Mol Endocrinol 1989;3:868-80.
7. Yamamoto KK, Gonzalez GA, Biggs WH, Montminy MR. Phosphorylation-induced binding and transcriptional efficacy of nuclear CREB. Nature 1988; 334:494-8.
8. Gonzalez GA, Yamamoto KK, Fischer WH, et al. A cluster of phosphorylation sites on the cyclic AMP-regulated nuclear factor CREB predicted by its sequence. Nature 1989;337:749-52.
9. Bokar JA, Roesler WJ, Vandenbark GR, Kaetzel DM, Hanson RW, Nilson JH. Characterization of the cAMP responsive elements from the genes for the α-subunit of glycoprotein hormones and phosphoenolpyruvate carboxykinase (GTP). J Biol Chem 1988;263:19740-7.
10. Andersen B, Kennedy GC, Hamernik DL, Bokar JA, Bohinski R, Nilson JH. Amplification of the transcriptional signal mediated by the tandem cAMP response elements of the glycoprotein hormone α-subunit gene occurs through several distinct mechanisms. Mol Endocrinol 1990;4:573-82.
11. Bokar JA, Keri RA, Farmerie TA, et al. Expression of the glycoprotein hormone α-subunit gene in the placenta requires a functional cyclic AMP response element, whereas a different cis-acting element mediates pituitary-specific expression. Mol Cell Biol 1989;9:5113-22.

12. Hostetler G, Eaton A, Carnes M, Gildner J, Brownfield MS. Immuno-cytochemical distribution of luteinizing hormone in the rat central nervous system. Neuroendocrinology 1987;46:185-93.
13. Hojvat S, Baker G, Kirsteins L, Lawrence AM. TSH in the rat and monkey brain. Neuroendocrinology 1982;34:327-32.
14. Gharib SD, Wierman ME, Shupnik MA, Chin WW. Molecular biology of the pituitary gonadotropins. Endocr Rev 1990;11:177-99.
15. Hamernik DL, Nett TM. Gonadotropin-releasing hormone increases the amount of messenger ribonucleic acid for gonadotropins in ovariectomized ewes after hypothalamic-pituitary disconnection. Endocrinology 1988;122:959-66.
16. Zoeller RT, Seeburg PH, Young WS III. In situ hybridization histochemistry for messenger ribonucleic acid (mRNA) encoding gonadotropin releasing hormone (GnRH); effect of estrogen on cellular levels of GnRH mRNA in female rat brain. Endocrinology 1988;122:2570-7.
17. Wray S, Zoeller RT, Gainer H. Differential effects of estrogen on luteinizing hormone-releasing hormone gene expression in slice explant cultures prepared from specific rat forebrain regions. Mol Endocrinol 1989;3:1197-206.
18. Karsch FJ, Cummins JT, Thomas GB, Clarke IJ. Steroid feedback inhibition of pulsatile secretion of gonadotropin-releasing hormone in the ewe. Biol Reprod 1987;36:1207-18.
19. Phillips CL, Lin LW, Wu JC, Guzman K, Milsted A, Miller WL. 17β-estradiol and progesterone inhibit transcription of the genes encoding the subunits of ovine follicle-stimulating hormone. Mol Endocrinol 1988;2:641-9.
20. Nett TE, Flores JA, Carnevali F, Kile JP. Evidence for a direct negative pituitary effect of estradiol at the level of the pituitary gland in sheep. Biol Reprod 1990; 43:554-8.
21. Mercer JE, Clements JA, Funder JW, Clarke IJ. Regulation of follicle-stimulating hormone and common α-subunit messenger ribonucleic acid by gonadotropin-releasing hormone and estrogen in sheep pituitary. Neuroendocrinology 1989;50: 321-6.
22. Kumar V, Green S, Stack G, Berry M, Jin JR, Chambon P. Functional domains of the human estrogen receptor. Cell 1987;51:941-51.
23. Klein-Hitpass L, Schorpp M, Wagner U, Ryffel GU. An estrogen-responsive element derived from the 5' flanking region of the Xenopus vitellogenin A2 gene functions in transfected human cells. Cell 1986;46:1053-61.
24. Diffley JFX, Stillman B. Purification of a cellular, double stranded DNA-binding protein required for initiation of adenovirus DNA replication by using a rapid filter-binding assay. Mol Cell Biol 1986;6:1363-73.
25. Fiddes JC, Goodman JM. The gene encoding the common alpha subunit of the four human glycoprotein hormones. J Mol Appl Genet 1981;1:3-18.
26. Keri RA, et al. Estradiol inhibits transcription of the human glycoprotein hormone alpha subunit gene despite the absence of a high affinity binding site for estrogen receptor. Mol Endocrinol 1991 (in press).

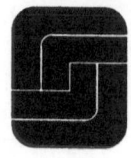

9

Expression of Recombinant Human FSH, LH, and CG in Mammalian Cells: A Model for Probing Functional Determinants

I. Boime, J. Keene, A.B. Galway, F.A.M. Fares, P. LaPolt, and A.J.W. Hsueh

The family of glycoprotein hormones includes pituitary thyrotropin (TSH), lutropin (LH), and follitropin (FSH) and placental chorionic gonadotropin (CG). TSH is critical for the maintenance of thyroid function; LH and FSH are needed for normal gonadal function, and CG is important for sustaining the corpus luteum during pregnancy. Each hormone is a heterodimer of 2 noncovalently associated subunits, α and β, that are encoded by separate genes located on different chromosomes in humans. The β-subunit confers the unique biological specificity for each hormone. Newly synthesized α- and β-subunits are rapidly assembled in the endoplasmic reticulum, and the oligosaccharides in the dimers undergo hormone-specific posttranslational modifications. Thus, the biological activity of these glycoprotein hormones can be regulated at several steps in the biosynthetic/secretory pathway.

The biologic activity of these hormones depends on the presence of intact dimers; free subunits are inactive. Although the β-subunit is hormone specific, there is more than 40% amino acid identity among the various β-subunits that is most apparent by the conserved positions of the 12 cysteine residues. This suggests a similar folding pattern that is consistent with their ability to assemble with a common α-subunit.

The structures of the gonadotropin-linked carbohydrate are unique (1). The subunits contain 1 or 2 asparagine-linked oligosaccharides (Fig. 9.1). The Asn glycosylation sites in the β-subunit are at analogous locations; FSH has 2 sites at Asn7 and Asn24; and for hCG the corresponding sites are at Asn13 and Asn30. Human LHβ has a single site at Asn30. The common human α-subunit has 2 sites, Asn52 and Asn78. The CGβ subunit is distin-

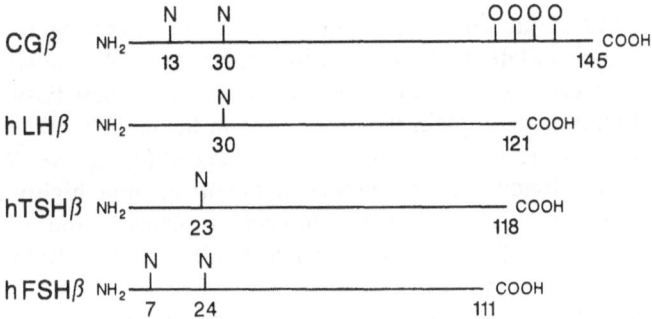

FIGURE 9.1. Positions of asparagine-linked carbohydrate (N) in the β-subunits of the glycoprotein hormone family.

guished by the presence of serine O-linked oligosaccharides attached to an extended carboxyterminus.

Figure 9.2 presents some of the major carbohydrate structures for each of the glycoprotein hormones. As discussed below, processing of the N-linked oligosaccharides of the gonadotropins (and TSH) is both tissue and dimer specific. Initially, the Asn-linked oligosaccharides are processed through a common pathway—that is, glucosidase and mannosidase trimming in the ER and cis Golgi (2, 3)—but there is a divergence in the final steps of oligosaccharide processing. The N-linked carbohydrate of CG terminates with

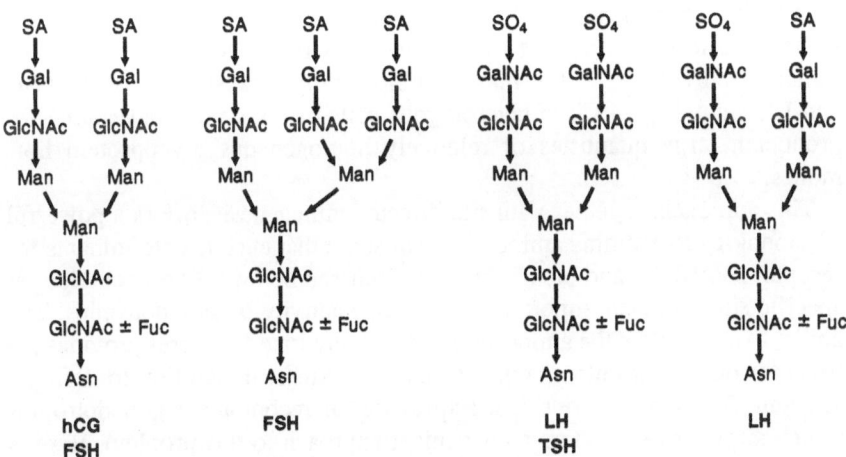

FIGURE 9.2. Major Asn-linked oligosaccharides associated with the glycoprotein hormones. (FUC = fucose; SA = sialic acid; GlcNAc = N-acetyl glucosamine; GalNAc = N-acetyl galactosamine.)

galactose and sialic acid (1), whereas LH bears N-acetylgalactosamine (GalNAc) and sulfate (1). The placenta lacks the sulfotransferase and GalNAc transferase found in the pituitary (1). However, these tissue-specific features do not alone explain the differences in the carbohydrates. For example, FSH and LH are synthesized in the same cell (4), and yet the former contains little sulfated oligosaccharides, but contains more highly branched sialylated structures (1). Since the amino acid sequence of the α-subunit is identical, the type of β-subunit must be a determinant in the oligosaccharide processing of the dimer (5).

FSH and LH are the pituitary hormones essential for follicular maturation and luteinization in the female and for testis maturation and spermatogenesis in the male. Purified FSH administered alone or in combination with semi-purified human menopausal gonadotropins containing a mixture of FSH and LH has been used to stimulate the development of ovarian follicles for in vitro fertilization (IVF) (7–10). Human FSH, partially purified from urine, is also used clinically to stimulate follicular maturation in anovulatory women with chronic anovulatory syndrome (11) or luteal phase deficiency (12). In males a combination of FSH and LH have been used in a variety of conditions related to male infertility.

Although a variety of treatment regimens have been tried and efforts made to titrate dosages in IVF protocols, multiple gestations still often occur (13). The glycoprotein hormones display significant charge heterogeneity due to structural differences in the Asn-linked carbohydrates (1, 14–16). Since these structural isoforms display different bioactivities, such species of FSH seen in commercial preparations (17) may contribute to the complications seen with human menopausal gonadotropin administration. It would be advantageous to have a source of homogeneous FSH and LH that could be standardized with respect to mass and bioactivity. Transfection of the FSH and LH subunit genes into heterologous cells offers a potential source for producing large quantities of relatively homogeneous glycoprotein hormones.

This approach, together with site-directed mutagenesis, offers a powerful methodology to examine amino acid sequences that encode determinants for receptor specificity and bioactivity. As discussed below, oligosaccharides at specific sites are also important for biologic activity of gonadotropins. The ability to manipulate the amino acid and carbohydrate structures provides the basis for designing potent agonists and antagonists, in addition to defining structure-function relationships. Expression of recombinant gonadotropins in heterologous cells offers a convenient approach to this problem. Here, a description of the components of the expression system is given, followed by a description of the hormones synthesized. Specific examples where gene manipulation was used to define structure function determinants in FSH, LH, and hCG are presented.

Expression System

hCG/LH

Gonadotropin subunit genes were inserted into a vector previously described (18). It contains an ampicillin resistance gene for screening in bacterial cells, a neomycin resistant gene for mammalian cell selection using the antibiotic G418, and a Harvey murine sarcoma virus long-terminal repeat (LTR), the promoter driving transcription of the inserted genes. This vector containing individual or both subunit genes was transfected into Chinese hamster ovary (CHO) cells. Such a system results in the production of 2–5 μg/mL of hCG in 10^6 cells per 24 h. The bioactivity of the recombinant hCG is comparable to hCG purified from pregnancy urine (19). The carbohydrate structures in these expressed hormones are similar to the purified material (20).

FSH

To achieve expression of human FSH dimer, a genomic clone containing the complete FSHβ coding sequence was transfected together with the α-subunit minigene into CHO cells, and stable lines expressing FSH dimer were selected (21). Recombinant FSH stimulated steroidogenesis comparable to purified human FSH isolated from pituitaries in an in vitro rat granulosa cell assay (22). The data indicated that the FSH line secreted ≈750 ng/mL/10^6 cells in 24 h.

As is the case with the other glycoprotein hormones, heterogeneity of FSH molecules manifests by different isoelectric points, primarily due to varying degrees of glycosylation. Some deglycosylated FSH molecules have reduced half-life in vivo (23, 24), while other immunoreactive basic FSH molecules may function as antagonists (25). The charge heterogeneity of the recombinant FSH was examined by chromatofocusing. When compared to a highly purified pituitary FSH preparation, the recombinant FSH eluted with an almost identical pH range (between 3.6 and 5.0), suggesting the presence of a molecule relatively homogeneous with respect to charge (21). Pituitary FSH displayed a heterogeneous profile of bioactive alkaline forms not seen in recombinant FSH (21). Thus, recombinant FSH is more homogeneous than pituitary-derived material, providing a basis for clinical use where the presence of heterogeneous species may be undesirable.

Changes in Asn-Linked Carbohydrate

Site-Directed Mutagenesis

Evidence from several laboratories showed that alterations in the carbohydrate structure result in derivatives with decreased ability to stimulate adenylate cyclase and steroidogenesis, but their receptor binding was unaffected. Thus, modification of oligosaccharides represents a potential source for generating receptor antagonists. Further studies were undertaken to define more fully the functional role of the oligosaccharides on hCG. Mutagenesis was chosen because of the disadvantages and problems associated with other methods to deglycosylate hormones (see references in 19). Site-directed mutagenesis results in derivatives containing no sugar at the site mutated, and individual glycosylation sites in those subunits containing more than one carbohydrate site can be examined. Thus, if there is a site-specific function of a carbohydrate unit, it should be detected.

Using clones expressing dimer mutants, the roles of the individual oligosaccharides on both α- and CGβ subunits in receptor binding and signal transduction were examined (19). To assess binding of the mutant hCG derivatives to the LH/hCG receptor, a murine Leydig tumor cell line, MA-10, was used (26–28). These experiments revealed that absence of N-linked carbohydrate on α, CGβ, or both has little effect on the binding of the mutant hormones to the murine LH/hCG receptor. In all cases, there was <40% variation in the affinity of the mutant versus wild-type hormones for the receptor. Thus, as reported by others (29–32), the N-linked oligosaccharides on hCG play a minor role in binding to the LH/hCG receptor, and there are no major differences in receptor affinity of mutants lacking oligosaccharides at the individual glycosylation sites.

These mutant hCG derivatives were examined for their effects on adenylate cyclase and steroidogenesis in mouse MA-10 cells (19). Site-directed mutagenesis uncovered a site-specific function of the hCG oligosaccharides. Absence of the N-linked oligosaccharide from the β-subunit or a single oligosaccharide from Asn78 of α did not affect the production of cAMP or steroidogenesis induced by these hCG variants. However, lack of the α-Asn52 oligosaccharide reduces both the steroidogenic and cAMP response. Furthermore, absence of this critical Asn52 oligosaccharide unit on α unmasks differences in the 2 N-linked oligosaccharides on β; the β-Asn13 oligosaccharide, but not the β-Asn30 oligosaccharide, plays a more important role in steroidogenesis. Finally, negligible stimulation of cAMP or steroid formation was obtained from dimers containing deglycosylated β-subunit combined with an α-subunit lacking either the Asn52 oligosaccharide or both oligosaccharides. These variants thus behave as competitive antagonists (Fig. 9.3) (19).

How does absence of the oligosaccharide at site I of α affect signal transduction? Absence of the oligosaccharide from this site may cause a conformational change elsewhere in one or both of the subunits, leading to a decrease in signal transduction without affecting receptor binding domains. This conformational change change in the α- and/or β-subunits could be further exaggerated by absence of the β-Asn13 oligosaccharide. The same spectra of bioactivity were seen with both the deglycosylated mutants of

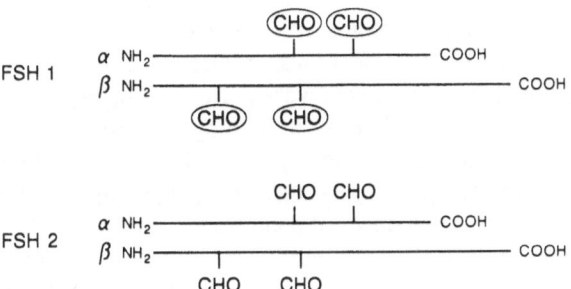

FIGURE 9.3. Variations in carbohydrate structure and the heterogeneity of gonadotropins.

the α-subunit and the β-subunit of FSH. Thus, although the conformation of the α-subunit is different for FSH and CG, the site-specific requirements for the α-Asn-linked oligosaccharides are maintained.

Mutant Cell Lines

Although the studies described above showed that the presence of carbohydrate at a particular site on a subunit influences bioactivity, they do not address how specific underlying oligosaccharides affect signal transduction. This issue is complicated by the oligosaccharide heterogeneity of the gonadotropins discussed above since these isoforms apparently have varied biologic activity. An alternative to the cumbersome chemical and enzymatic methods for generating changes in the oligosaccharides is to transfect the genes into CHO mutant cell lines that have a block in one or more steps of the carbohydrate-processing pathway (33–35). This represents a potentially effective method for generating homogeneous populations of structures with specific changes in the carbohydrate structure that would otherwise be difficult to obtain in sufficient quantities by other methods.

Thus, having mutant cell lines, one can examine the effects of the underlying carbohydrate structure on hormone function/stability. The in vitro and in vivo bioactivity of recombinant hCG and FSH produced by 2 CHO mutant cell lines was determined (36, 37). The lines included cells deficient in the glycosylation enzyme N-acetylglucosamine transferase-I (NAGT–) resulting in glycoproteins with asparagine-linked $(GlcNAc)_2$ (mannose)$_5$ oligosaccharides or mutant cells defective in sialic acid transport into the Golgi (ST–). In the latter, glycoproteins are secreted lacking terminal sialic acids. The binding of these derivatives to the LH/CG receptor did not differ significantly from purified CG, but the ability of the mutant hormones to stimulate cAMP biosynthesis in vitro was reduced compared to wild-type CG. Since the amino acid sequence of CG from the mutant and wild-type cells is identical, these data indicate that the oligosaccharide structure, while not influencing receptor binding, had some effect on signal transduction.

The corresponding experiments were performed using these mutant lines expressing FSH (37). In vitro receptor binding and aromatase activity of the variants were comparable to wild type. (Cyclic AMP production was not examined.) The in vivo potency was tested by injecting immature estrogen-treated rats with increasing doses of conditioned medium derived from CHO cells transfected with FSH genes, followed by determination of granulosa cell aromatase activity in vitro. Injection of recombinant WT FSH induced high levels of aromatase activity in the granulosa cells, but comparable amounts of either recombinant FSH variants did not increase detectable activity. The lack of in vivo activity of these variants was associated with rapid clearance in serum.

It is apparent that subtle changes in oligosaccharide structure can effect the biologic responses of gonadotropins; thus, posttranslational processing of oligosaccharides represents a major step in controlling gonadotropin bio-activity.

O-Linked Carbohydrate

As discussed above, the CGβ subunit contains a hydrophilic carboxyterminal extension with 4 serine O-linked oligosaccharides (Fig. 9.1). It was proposed that the longer half-life of CG compared to LH is due to the presence of this O-linked region. Site-directed mutagenesis and gene transfer techniques were used to examine the role of the CGβ O-linked oligosaccharides. A CGβ analog lacking the carboxyterminal amino acids 115–145 was cotransfected into CHO cells with the α-subunit (38). The efficiency of combination with this derivative was comparable to native β, and the resulting dimer was secreted at the same rate. The carboxyterminal extension played a minor role in receptor binding and signal transduction in vitro (39). However, in an in vivo rat ovulation assay, CG dimer containing the truncated β-subunit was 3-fold less active than native CG. These findings indicated that the carboxyterminal extension of CGβ and the associated O-linked oligo-saccharides are not important for receptor binding or in vitro signal transduc-tion, but are critical for maximal in vivo activity.

One major issue regarding the clinical use of FSH is its relatively short half-life in the circulation (40, 41). In an attempt to enhance its potency, the DNA sequence encoding the carboxyterminal extension of CGβ could be fused to the 3' end of the FSHβ coding sequence. The prediction is that the FSH-CGβ fusion protein will retain the same biologic activity as native FSH, but will have a prolonged circulating half-life. If so, this represents an obvious candidate for a long-acting agonist. Alternatively, deglycosylated mutants of this chimera can be engineered and together with deglycosylated α-subunit, could result in longer-acting antagonists.

In summary, recombinant DNA technology can be used not only to express the human gonadotropins in eukaryotic cell lines in relatively abundant amounts, but also as a source for more homogeneous material without the heterogeneity generated by in vivo metabolism. This approach could also provide clinical application of a more standardized and readily available produce than that currently obtained from urinary sources. In addition, this technology permits the design of potential therapeutically active agonists and antagonists by altering key protein and carbohydrate regions in the α- and β-subunits.

References

1. Baenziger J. In: Chin W, Boime I, eds. Glycoprotein hormones. Norwell, MA: Serono Symposia USA, 1990:11-8.
2. Hubbard C, Ivatt R. Annu Rev Biochem 1981;50:555-83.
3. Kornfeld S, Kornfeld R. Annu Rev Biochem 1985;54:631-64.
4. Childs G, Ellison D, Unabia G. In: Chin W, Boime I, eds. Glycoprotein hormones. Norwell, MA: Serono Symposia USA, 1990:1-10.
5. Corless C, Matzuk M, Ramabhadran T, Krichevsky A, Boime I. J Cell Biol 1987; 104:1173-81.
6. Grotjan E, DesJarlais S, Rand S. In: Chin W, Boime I, eds. Glycoprotein hormones. Norwell, MA: Serono Symposia USA, 1990:27-36.
7. Jones GS, Acosta A, Garcia JE, Bernardus RE, Rosenwaks Z. Fertil Steril 1985; 43:696-702.
8. Albert PJ, Schläfke J, Kaesemann H, Gille J. Arch Gynecol Obstet 1987;241:53-6.
9. Russell JB, Polan ML. In: DeCherney AH, Polan ML, Lee RD, Boyers SP, eds. Decision making in fertility. Toronto: BC Decker, 1988:198-9.
10. Jones HW, Jr. In: Behrman SJ, Kistner RW, Patton GW, eds. Progress in infertility. Boston: Little, Brown, 1988:543-61.
11. Worley RJ. In: Garcia C-R, Mastroianni L, Amerlar RD, Dubin L, eds. Current therapy of infertility-3. Toronto: BC Decker, 1988:106-10.
12. Lightman A, Jones, EE, Boyers SP. In: DeCherney AH, Polan, ML, Lee RD, Boyers SP, eds. Decision making in infertility. Toronto: BC Decker, 1988:32-3.
13. Karafiol PE, Rosenfeld DL, Pek H, Goldman MA, Bronson RA. J Reprod Med 1982;27:367-70.
14. Chappel SC, Ulloa-Aguirre A, Coutifaris C. Endocr Rev 1983;4:179-211.
15. Wide L. Acta Endocrinol 1987;115:7-15.
16. Foulds LM, Robertson DM. Mol Cell Endocrinol 1983;31:117-30.
17. Harlin J, Khan SA, Diczfalusy E. Fertil Steril 1986;46:1055-61.
18. Matzuk MM, Kornmeier CM, Whitfield GK, Kourides IA, Boime I. Mol Endocrinol 1988;2:95-100.
19. Matzuk MM, Boime I. Biol Reprod 1989;40:48-53.
20. Smith P, Kaetzel D, Nilson J, Baenziger J. J Biol Chem 1990;265:874-81.
21. Keene JL, Matzuk MM, Otani T, et al. J Biol Chem 1989;264:4769-75.
22. Jia XL, Hsueh AJW. Endocrinology 1986;119:1570-7.

23. Morell AG, Irvin RA, Sternlieb I, Scheinberg IH, Ashwell G. J Biol Chem 1968; 243:155-9.
24. Bahl OP, Thotakura NR, Anumula KR. In: Saxena BB, Catt KJ, Birnbaumer L, Martini L, eds. Hormone receptors in growth and reproduction. New York: Raven Press, 1984:165-84.
25. Dahl KD, Bicsak TA, Hsueh AJW. Science 1988;239:72-4.
26. Segaloff DL, Puett D, Ascoli M. Endocrinology 1981;18:632-8.
27. Buethen K, Ascoli M. J Biol Chem 1984;259:15078-84.
28. Perein ME, Segaloff DL, Ascoli M, Eckstein F. J Biol Chem 1987;262:6093-100.
29. Manjunath P, Sairam MR. J Biol Chem 1982;257:7109-15.
30. Goverman JM, Parsons TF, Pierce JG. J Biol Chem 1982;257:15059-64.
31. Chen HC, Shimohigashi Y, Dufau ML, Catt KJ. J Biol Chem 1982;257:14446-52.
32. Kalyan NK, Bahl OP. J Biol Chem 1983;258:67-74.
33. Gottlieb C, Baenziger J, Kornfeld S. J Biol Chem 1975;250:3303-9.
34. Deutscher S, Newaybid N, Stanley P, Briles E, Hirschberg C. Cell 1984;39:295-9.
35. Stanley P. Trends Genet 1987;3:77-81.
36. Keene J, Matzuk M, Boime I. Mol Endocrinol 1989;3:2011-17.
37. Galway A, Hsueh A, Keene J, Yamoto M, Fauser B, Boime I. Endocrinology 1990; 127:93-100.
38. Matzuk M, Hsueh AJW, Lapolt O, Tsafriri A, Keene J, Boime I. Endocrinology 1990;126:376-83.
39. Wide L. Acta Endocrinol 1986;112:336-44.
40. Amin H, Hunter W. J Endocrinol 1970;48:307-13.

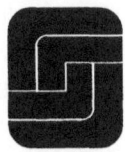

10

Glycoprotein Hormone Receptors: A Particular Class of G-Protein-Coupled Receptors

ROLF SPRENGEL AND THOMAS BRAUN

Molecular cloning and functional expression studies of receptor-encoding cDNAs identified the glycoprotein hormone receptors for lutropin and choriogonadotropin (LH/CG), follicle stimulating hormone (FSH), and thyroid stimulating hormone (TSH) as single polypeptides containing a large putative extracellular domain with 14 leucine-rich repeats and 7 transmembrane-spanning segments (7 TM)—the hallmark of G-protein-coupled receptors (1–6). Like the G-protein-coupled receptors, the glycoprotein hormone receptors mediate the physiological effect of their hormones via the G_s-protein to activate adenyl cyclase in their respective target cells (7, 8). The activation might follow a common mechanism of action characteristic for G-protein-coupled receptors. For many receptors of this kind, the membrane-spanning regions seem to form a binding pocket for the ligand (9). After ligand binding, a conformational change of the receptor molecule might promote its interaction with a G-protein, leading to the activation or inhibition of the signal cascade.

For the glycoprotein hormone receptors, the mechanism of ligand binding and receptor activation seems to be different. These receptors interact with large heterodimeric glycoprotein hormones 28–38 kD in size (10, 11), too large to fit into the space defined by the 7 TM. Hence, we speculated that the hormones bind specifically to the large aminoterminal extracellular domain of the receptor (2). To evaluate functions of the different receptor regions, we compared the primary sequences of glycoprotein hormone receptors and analyzed recombinantly expressed truncated LH/CG-R molecules comprising different lengths of the extracellular and membrane-spanning parts.

Materials and Methods

Hormone

Highly purified hCG (CR-123; 12,780 IU/mg) was a generous gift from the National Hormone and Pituitary Program of the NIDDK (NIH). For competition experiments, hCG (5000 IU/mg) was purchased from Sigma.

Plasmid Constructions

The expression vector pCLHR (2), which contains the entire LH-R coding sequence on a 2622-bp EcoRI restriction fragment, was used for oligonucleotide-specific mutagenesis (Amersham oligonucleotide-directed mutagenesis system) to introduce unique EcoRV restriction sites at two different positions within the LHR cDNA. The 45-mer olignucleotide LH336 (5'CACATTGGAGTGTCTTGTTTGAACAGTTGCCGATATCATAATCCCA 3') was used to introduce an EcoRV restriction site at position Asp 310, and the 27-mer oligonucleotide LH232 (5'CAATTTGGTGGAAGAGATATCCAGGAT 3') was used to introduce this site at position Asp 206.

For isolation of DNA fragments encoding part of the extracellular domain, the EcoRI restriction site in the 5' polylinker sequence, the mutagenesis-derived EcoRV restriction sites, and the EcoNI restriction site (nucleotide position 1096 [2]) were used. Fragments were ligated into the same expression vector used for LHR expression except that translational stop codons were introduced in all 3 reading frames at the 3' end of the cDNA insertion site.

Plasmids pLHR-C340, pLHR-C311, and pLHR-C207 were obtained by deleting sequences between the translational start codon and the EcoRV or EcoNI restriction sites within the mutated pLHR expression plasmid. The NcoI restriction site cutting at the start codon was used as the 5' deletion point. The ATG start codon of the LHR is used to express the aminoterminal receptor deletions. All plasmid constructs were verified by sequence analysis (30). Expression plasmid pLHR-S9 contains an LHR cDNA insert isolated from a rat ovarian cDNA library (2). This cDNA clone carries a deletion of 180 nucleotides (positions 690–879 [2]). The sequence of the rest of the cDNA is identical with the published LHR-cDNA (2).

Functional Expression of Truncated Receptor Molecules

Exponentially growing human embryonic kidney cells 293 (ATCC CRL 1573) were transiently transfected with the expression vector encoding LH-R deletion mutants (31). After 48 h, cells were harvested and subjected to binding studies or hormone stimulation. For binding studies, transfected cells were homogenized in an ultratorrax using a buffer containing 125-mM Tris/Cl pH 7.5, 5-mM EDTA. After separation (100,000 × g, 1 h) supernatant and crude membranes were diluted in 125-mM Tris/Cl pH 7.5 EDTA, 0.1% BSA. Samples from each fraction were incubated in a final volume of 300 µL for 12 h at 4°C with [^{125}I]-labeled hCG prepared as described elsewhere (2). Thereafter, 3 mL of ice-cold PBS containing 0.1% BSA was added to each tube, and receptor-bound hormone and free hormone were separated by filtration over GF/C filters presoaked in 0.3% polyethylenimine. The filters were washed twice with 3-mL PBS, 0.1% BSA. Unspecific binding was determined in the presence of 1 µg of hCG per assay and was generally 1%–3% of total radioactivity added.

To determine hormone-stimulated cAMP production, cells were harvested and 5×10^5 viable cells were stimulated for 30 min at 37°C in 0.5-mL PBS, with and without hCG (2.6 nM). The reaction was stopped by adding 100-µL 3.9 M perchloric acid. Cell debris was removed by centrifugation, and 200 µL of the supernatant was neutralized by adding potassium carbonate to a final concentration of 0.2 M. After 30-min incubation on ice, precipitated salt was removed by centrifugation, and 200 µL of supernatant was equilibrated using 50-µL sodium-acteate buffer (pH 6.0), and 1 and 5 µL were assayed for cAMP using an Amersham kit.

Ligand Blotting

For ligand blotting, membrane proteins were prepared as described above, solubilized in PBS, 1% Triton X-100 and subjected to SDS-PAGE under nonreducing conditions without prior heating. After electroblotting to an immobylon nylon membrane, incubation with [^{125}I]hCG and washing were performed as described elsewere (26).

Results and Discussion

Primary Structure of Glycoprotein Hormone Receptors

Conserved and receptor-specific regions of the glycoprotein hormone receptors can be identified by comparing primary peptide sequences of FSH-R (1), LH/CG-R (2), and TSH-R (Fig. 10.1) (4). All receptors are similar in size and are synthesized as precursor molecules with an aminoterminal signal peptide. The mature receptors are composed of a less conserved aminoterminal extracellular domain and a better-conserved transmembrane domain. The extracellular domain can be viewed as consisting of 14 tandem arrays of imperfectly replicated units with a common underlying motif (V,L,I)xx(V,L,I)PxxAFxx(V,L,I)xx(V,L,I)xx(V,L,I)x(V,L,I)x(N) (Fig. 10.2). This motif is also found in other proteins and is known as a *leucine-rich repeat* (12), having a characteristic amphipatic sequence and leucin, valine, and isoleucine as the predominant amino acids.

```
d-TSHR        KG PSPP E HQEDDFRVT K IHRIP...T  PSTQT K
r-LH/CG   RELSGSR PE.P D APDGA R.. PGPRAGLAR......... SL
r-FSHR        CHHWLCHCSNRVFL...CQDSKVTEIPTDLPRNAIELRF

 39  IE Q KT  SRA SNLP■NISR YL IDAT QRL SHS Y■ S MTH E R
 35  TYLP VK   SQA R LNEVV      S S  R   NA D L■ S LL Q
 37  VLTK LRVIPKGSFAGFGDLEKIEISQND VLEVIEADVFSNLPKLHEIRIE

 89  NTRS TS D D LKE  L KF G F  LGVF D T VY TDVFFI E T
 85  NTK    E G T   RK S C   RT D T S SEFNFI E C
 87  KANN LLYINPEAFQNLPSLRYLLISNTG IKHLPAVHKIQSLQ.KVLLDIQ

139   PY MASIPA A Q C■ TLT K YN  FTS QGH    K AVY NK
135   LH TTIPG A Q MN■   T K YG  F  VQSH    T IS E KE
136  DNIN IHIVARNSFMGLSFESVILWLSKNG IEEIHNCAF■NGTQLDEL■LSD

189  K Y SAIDK A G VY    TL  V Y S TA  SK   H E I N WT
185  I Y  KMHSGA     .T  S    S LQA  S   SIQT I L S S
186  NNN LEELPNDVFQGA.SGPVILDISRTK VHSLPNHGLENLKKLRARSTYR

239     LSLS LH TR D S      K QPKI GI.LESLM E SI S
234    T  SKE  TS LV T      R  PK E ■FSFSIFE F KQC.
235  LKKL PNLDKFVTLMEAS LTYPSHCCAFANL..KRQISELHPIC■KSILRQ

289  RQRKSVNTLNGPFDQEYEEYLGDSHAGYKDNSQFQDT SNSH YVFFEEQ
283  ..........................EST RKA ■ TL SAIFEEN
283  ..................DIDDMTQIGDQRVSLIDDEPSYG...KGS

339  EDEILGFGQELKNPQEETLQAFDSHY  TV GGNE MV T  S E
303  ELSG...................WDY  GF SPK.TLQ A E
309  DMMY................NEFDYDLCNEVVD VTCSPKPDAFNPCE

                      TM I
389     KF  IVV  V L  LL  VF  I L  H
333     AF      L N   F L   F L  R              S
340  DIMGYNILR VLIWFISILAITGNTTVLVVLTTS QYKLTVPR FLMCNLAFA

    TM II                                   TM III
439  F M M      LY H E Y H      P  N T
383  F M L      SQ  G Y H       S  G
390  DLCIGIYLLLIASV DIHTKSQYHNYAIDWQTGAGCD AAGFFTVFASELSV

                          TM IV
489     V      YA  F  R DR IR   YAI  G  VCC LL  L LV
433     V         Y V DQ LR   IPI LG  L STLI TM LV
440  YTLTAITL ERWHTITHAMQLECKVQLRH AASVMVLGWTFAFAAALFPIFG

                              TM V
539     A          TET  A LA IILV L  IV  IIV S  V K  I◯
483  N          VE T  V ILSI I   V    A  I R   FA Q
490  ISSYMKVSICLPMDIDSPLSQ LYVMALLVLNVLAFVVICGCYT HIYL TVR

                          TM VI
589  QYNPGDK      V      M      Y L  LM NK      TNS
533  ELTAPNK   K  I      T           AF NK      TNS
540  NPTIVS SSSDTKIAKR MATLIFTDFLCMAPISFFAISASL KVPLITVSKA

        TM VII
639      L          A Q V      ICKR   A  GQ
583      V          A Q  LL   R  CKRR EL  RK
590  K ILLVLFYP INSCANPFLYAIFT KNFRRDFFILLSKFGCYEMQAQIYRTE

689  RV◯PKNS.. GIQIQKVTRDMRQ LPNMQDEYELLENSHLTPNKQGQISK
633  EF ◉TS..NC NGFPG SKPSQA TLKLSTV CQ PIPPRALTH
640  TSSATHNFHARKSHCSSAPRVTNS YVLVPLNHSSQN

737  EYNQTVL
```

It was speculated that leucine-rich repeats may allow the formation of a protein domain specialized for protein-protein interaction (2, 12). Thus, recent studies suggested that leucine-rich repeat regions are required for complex formation between yeast adenyl cyclase and ras (13) and mediate the homophilic interaction between the cell adhesion molecule chaoptin (14). In the glycoprotein hormone receptors, the leucine-rich repeat structure is obvious in repeats 1–11, whereas repeats 12 and 13 do not show the conserved motif. Repeats 12 and 13 are highly variable in length and sequence and could function as hinge regions followed by a highly conserved repeat (repeat 14) directly preceding the first transmembrane segment.

The previously noted similarity between a segment of soybean lectin and repeats 8–11 of the rat LH/CG-R (2) is not seen in the FSH-R and TSH-R sequences. In each glycoprotein hormone receptor, the extracellular domain contains several putative N-linked glycosylation sites. The FSH-R contains 3, LH/CG-R, 6, and TSH-R, 5, potential sites. Two of the sites are conserved among the three receptors and may be important in receptor function. The alignment further reveals 8 conserved cysteine residues (Fig. 10.1). Therefore, the formation of disulfide bonds might be crucial for the conformational integrity of the large extracellular domain.

The carboxyterminal half of the glycoprotein receptor polypeptides contains 7 hydrophobic segments of membrane-spanning length (TM regions) and displays sequence homology to all members of the G-protein-coupled receptor family (2). Although the overall sequence similarity is low, certain amino acid residues are indeed conserved in all members of the adrenergic, muscarinic and tachykinin receptors (15); for example, the aspartic acid residue within TMII and the asparagine in TMVII. The conserved proline residues in TMIV, TMVI, and TMVII were suggested to induce bends in transmembrane helices to facilite the interaction of adjacent helices (16). Two cysteine residues thought to form a disulfide bridge between the second and

---

◀ FIGURE 10.1. Sequence alignment of the mature receptors for glycoprotein hormones. The rat FSH-R sequence is shown as the lower sequence, and substitutions in the rat LH/CG-R (middle line) and the dog TSH-R (top line) are presented above. Dots denote insertions introduced for optimal alignment. Transmembrane regions TMI to TMVII are boxed. In the extracellular domain, repetitive units are seperated by vertical lines, conserved cysteine residues are denoted by black ovals, and potential N-linked glycosylation sites are indicated as shaded boxes. Potential phosphorylation sites in the third cytoplasmic loop and in the carboxyterminal region are indicated by open ovals (Ser and Thr residues of consensus protein kinase C phosphorylation sites), by shaded ovals (Tyr residues within tyrosine kinase recognition sequences), and underlined (Ser residues, calmodulin-dependent phosphorylation sites). The first amino acid of the putative mature receptors is numbered as 1.

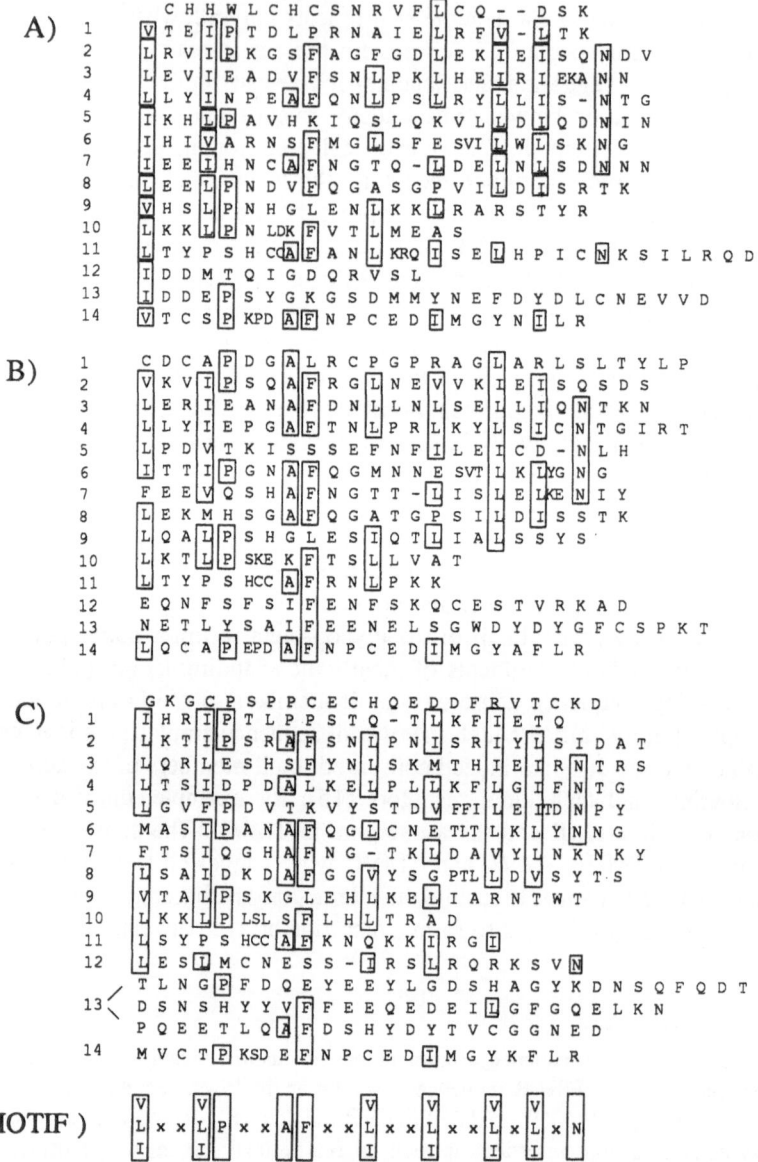

FIGURE 10.2. Alignment of the repeat units in the extracellular domains of FSH-R (*A*), LH/CG-R (*B*), and TSH-R (*C*). The motif present in most repeats is shown in the bottom line. Amino acid residues that conform to the consensus motif are boxed.

third extracellular loops (17) are also present in the glycoprotein hormone receptors. A third conserved cysteine residue, which immediately follows TMVII and has been implicated as the residue that is palmitoylated to anchor the receptor to the plasma membrane (18), is also found in FSH-R, TSH-R and LH/CG-R.

In the glycoprotein hormone receptors, the third intracellular loop flanked by TMV and TMVI is short and quite divergent, as seen for other subtypes of G-protein-coupled receptors (19). In some of these receptors, the region bordered by, and comprising part of, TMV and TMVI appears to be involved in the coupling to G-protein (20, 21). For β-adrenergic receptors, a sequence of 8–10 amino acids at the C-terminal end of this intracellular loop might interact with G-protein via an amphiphilic α-helical structure (9). A similar sequence at an analogous position is well conserved in the glycoprotein hormone receptors, and a helical wheel analysis perfomed on the conserved 8-residue sequence reveals that the hydrophilic side chains are located on one face and the hydrophobic ones on the opposite face of the helix.

As described for the other members of the G-protein-coupled receptor family, TMVII is followed by an intracellular carboxyterminal tail, variable in length and sequence. Phosphorylation of amino acid residues in this part of the receptor is important for cellular regulation of receptor activity, as demonstrated for β-adrenergic and muscarinic receptors (22, 23). This carboxyterminal tail of the three glycoprotein receptors contains serine, threonine, and tyrosine residues where phosphorylation might occur. However, only LH/CG-R and TSH-R contain Ser, Thr, and Tyr residues as part of consensus protein kinase C and tyrosine kinase phosphorylation site (Fig. 10.1).

Expression and Binding Studies of Truncated Receptor Molecules

The sequence comparison of LH/CG-R, FSH-R, and TSH-R has identified the extracellular domain as a putative hormone binding site and the membrane-spanning domains as being important for signal transduction and coupling to G_s protein. For a clear understanding of the function of the different receptor domains, truncated LH/CG-R molecules comprising different parts of the receptor were expressed in a cell culture system and functionally analyzed. The different deletion mutants are shown in Figure 10.3. Using oligonucleotide-specific mutagenesis (24), single restriction sites were introduced at different positions of the rat LH/CG-R sequence, and restriction fragments encoding aminoterminal or carboxyterminal LH/CG-R parts were incorporated in a eukaryotic expression vector (25).

The carboxyterminal mutant LHR-N339 encodes the entire extracellular domain up to TMI. A further deletion is introduced in mutant LHR-N310

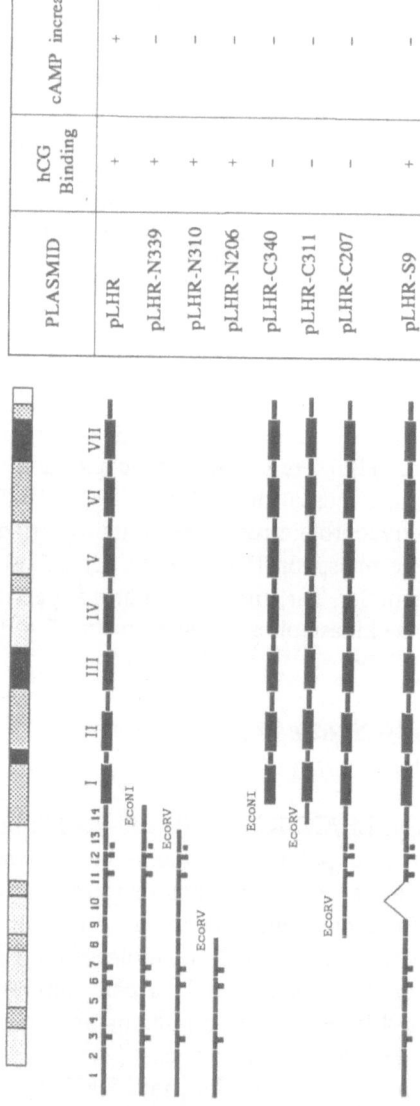

PLASMID	hCG Binding	cAMP increase
pLHR	+	+
pLHR-N339	+	−
pLHR-N310	+	−
pLHR-N206	+	−
pLHR-C340	−	−
pLHR-C311	−	−
pLHR-C207	−	−
pLHR-S9	+	−

FIGURE 10.3. Schematic representation and activity of truncated LH/CG-R molecules expressed in embryonic kidney cells. The shaded box at the top represents conserved (darkly shaded) and variable (lightly shaded) regions in three glycoprotein hormone receptors. The LH/CG-R is subdivided into 14 imperfectly duplicated units comprising the extracellular domain and 7-TM segments. Potential N-linked glycosylation sites are indicated by black dots. The columns at the left indicate the name of the plasmid encoding the truncated receptors and the ability of the transfected cells to bind [^{125}I]hCG and to enhance cAMP synthesis after stimulation with hCG.

encompassing conserved repeat 14. The shortest mutant, LHR-N206, lacks a region with homology to soybean lectin. LHR-N206 encodes only repeats 1–8 of the extracellular domain.

The aminoterminal mutant LHR-C340 encodes the membrane-spanning part, and in mutant LHR-C311, repeat 14 is still linked to the 7-TM segments. Mutant LHR-C207 expresses the TM segments together with the highly variable region of the extracellular domain (repeats 11–13), which contains the lectin homology region. In addition, deletion mutant LHR-S9 was inserted into a eukaryotic expression vector. LHR-S9 represents an LH/CG-R molecule lacking repeats 11–13 (AA positions 206–269). The deleted part covers the lectin homology region and a conserved stretch of 10 amino acid residues, including 2 adjacent cysteines.

Hormone Binding of Truncated Receptors

For functional analysis of the different receptor molecules, cultured human embryonic kidney 293 cells were transfected with either plasmids encoding native receptors or plasmids expressing the truncated receptor molecules. Crude cell extracts from these cells were prepared and analyzed for specific binding of [^{125}I]hCG. As shown in Figure 10.3, receptor molecules containing the aminoterminal part of the LH/CG receptor can bind [^{125}I]hCG, indicating that the hormone binding region of the LH/CG receptor is localized within repeat modules 1–8 of the extracellular receptor domain. This result is confirmed by truncated receptor molecules that lack extracellular repeats 1–11.

Cells expressing plasmids pLHR-C365, pLHR-C336, and pLHR-C232 show no specific hCG binding. Hormone-specific binding of the extracellular domain is further demonstrated by ligand blotting (26). For this, solubilized membranes from stable cell lines expressing LH/CG-R and mutant LHR-N364 were resolved by SDS-PAGE and analyzed by ligand blotting. Single bands with predicted sizes were detected for the LH/CG-R and LHR-N339, clearly demonstrating that the extracellular domain carries sufficient information needed for hormone-specific binding (Fig. 10.4).

Signal Transduction of Truncated LH/CG Receptors

To analyze if the truncated receptor molecules can stimulate adenyl cyclase, we tested transfected cells for their ability to respond to hCG with an increase in cAMP levels. Intact cells expressing deleted LH/CG-R molecules do not respond to hCG, whereas cells containing native LH/CG-R display a hormone-dependent increase in intracellular cAMP (Fig. 10.3). This indicates that the hormone binding domain must be expressed together with the

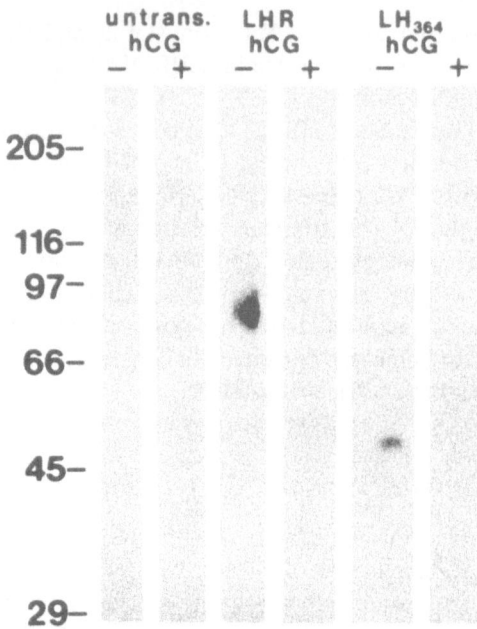

FIGURE 10.4. Receptor analysis in a ligand blot. Solubilized membranes from cells expressing complete LH/CG-R (LHR), carboxyterminal mutant LHR-N339 (LH$_{364}$), and no LH/CG-R were resolved by SDS-PAGE and electroblotted on nylon membranes. Nylon stripes were incubated in a buffer containing [^{125}I]hCG in competition (+) and without competition (–) with unlabeled hCG, as described in reference 26. After washing, receptor/hormone complexes were visualized by autoradiography. Molecular weight standards (kD) are indicated at the left.

TM segments in order to get functionally active receptor. Furthermore, both domains must be expressed on one molecule since cells cotransfected with an aminoterminal mutant and a corresponding carboxyterminal mutant (e.g., LHR-N364 and LHR-C365) show hCG binding, but no stimulation of adenyl cyclase.

Interestingly, mutant LHR-S9, which has repeats 9–11 deleted, can bind hCG, but does not transduce the signal after hormone binding. In a ligand blotting experiment, we were able to show that LHR-S9 is rapidly degraded in cells (data not shown), indicating that amino acids of repeats 9–11 are important for correct folding of the receptor. Repeat 11 contains a stretch of 10 conserved amino acid residues, including 2 adjacent cysteines (Fig. 10.1). These 2 cysteine residues might contribute to the formation of a functionally active LH/CG-R structure.

Summary

Our experiments identify leucine-rich repeats 1–8 of the large extracellular domain of LH/CG-R as the hormone binding site. Since the remaining leucine-rich repeats cannot be deleted without losing functional activity of the receptor, it is likely that the amphiphilic nature of the leucine-rich repeats confers the dual property of interacting with hormone and TM regions, leading to receptor activation. The 7-TM segments of the receptor may not contribute to hormone binding, but seem to be needed in signal transduction. Hence, for glycoprotein hormone receptors, ligand binding and signal transduction might be two spatially separated processes, which reflects a new design in the G-protein receptor family. A two-step mechanism necessary for receptor activation is supported by previous results, demonstrating that deglycosylated hormone binds with high affinity to the receptor, but elicits little or no activation of adenyl cyclase (27–29). After hormone binding (step 1), the carbohydrate moieties, especially those of the hormonal α-subunit, may direct residues of the extracellular domain to essential sites in the transmembrane segments or contact defined sites in the membrane-contained part of the receptor (step 2) to induce a conformational change in the tertiary receptor structure. This change, in turn, allows the G-protein to interact with the receptor. Chimeric receptor molecules between the different gonadotropin receptors might provide a useful tool to investigate the mechanism(s) in hormone-bound receptor G-protein activation in more detail.

References

1. Sprengel R, Braun T, Nikolics K, et al. The testicular receptor for follicle stimulating hormone: structure and functional expression of cloned cDNA. Mol Endocrinol 1990;4:525-30.
2. McFarland KC, Sprengel R, Phillip H, et al. Lutropin-choriogonadotropin receptor: an unusual member of the G protein-coupled receptor family. Science 1989; 245:494-9.
3. Loosfelt H, Misrahi M, Atger M, et al. Cloning and sequencing of porcine LH-hCG receptor cDNA: variants lacking transmembrane domain. Science 1989; 245:525-8.
4. Parmentier M, Libert F, Maenhaut C, et al. Molecular cloning of the thyrotropin receptor. Science 1989;246:1620-2.
5. Libert F, Lefort A, Gerard CM, et al. Cloning, sequencing and expression of the human thyrotropin (TSH) receptor: evidence for binding of autoantibodies. Biochem Biophys Res Comm 1989;5:1250-5.
6. Nagayama Y, Kaufman KD, Seto P, et al. Molecular cloning, sequence and functional expression of the cDNA for the human thyrotropin receptor. Biochem Biophys Res Comm 1989;165:1184-90.
7. Hunzicker-Dunn M, Birnbaumer L. The involvement of adenylate cyclase and

cyclic AMP-dependent protein kinase in luteinizing hormone actions. In: Ascoli M, ed. Luteinizing hormone action and receptors. Boca Raton, FL:1985:57.

8. Reichert LE, Jr, Dattatreyamurty B. The follicle-stimulating hormone (FSH) receptor in testis: interaction with FSH, mechanism of signal transduction, and properties of the purified receptor. Biol Reprod 1989;40:13-26.

9. Strader CD, Sigal IS, Dixon RA. Structural basis of β-adrenergic receptor function. FASEB J 1989;3:1825-32.

10. Pierce JG, Parsons TF. Glycoprotein hormones: structure and function. Annu Rev Biochem 1981;50:465-95.

11. Ryan RJ, Charlesworth MC, McCormick DJ, et al. The glycoprotein hormones: recent studies of structure-function relationships. FASEB J 1988;2:2661-9.

12. Patthy L. Detecting homology of distantly related proteins with consensus sequences. J Mol Biol 1987;198:567-77.

13. Field J, Xu H-P, Michaeli T, et al. Mutations of the adenyl cylase gene that block ras function in saccharomyces cerevisea. Science 1989;247:464-7.

14. Krantz DE, Zipursky SL. *Drosophila chaoptin*, a member of the leucine-rich repeat family, is a photoreceptor cell-specific adhesion molecule. EMBO J 1990; 9:1969-77.

15. Shigemoto R, Yokota Y, Tsuchida K, et al. Cloning and expression of a rat neuromedin K receptor cDNA. J Biol Chem 1990;265:623-8.

16. O'Dowd BF, Lefkowitz RJ, Caron MG. Structure of the adrenergic and related receptors. Annu Rev Neurosci 1989;12:67-83.

17. Dixon RAF, Sigal IS, Candelore MR, et al. Structural features required for ligand binding to the β-adrenergic receptor. EMBO J 1987;6:3269-75.

18. O'Dowd BF, Hanatowich M, Caron MG, et al. Palmitoylation of the human β_2-adrenergic receptor. J Biol Chem 1989;264:7564-9.

19. Peralta EG, Ashkenazi A, Winslow JW, et al. Distinct primary structures, ligand-binding properties and tissue-specific expression of four human muscarinic acetylcholine receptors. EMBO J 1987;6:3923-9.

20. Kobilka BK, Kobilka TS, Daniel K, et al. Chimeric α2-, β2-adrenergic receptors: delineation of domains involved in effector coupling and ligand binding specificity. Science 1988;240:1310-6.

21. Dixon RAF, Sigal IS, Rands E, et al. Ligand binding to the β-adrenergic receptor involves its rhodopsin-like core. Nature 1987;326:73-7.

22. Palczewski K, McDowell JH, Hargrave PA. Rhodopsin kinase: substrate specificity and factors that influence activity. Biochemistry 1988;27:2306-13.

23. Benovic JL, Strasser RH, Caron MG, et al. Beta-adrenergic receptor kinase: identification of a novel protein kinase that phosphorylates the agonist-occupied form of the receptor. Proc Natl Acad Sci USA 1986;83:2797-801.

24. Sayers JR, Schmidt W, Eckstein F. 5'-3' exonucleases in phosphothioate based oligonucleotide-directed mutagenesis. Nucleic Acids Res 1988;16:791-802.

25. Gorman CM, Gies D, McCray G, et al. The human cytomegalovirus major immediate early promoter can be trans-activated by adenovirus early proteins. Virology 1989;171:377-85.

26. Keinänen KP, Kellokumpu S, Rajaniemi HJ. Visualization of the rat ovarian lutropin receptor by ligand blotting. Mol Cell Endocrinol 1987;49:33-8.

27. Sairam MR. Role of carbohydrates in glycoprotein hormone signal transduction. FASEB J 1989;3:1915-26.
28. Matzuk MM, Keene JL, Boime I. Site specificity of the chorionic gonadotropin N-linked oligosaccharides in signal transduction. J Biol Chem 1989;264:2409-14.
29. Dahl KD, Bicsak TA, Hsueh AJW. Naturally occuring antihormones: secretion of FSH antagonists by women treated with a GnRH analog. Science 1988;239:72-4.
30. Sanger F, Nicklen S, Coulson AR. DNA-sequencing with chain-terminating inhibitors. Proc Natl Acad Sci USA 1977;74:5463-7.
31. Chen C, Okayama H. High efficiency transformation of mammalian cells by plasmid DNA. Mol Cell Biol 1987;7:2745-51.

Part III

Molecular Mechanisms of FSH Action in the Ovary

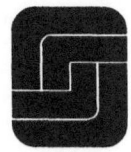

11

Diverse Mechanisms Regulating Gene Expression in Granulosa Cells

JoAnne S. Richards, Richard C. Kurten, Susan L. Fitzpatrick, Ria B. Oonk, and Winona L. Wong

Growth of the ovarian follicle to the preovulatory (PO) stage of development involves specific, sequential changes in the response of granulosa cells to the pituitary gonadotropin, FSH (18, 43, 45). For example, whereas FSH can stimulate mitogenic responses in granulosa cells of small follicles (39), FSH alone (or in combination with steroids) induces expression of specific genes in granulosa cells in large follicles, leading to a highly differentiated state required for ovulation and luteinization (17, 18, 43, 45). Changes in the response of granulosa cells of small and large follicles to FSH are not associated with changes in the number of FSH receptors per cell (42). Rather, follicles acquire enhanced stimulation of adenyl cyclase by FSH (21) and increased responsiveness to the intracellular second messenger, cAMP (43).

Some of the genes that are differentially regulated by FSH/cAMP as follicles develop and ovulate include RIIβ, the regulatory subunit of A-kinase type II (12, 40, 41, 48–50); aromatase cytochrome P450 ($P450_{arom}$) (14–17); cholesterol side-chain cleavage cytochrome P450 ($P450_{scc}$) (9, 33–35); LH receptor (25, 52); and prostaglandin synthase (PGS) (11, 55, 56). Features of some of these genes and their regulation by cAMP are discussed below and summarized in Figure 11.1.

Cyclic AMP-Dependent Protein Kinase

It is now well established that cAMP exerts regulatory effects on cell function by activating cAMP-dependent protein kinases, leading to phosphorylation of specific intracellular proteins. Four distinct genes that encode the regulatory R-subunits (RIα, RIβ, RIIα, and RIIβ) and two genes that encode the catalytic C-subunits (Cα and Cβ) have been identified in mammalian cells (19, 20, 28). A third gene for a C-subunit (Cq) may be expressed

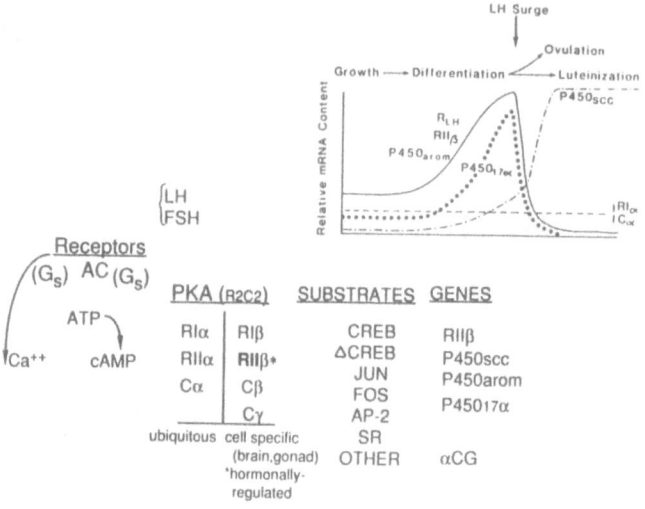

FIGURE 11.1. Schematic of the A-kinase pathway.

specifically in the testis (1). Whereas RIα, RIIα, and Cα are ubiquitous, RIβ, RIIβ, and Cβ are expressed in a tissue-specific manner. RIβ and Cβ are expressed only in the brain. RIIβ is hormonally regulated in gonadal cells (37, 40, 41, 48), developmentally regulated in the brain (27, Kurten, unpublished) and adipocytes (24), and regulated by cAMP in erythroleukemic cells (Fig. 11.2) (51). In cells that co-express RII subunits (RIIα or RIIβ) along

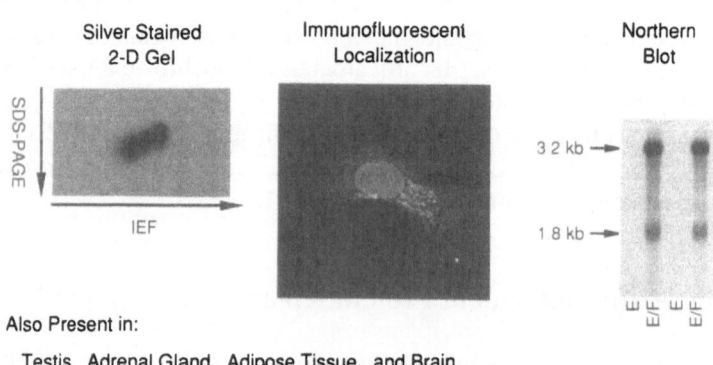

Also Present in:

Testis, Adrenal Gland, Adipose Tissue, and Brain

Absent in:

Liver, Heart, and Skeletal Muscle

FIGURE 11.2. Composite of RIIβ structure, localization, and regulation in GC.

with RI subunits (RIα or RIβ), the RII subunit confers the dominant holo-enzyme phenotype (12, 28, 36). These results suggest that expression of C-subunit is limiting and that the RII subunits preferentially form a more stable complex with C-subunits (36).

In developing follicles of the rat ovary, RIIβ is not only the dominant subunit, it is hormonally regulated (48). As shown in Figure 11.2, purified ovarian RIIβ exists as 3 isoelectric variants ($M_r = 51$–$52{,}000$) (19, 20, 48). Using affinity-purified antibodies, RIIβ has been colocalized with C-subunit to a perinuclear region in cultured rat granulosa cells (GC). RIIβ is encoded by a single gene that produces 2 transcripts (3.2 and 1.8 kb) arising from the use of distinct polyadenylation sites (19). RIIβ mRNA is low in GC of small follicles isolated from hypophysectomized rats treated with estradiol (E) (Fig. 11.2). RIIβ mRNA is induced in GC by the synergistic actions of E and FSH (12, 19, 40, 41, 50). Similarly, the RIIβ mRNA and protein are abundant in GC of PO follicles in vivo (12) and can be induced in GC in vitro by E and FSH (40, 41). The increase in RIIβ mRNA is dependent, in part, on increased transcription of the RIIβ gene (12). RIIβ mRNA and protein are reduced as a consequence of the ovulatory LH surge and luteinization (12) and are not regulated by cAMP in luteinized GC in cultures (34). However, even low levels of RIIβ present in rat luteal cells appear to maintain the dominant holoenzyme phenotype in the corpus luteum despite more abundant synthesis of RIα in this tissue (DeManno and Hunzicker-Dunn, this symposium).

To determine the mechanisms by which FSH and E regulate expression of RIIβ, we have isolated a 12-kb genomic clone containing 8 kb of 5' flanking DNA, the first exon, and 3 kb of intronic DNA. A sequence of 400-bp 5' flanking DNA characterized the promoter. There is no TATA box or CAAT box. The region was 79% GC rich. No cAMP response element (CRE) is present. However, there are several putative Sp1 sites (GC boxes) and 2 putative AP2 consensus sites. Primer extension analyses revealed multiple (at least 3) transcription initiation sites between −100 to −130 bp upstream from the ATG translational start cordon. These features of the RIIβ promoter place it in the "housekeeping" class of genes. However, because RIIβ is expressed in a tissue-specific manner and is hormonally regulated, RIIβ does not appear to qualify strictly as a constitutively expressed gene product.

To determine if the RIIβ promoter could confer cAMP regulation to a reporter gene, 4.5 kb of RIIβ 5' flanking DNA were fused to the chloramphenicol acetyltransferase (CAT) gene and transfected into primary cultures of rat GC in which forskolin is known to increase expression of the endogenous gene (23). As control vectors, αCG˙CAT, hMTIIα˙CAT, and SV40˙ENH/CAT were tested in parallel cultures. The αCG promoter contains the CRE consensus sequence regulated by the CREB/ATF protein families (10, 57); the hMTIIα promoter contains 3 AP2 sites activated by

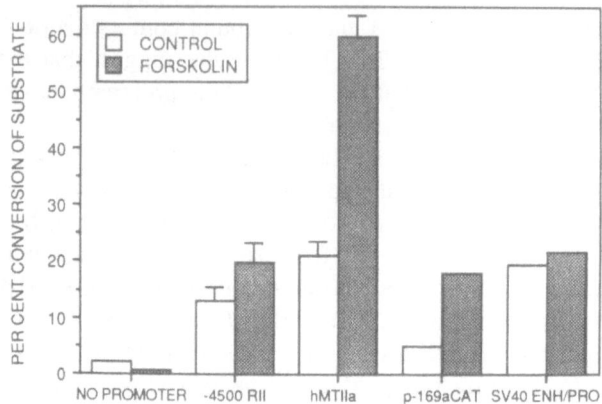

FIGURE 11.3. Expression of chimeric genes in primary cultures of rat GC.

AP2 activator protein 2 (31, 54). The SV40 enhancer contains AP2 and Sp1 binding sites (31). Basal expression of these chimeric genes would provide evidence that the transfections of GC were successful and that specific transcriptional proteins were present in GC. Activation of expression of these chimeric genes by cAMP would provide suggestive evidence that cAMP can regulate CREB (10, 57) and AP2 (31, 54) activity in GC.

As reported previously (23), αCG'CAT is regulated by cAMP, indicating that CREB is present and functionally active in GC (Fig. 11.3). The hMTIIα'CAT plasmid exhibited high basal activity and was also stimulated markedly by cAMP, suggesting that AP2 is present in primary cultures of GC and regulated by cAMP. The lack of response of SV40EN promoter and the marginal response of the RIIβ promoter suggest that the activity of AP2 may be modified by other contextual sequences of these promoters. In the SV40 enhancer, AP2 sites have been mapped close to a series of Sp1 sites. Likewise, the putative AP2 sites of the RIIβ gene are upstream of a GC-rich region also containing multiple putative Sp1 sites. Alternatively, the lack of a more dramatic response of the RIIβ promoter to cAMP may indicate that silencer regions are also present in the 4.5-kb 5' flanking region. This would not be unexpected since cAMP can also reduce RIIβ expression in GC at certain stages of development (12, 48). In fact, a 400-bp fragment (−400 RII'CAT) of the RIIβ promoter gave a greater cAMP response than the −4500-bp region (not shown). However, further analyses will be needed to determine unequivocally if the putative AP2 sites and the Sp1 sites in the 400-bp fragment alone are sufficient for basal and cAMP-regulated expression of the RIIβ gene in GC or if other transcriptional elements are involved.

Aromatase Cytochrome P450

The aromatase cytochrome P450 ($P450_{arom}$) enzyme catalyzes the conversion of androgens to estrogens. Protein purification (32), cloning of human (2–4), chicken (29), and rat (14, 16, 26) cDNA clones, and expression vectors containing recombinant human (38) or chicken cDNAs (29) confirm that a single protein catalyzes all 3 hydroxylation reactions required for aromatization of the A-ring. Furthermore, aromatase appears to be encoded by a single gene. The 3 mRNA transcripts (3.2, 2.6, and 1.9 kb) present in rat ovarian GC and luteal cells appear to be derived by alternate splicing events (26). The 3.2-kb mRNA encodes the aromatase enzyme. The 2.6 and 1.9 kb mRNAs lack the 3' heme-containing sequences and instead contain unspliced intronic sequence followed by a poly(A) tail (26). Whether or not protein is translated from these alternate messages remains to be determined.

Aromatase mRNA, protein, and activity are increased during the development of PO follicles in vivo (14–16) and are subsequently reduced as a consequence of the LH surge and luteinization (14–16, 22) in a pattern remarkably similar to that for RIIβ (Fig. 11.1). To determine the effects of FSH and steroids on expression of aromatase in rat GC, we have used both in vivo and in vitro approaches. Hypophysectomized rats were treated with E, FSH (1 μg twice daily × 2 days), or both hormones. At this dose, FSH alone did not increase aromatase mRNA. However, when this dose of FSH was combined with E-treatment, aromatase mRNA was markedly induced. When higher doses of FSH (5, 10, and 50 μg) were administered alone to hypophysectomized rats in a similar treatment regimen, $P450_{arom}$ mRNA was induced in GC. These increases were associated with increased uterine weight (ballooning), indicating that the higher dose of FSH stimulated endogenous E-production. The greatest level of aromatase mRNA (after 2 days of treatment) was observed using 5- and 10-μg FSH alone. Large, healthy, antral follicles were observed in histological sections of the ovaries of these rats. The highest dose of FSH (50 μg) induced lower amounts of aromatase and was associated with morphological signs of follicular luteinization.

To examine the direct effects of FSH on aromatase expression, GC were isolated from immature rats and cultured in serum-free medium. Cells isolated from rats at day 24 of age and cultured in medium alone exhibited no detectable aromatase transcripts, but did show a small response to FSH alone (50 ng). Presence of E (10 nM) enhanced the response of GC to FSH during 48 h of culture. Cells isolated from rats at day 26 of age showed greater induction of aromatase mRNA by FSH alone or FSH plus E. Cells isolated from rats that had been primed with E in vivo showed a maximal response to FSH alone (Fig. 11.4).

Taken together, these results indicate that the ability of FSH to induce

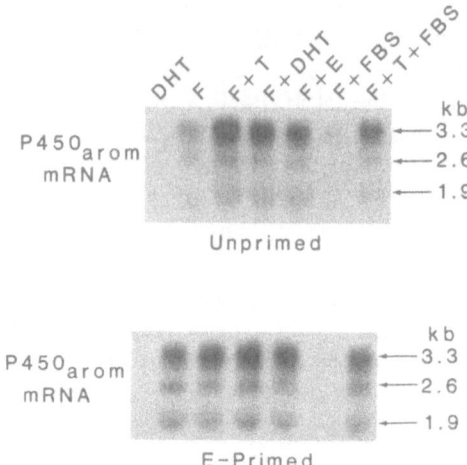

FIGURE 11.4. Induction of aromatase mRNA by FSH (F) and steroids in GC isolated from unprimed or E-primed immature rats and cultured in serum-free conditions or with 5% FBS.

aromatase mRNA in GC in serum-free cultures is dependent on the hormonal milieu from which the cells have been derived and that FSH alone can stimulate low steady state levels of aromatase mRNA. In contrast, the ability of FSH alone to increase aromatase was markedly reduced if the GC were cultured in the presence of 5% FBS (Fig. 11.4) (17). However, if steroids (T or E) were added to the serum-containing medium, the ability of FSH to induce aromatase was restored, and the level of induction was associated with the ability of FSH to stimulate cAMP (Fig. 11.4).

Whereas steroids (T and E) and FSH induce aromatase expression in GC during the development of PO follicles, the LH surge in vivo decreases $P450_{arom}$ mRNA in a rapid time-dependent manner prior to ovulation. To determine if we could mimic this effect in vitro, GC were cultured in the presence of E and FSH for 48 h. At that time, either LH (500 ng/mL) or LH and cycloheximide (25 μg/mL) were added to the cultures. Whereas aromatase mRNA was maintained by continuous presence of E and FSH, aromatase mRNA was markedly reduced within 6 h by the ovulatory levels of LH. Surprisingly, aromatase mRNA was far greater than controls (FSH plus E alone) if cycloheximide was added alone or with LH for 6 h. These results suggest that the steady state levels of $P450_{arom}$ mRNA are submaximal in the presence of ongoing protein synthesis. Thus, whereas low concentrations of FSH (cAMP) are required to induce expression of the aromatase gene in GC, high concentrations of FSH/LH (cAMP) are inhibitory both in vivo and in vitro. This inhibitory effect appears to require protein synthesis.

To determine the molecular mechanisms mediating expression of the aromatase gene during GC differentiation, genomic clones containing 5' flanking sequences have been isolated. Nucleotide sequence analysis reveals that the aromatase promoter contains a TATA box, CAAT box, 2 CRE-like sequences (2 mismatches each), and a GT-rich sequence. Whereas comparison of the rat and human cDNAs shows 80% similarity in their nucleotide sequences, the human aromatase promoter (30) shows no sequence homology with that of the rat. Furthermore, the human aromatase promoter lies 5' to a large intron (30), whereas the rat aromatase promoter is directly 5' of the first exon (16). This has been verified by primer extension analyses. Using this 5' fragment of the rat aromatase gene, we hope to determine if tissue-specific and cAMP regulatory regions are present in the aromatase promoter and are functional in GC transfected with chimeric genes.

Cholesterol Side-Chain Cleavage Cytochrome P450

The cholesterol side-chain cleavage cytochrome P450 ($P450_{scc}$) enzyme converts cholesterol to pregnenolone and is a key rate-limiting step in ovarian cell biosynthesis of progesterone (53). We have documented that different molecular mechanisms regulate $P450_{scc}$ in GC of PO follicles prior to and after LH/hCG induction of luteinization (Fig. 11.2). $P450_{scc}$ mRNA is negligible in theca cells and GC of small antral follicles and is low but present in both cell types of PO follicles (9). Initial induction of $P450_{scc}$ in rat GC in vivo and in vitro is dependent on the synergistic actions of estradiol and FSH (9, 15, 34, 39). However, the most dramatic increase in $P450_{scc}$ mRNA occurs in response to the LH surge (Fig. 11.2) (33–35). Once $P450_{scc}$ is induced by the LH surge, elevated expression of $P450_{scc}$ mRNA then appears to be constitutively maintained in corpora lutea throughout gestation, irrespective of changes of pituitary and placental hormones (9, 14, 15). A similar pattern is observed for $P450_{scc}$ enzyme content (9, 14, 15).

The constitutive expression of $P450_{scc}$ mRNA and protein in corpora lutea during gestation is supported directly by in vitro studies. Specifically, forskolin stimulation of cAMP is obligatory to maintain $P450_{scc}$ mRNA and progesterone biosynthesis in cultures of GC isolated from small antral (23) or PO follicles (33–35, 46). In contrast, once $P450_{scc}$ and progesterone biosynthesis are induced as a consequence of the LH/hCG surge in vivo, they are constitutively maintained by luteinized GC in vitro in the absence of hormones for as long as 14 days and are no longer regulated by forskolin stimulation of cAMP (33–35, 46). Time course studies have revealed that exposure to elevated concentrations of hCG in vivo for only 5–7 h is sufficient for PO GC to undergo a functional transition, establishing the stable luteal cell phenotype in vitro (34).

We have recently reported the complete nucleotide sequence and genomic structure for rat P450$_{scc}$ (33–35). Rat P450$_{scc}$ cDNA and protein sequences are highly homologous to those of bovine and human P450$_{scc}$, especially in regions (putative heme and steroid domains) presumed to be relevant for enzyme activity. More recently, we have reported that the promoter region of the rat P450$_{scc}$ gene is highly homologous to promoters of the mouse, human, and bovine P450$_{scc}$ genes from the transcriptional start site to approximately –100 bp upstream (35). Rat and mouse 5' flanking regions exhibit additional regions of high homology for –900 bp upstream (35).

Chimeric genes containing rat (–940 bp) and mouse (–1500 bp) 5' flanking sequences, fused to the human growth hormone reporter gene, were used to transfect primary cultures of rat GC. Both rat and mouse sequences conferred cAMP regulation of GH expression (mRNA and protein) in these GC (35). Whereas basal expression of the rat P450$_{scc}$˙GH gene was lower than that of the mouse P450$_{scc}$˙GH gene, the stimulation by cAMP was greater. Although CRE-like sequences are present in the rat promoter, none of these is conserved in the mouse. No CRE-like sequences have been reported for human or bovine genes. Thus, other sequences and proteins must be involved in cAMP regulation of these genes.

Prostaglandin Endoperoxide H Synthase

Prostaglandin production by PO follicles is obligatory for ovulation, is induced by the FSH/LH surge, and is transient (7, 44). The transient induction of prostaglandin endoperoxide H synthase (PGS) represents a pattern of expression that is unique and may involve a novel mechanism of cAMP action in the ovary (55, 56). Specifically, hormone-induced synthesis of prostaglandins is associated with a dose- and time-dependent induction of the PGS enzyme in PO follicles (11). Maximal increases in PGS content occur 7 h after administration of an ovulatory dose of hCG in vivo (11) or in response to high amounts of LH (1 µg), FSH (500 ng), and forskolin (10 µM) in vitro (55, 56). Induction of PGS in follicles in vitro by either FSH/LH or forskolin is inhibited by α-amanitin or cycloheximide, suggesting that the appearance of the enzyme in GC is dependent on a transcriptional event, possibly involving activation of the PGS gene itself (55, 56).

Recently, we have raised 2 new antibodies in rabbits against sheep seminal vesicle PGS. One antibody (anti-PGS-3) recognizes a form of PGS localized to and expressed in theca cells and luteal cells but not in GC. A second antibody (anti-PGS-2), like our original antibody (anti-PGS-1 [11]), preferentially recognizes the PGS enzyme, which is hormonally induced in GC. The enzyme in GC has a slightly higher molecular weight based on SDS-PAGE. These results provide the first immunological evidence that there are at least 2 isoforms of PGS in the rat ovary. One appears to be constitutively expressed and may be associated with fibroblasts and/or endothelial cells and is not expressed in GC. The induced form appears specific for GC of the ovary and may be induced in other epithelial cells as well. Purification and cloning of the induced form will be required to verify that it is the product of a single gene.

Summary

The response of GC to FSH and activation of the A-kinase pathway changes during the development of PO follicles, ovulation, and luteinization (Fig. 11.1). The expression of some genes is increased in response to low levels of FSH alone or FSH in the presence of steroids (E and T). These genes include RIIβ, aromatase, and the LH receptor. Expression of these same genes is rapidly reduced as a consequence of the FSH/LH surge. In contrast, increased expression of other genes requires high concentrations of FSH/LH stimulating elevated intracellular levels of cAMP. $P450_{scc}$ is an example of a gene that is transcriptionally turned on by the LH surge and is subsequently expressed in a constitutive, hormone-independent manner. PGS (not shown in Fig. 11.1) is an example of a protein that is transiently and selectively expressed in GC of PO follicles in response to elevated cAMP.

The molecular basis for the diverse responses of these genes to FSH and cAMP and the manner by which these responses are modified by steroids and other regulatory factors remain to be determined. Cis-acting DNA fragments of RIIβ, $P450_{scc}$, and $P450_{arom}$ do not share sequence similarities and do not contain the consensus CREs so well characterized in other genes, such as αCG (10). Nor do these cis-acting DNA fragments contain consensus regulatory sequences for E-receptor or P-receptor. However, using the αCG˙CAT reporter gene and the hMTIIα˙CAT gene, we have documented that GC have proteins capable of interacting with CRE and AP2 sequences. The intracellular cascade leading to increased or decreased transcription of genes in PO follicles may involve induction and/or modification of other transcriptional regulatory molecules. Further studies are needed to identify the diverse mechanisms by which FSH and cAMP regulate ovarian GC differentiation and gene expression.

References

1. Beebe SJ, Oyen O, Sandbert M, Froysa A, Hansson V, Jahnsen T. Mol Endocrinol 1990;4:465-75.
2. Chen S, Besman MJ, Sparkes RS, et al., DNA 1987.

3. Chen S, Shively JE, Nakajin S, Shinoda M, Hall PF. Biochem Biophys Res Comm 1986;135:713-9.
4. Corbin CJ, Graham-Lorence S, McPhaul M, Mason JI, Mendelson CR, Simpson ER. Proc Natl Acad Sci USA 1988;85:8948-52.
5. Dewitt DL, Smith WL. Proc Natl Acad Sci USA 1988;85:1412-6.
6. Diamond MI, Miner JN, Yoshinaga SK, Yamamoto KR. Science 1990;249: 1266-72.
7. Espey LL. Biol Reprod 1980;22:73-106.
8. Evans CT, Ledesma DB, Schulz TZ, Simpson ER, Mendelson CR. Proc Natl Acad Sci USA 1986;83:6387-91.
9. Goldring NG, Durica J, Lifka J, et al. Endocrinology 1987;120:1942-50.
10. Habener JF. Mol Endocrinol 1990;4:1087-94.
11. Hedin L, Gaddy-Kurten G, Kurten R, DeWitt DL, Smith WL, Richards JS. Endocrinology 1987a;121:722-31.
12. Hedin L, McKnight GS, Lifka J, Durica JM, Richards JS. Endocrinology 1987b; 120:1928-35.
13. Hedin L, Rodgers RJ, Simpson ER, Richards JS. Biol Reprod 1987c;38:211-23.
14. Hickey GJ, Chen S, Besman MJ, et al. Endocrinology 1988;122:1426-36.
15. Hickey GJ, Richards JS. Endocrinology 1989;125:1673-82
16. Hickey GJ, Krasnow JS, Beattie WG, Richards JS. Mol Cell Endocrinol 1990; 4:3-12.
17. Hillier SG, de Zwart FA. Endocrinology 1981;109:1303-4.
18. Hsueh AJW, Adashi EY, Jones PBC, Welsh TH, Jr. Endocr Rev 1984;5:76-127.
19. Jahnsen T, Hedin L, Kidd VJ, et al. J Biol Chem 1986a;261:12352-61.
20. Jahnsen T, Hedin L, Lohmann SM, Water U, Richards JS. J Biol Chem 1986b; 261:6637-9.
21. Jonassen JA, Bose K, Richards JS. Endocrinology 1982;111:74-9.
22. Krasnow JS, Hickey GJ, Richards JS. Mol Cell Endocrinol 1990;4:13-21.
23. Kurten RC, Richards JS. Endocrinology 1989;125:1345-57.
24. Kurten RC, Navre M, Gaddy-Kurten D, et al. Endocrinology 1988;123:2408-18.
25. LaPolt PS, Oikawa M, Jia X-C, Dargon C, Hsweh AJW. Endocrinology 1990; 126:3277-9.
26. Lephart ED, Peterson KG, Noble JF, George FW, McPhaul MJ. Mol Cell Endocrinol 1990;70:31-40.
27. Lohmann SM, Walter U. Adv Cyclic Nucleotide Protein Phosphorylation Res 1984;18:63-117.
28. McKnight GS, Clegg GH, Uhler MD, et al. Recent Prog Horm Res 1988;44: 307-35.
29. McPhaul MJ, Noble JF, Simpson ER, Mendelson CR, Wilson JD. J Biol Chem 1988;263:16358-63.
30. Means GD, Mahendroo MS, Corbin CJ, et al. J Biol Chem 1989;264:19385-91.
31. Mitchell PPJ, Wang C, Tjian R. Cell 1987;50:847-61.
32. Nakajin S, Hall PF. J Biol Chem 1981;256:3871-6.
33. Oonk R, Jansen R, Hickey GJ, Beattie WG, Richards JS. In: Hirshfield A, ed. VII Ovarian Workshop, Serono Symposia, USA.
34. Oonk RB, Krasnow JS, Beattie WG, Richards JS. J Biol Chem 1989;264: 21934-42.

35. Oonk RB, Parker KL, Gibson JL, Richards JS. J Biol Chem 1991 (in press).
36. Otten AD, McKnight GS. J Biol Chem 1989;264:20255-60.
37. Oyen D, Froysa A, Sandberg M, et al. Biol Reprod 1987;37:947-56.
38. Pompon D, Liu RY-K, Besman MJ, Wang P-L, Shively JE, Chen S. Mol Cell Endocrinol 1989;3:1477-87.
39. Rao MC, Richards JS, Midgley AR, Jr, Reichert LE, Jr. Endocrinology 1978; 101:512-23.
40. Ratoosh SL, Lifka J, Hedin L, Jahnsen T, Richards JS. J Biol Chem 1987;262: 7306-13.
41. Ratoosh SL, Richards JS. Endocrinology 1985;117:917-27.
42. Richards JS, Ireland JJ, Rao MC, Bernath GA, Midgley AR, Jr, Reichert LE, Jr. Endocrinology 1976;99:1562-70.
43. Richards JS. Physiol Rev 1980;60:51-89.
44. Richards JS, Bogovich K. Endocrinology 1982;111:1429-38.
45. Richards JS, Hedin L. Annu Rev Physiol 1988;50:441-63.
46. Richards JS, Hedin L, Caston L. Endocrinology 1986;118:1660-8.
47. Richards JS, Hickey GJ, Chen S, et al. Steroids 1987a;50:391-409.
48. Richards JS, Jahnsen T, Hedin L, et al. Recent Prog Horm Res 1987b;43:231-76.
49. Richards JS, Kirchick HJ. Biol Reprod 1984;30:737-51.
50. Richards JS, Rolfes AI. J Biol Chem 1980;255:5481-9.
51. Schwartz DA, Rubin CS. J Biol Chem 1985;260:6296-303.
52. Segaloff DL, Wang H, Richards JS. Mol Cell Endocrinol 1990.
53. Waterman MR, Simpson ER. Mol Cell Endocrinol 1985;39:81-9.
54. Williams T, Admon A, Luscher B, Tjian R. Genes Dev 1988;2:1557-69.
55. Wong WYL, Richards JS. [Abstract #375]. 23rd annu meet Soc Study Reprod. Knoxville TN.
56. Wong WYL, DeWitt D, Smith WL, Richards JS. Mol Cell Endocrinol 1989; 3:1714-23.
57. Yamamoto KK, Gonzalez GA, Menzel P, Rivier J, Montminy MR. Cell 1990; 60:611-7.

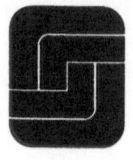

12

FSH Regulation of cAMP-Dependent Protein Kinase Regulatory Subunits in Rat and Porcine Ovarian Tissues

DEBORAH A. DEMANNO AND MARY HUNZICKER-DUNN

Follicle stimulating hormone (FSH) is essential for ovarian folliculogenesis. In the ovary, high-affinity FSH receptors on granulosa cells (GC) are the specific targets for FSH (1, for review). The end point of FSH action is the induction and/or regulation of multiple physiological responses that result in follicle development and eventually ovulation, the discussions of which are well covered by other authors in this symposium.

The focus of this paper is the early components of the FSH signal transduction pathway. Thus far, the only known second messenger for FSH is cAMP, and the only known function of cAMP is the regulation of cAMP-dependent protein kinases (A-kinases). A-kinases are tetrameric holoenzymes comprised of 2 catalytic (C) subunits and 2 regulatory (R) subunits in a dimer. Each R-subunit binds 2 molecules of cAMP, causing the dissociation of the active C-subunits. The C-subunits then catalyze the phosphorylation of serine or threonine residues on substrate proteins (2). Presumably, these as yet unknown substrate proteins play roles in genomic activation. A-kinases were originally classified as type I or type II based upon their order of elution from DEAE-cellulose (3). The distinction in holoenzymes results from the two types of R-subunits, RI and RII, which differ in several physical and biochemical properties including isoelectric point (2, 3). More recently, isoforms of both RI and RII have been described and are summarized in Table 12.1. In addition, at least 2 C-subunit genes have been identified; $C\alpha$ is the subunit for both types I and II A-kinases, while the function of $C\beta$ is unknown (4).

Of particular interest is $RII\beta$, which has been shown to be hormonally regulated in GC of rat preovulatory (PO) follicles in contrast to $RI\alpha$ and $RII\alpha$, which are expressed in a constitutive manner in these cells (18, 19). $RII\beta$ mRNA is induced by estradiol and FSH or cAMP, resulting in a 10-fold

TABLE 12.1. Regulatory subunit isoforms.

Subunit	Isoform	M_r ($\times 10^{-3}$)	Tissue distribution	Reference
RI	RIα	47–49	Ubiquitous	5
	RIβ	53	Brain and testis (round spermatids)	6, 7
RII	RIIα	54–56	Ubiquitous	8, 9
	RIIβ	52	Brain, adipose, adrenal, ovarian granulosa cells, and Friend erythroleukemic cells	10–17

increase in RIIβ protein that decreases with luteinization (18–26). The increase in RIIβ occurs without an accompanying increase in C-subunit protein (18, 20).

In an effort to determine the potential physiological significance of the increase in C-subunit-free RIIβ (free RIIβ), we compared the rat PO follicle model with that of another species, the pig. A-kinases in soluble extracts were resolved using DEAE-cellulose chromatography in order to examine subunit associations.

Methods and Materials

Animals

Preovulatory follicle-enriched ovaries were obtained from PMSG-treated 24- to 28-day-old rats, as previously described (27). Pig ovaries were obtained from a local slaughterhouse and transported on ice to the laboratory. The walls of PO follicles (6–10 mm in diameter) were dissected and cooled to 4°C in an iced buffer (buffer A) previously described (27).

Soluble Extracts

All procedures were performed at 4°C. Rat ovaries were homogenized in buffer A as described (27). Pig PO follicles were homogenized in buffer A at a wet weight: buffer volume ratio of 1:36 using 15 strokes of a ground-glass homogenizer. Supernatant fractions of either tissue were obtained by centrifuging the homogenate 105,000 × g for 70 min. Soluble protein in the supernatants was determined using the technique of Lowry, et al. (28) with crystalline BSA as standard.

DEAE-Cellulose Chromatography

Protein kinases in the soluble extracts were separated using DEAE-cellulose chromatography as described (27), with one modification. The final benzamidine concentration in collected DEAE fractions of pig PO follicle samples was 50 mM, while it was 25 mM for rat follicle fractions.

Protein Kinase and [^{3}H]cAMP Binding Assays

Protein kinase activity was determined in the absence and presence of 0.5-μM cAMP using 100 μg of protamine sulfate as substrate and 38-μM [^{32}P$_γ$]ATP, as previously described (29, 30). Where indicated, protein kinase activity was assayed using 71.5-μM Kemptide as substrate in the presence of 31-mg BSA. Labeled Kemptide was quantitated on P-81 filters as described by Roskoski (31). [^{3}H]cAMP binding activity was determined by the method of Corbin, et al. (32) with modifications as previously described (27). The incubation conditions used for rat follicle samples (5 min at 30°C followed by 1 hr at 4°C) detects 50% of total binding sites in cytosols (27). Porcine follicle samples for assay were incubated at 30°C for 30 min. This protocol detects 100% of RI and 60% of RII binding sites in porcine follicle DEAE fractions (DeManno, personal observation).

Identification of RII Subunits

To photoaffinity-label R-subunits, aliquots of column fractions were incubated with 1-μM 8-N$_3$[^{32}P]cAMP following the protocol of Hunzicker-Dunn (33) with two modifications. First, 5-mM EGTA was included in the incubation to inhibit proteolysis. Second, the reaction was incubated at 30°C for 30 min in the dark. Following UV irradiation, the reaction was stopped (33), and proteins were separated on SDS-polyacrylamide gel electrophoresis (SDS-PAGE) as described (34) using a 10.5% acrylamide resolving gel and 5% acrylamide stacking gel. Gels were processed for autoradiography (33), and labeled bands were identified on autoradiographs as R-subunits by their migration relative to protein standards and by the loss of label in samples incubated with 0.1-mM cAMP. To phosphorylate RII, aliquots of column fractions were incubated with [^{32}P$_γ$]ATP as described (30). The reaction was stopped, and samples were treated for SDS-PAGE as described above. Phosphorylated RII was identified on autoradiographs by its migration relative to protein standards and to 8-N$_3$[^{32}P]cAMP-labeled RII.

Sucrose Density Gradient Centrifugation

DEAE-cellulose column fractions were pooled and concentrated 10-fold using a Centriprep 30 concentrator (Amicon; Danvers, MA). A 300-μL aliquot of the concentrated sample, together with protein standards (15-mg/mL hemoglobin and 30 mg/mL rabbit muscle phosphorylase b), was centrifuged in a Beckman SW 40 Ti rotor at 40,000 rpm for 20 hr at 4°C in a 5.5%–15% sucrose gradient containing 42-mM BME, 2-mM EGTA, and 50-mM benzamidine. After centrifugation, 400-μL fractions were collected;

aliquots were assayed for A-kinase activity (60 µL) with Kemptide as substrate in the presence of cAMP for 15 min and for [^{3}H]cAMP binding activity (100 µL) as described above. Aliquots of selected fractions were labeled with 8-N$_3$[^{32}P]cAMP or [^{32}P$_\gamma$]ATP and separated on SDS-PAGE as described above. Each fraction was also assayed using the Bio-Rad protein assay to determine the position of protein standards.

Materials

DEAE-cellulose and P-81 cellulose phosphate paper were obtained from Whatman (Hillsboro, OR). [^{32}P$_\gamma$]ATP, ammonium salt (spec. act. 3000 Ci/mM) was purchased from Dupont-New England Nuclear (Boston, MA) while 8-N$_3$[^{32}P]cAMP (spec. act. 25–100 Ci/mM) and [2,8-^{3}H]cAMP, sodium salt (spec. act. 15–40 Ci/mM) were purchased from ICN Radiochemicals (Irvine, CA). Electrophoresis and protein assay reagents were obtained from Bio-Rad (Richmond, CA). X-ray film (XAR-5) was supplied by Eastman Kodak (Rochester, NY) and Boehringer Mannheim (Indianapolis, IN) supplied SDS-PAGE standards and ultrapure sucrose. All other chemicals were purchased from Sigma (St. Louis, MO). Final concentrations are indicated throughout.

Results and Discussion

The DEAE elution profile of A-kinase and [^{3}H]cAMP binding activities in soluble extracts of rat PO follicle-enriched ovaries shown in Figure 12.1A exhibited 2 distinct peaks, here labeled 2 and 3. The A-kinase holoenzymes and subunits in this tissue have previously been characterized (27, 30). Peak 2 and the shoulder following it consist of type II holoenzymes. The RII subunits associated with peak 2 have an apparent molecular weight (M$_r$) of 52,000 on SDS-PAGE (RII$_{52}$; results not shown). Free-RI subunits co-eluted with the type II holoenzyme in peak 2. Eluting in peak 3 are free-RII$_{52}$ subunits, as well as a minor amount of RII subunits with M$_r$ 54,000 (RII$_{54}$; results not shown). It should be noted that the level of [^{3}H]cAMP binding activity depicted in Figure 12.1A is underestimated by at least 50% due to the binding assay conditions used (see Methods). In addition to having a lower M$_r$, the RII$_{52}$ subunits crossreact with antibodies that preferentially react with RIIβ and do not exhibit a shift in size upon phosphorylation (results not shown). Thus, the RII$_{52}$ subunits resolved on DEAE-cellulose in this tissue correspond to RIIβ (4, 25). The resolution on DEAE of A-kinase holoenzymes and subunits supports the results of studies on rat PO follicle cytosols in which FSH and estradiol induced a 10-fold increase in RIIβ subunits without a coincident increase in C-subunits (20).

Soluble extracts of porcine preovulatory follicles, separated on DEAE-

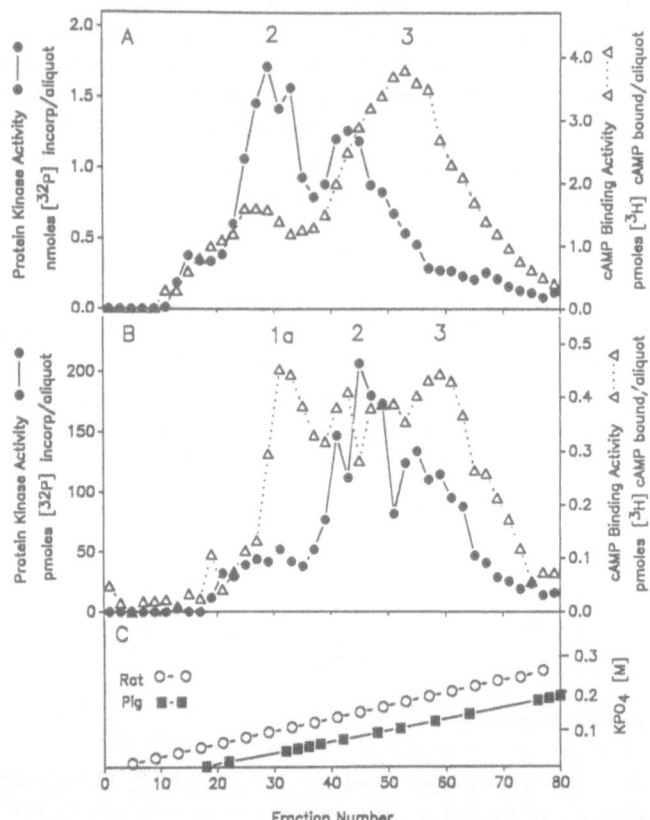

FIGURE 12.1. Resolution of A-kinases in soluble extracts prepared from ovaries of PMSG-treated immature rats and porcine PO follicles. *A*: Soluble extract (109-mg protein) prepared from ovaries of PMSG-primed rats was applied to a DEAE-cellulose column, and A-kinases were eluted with a linear salt gradient. Aliquots of column fractions were assayed for A-kinase activity in the presence of 0.5-μM cAMP and for [³H]cAMP binding activity. Equivalent DEAE-cellulose profiles were obtained in more than 15 separate experiments. Reprinted with permission from Hunzicker-Dunn, Maizels, Kern, Ekstrom, and Constaninou (27). *B*: Soluble extract (29.3-mg protein) prepared from porcine PO follicles was separated on DEAE-cellulose and assayed as described above. Note difference in units of A-kinase activity (left ordinate) relative to (*A*). Equivalent DEAE elution profiles were obtained in 7 additional experiments. *C*: Potassium phosphate concentration gradients for DEAE elution profiles in (*A*) and (*B*).

cellulose, exhibited 3 distinct peaks: 1a, 2, and 3 (Fig. 12.1B). Peak 2 denotes A-kinase activity with coincident [³H]cAMP binding activity that eluted with 0.1-M salt, characteristic of a type II A-kinase (2). The peaks of [³H]cAMP binding activity with reduced kinase activity that eluted before peak 2 (peak 1a) and after peak 2 (peak 3) are in the correct elution positions for

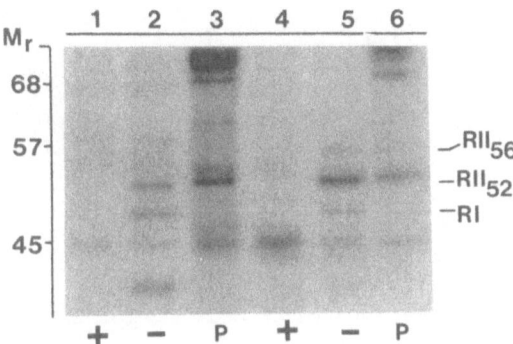

FIGURE 12.2. Identification of R-subunits in porcine PO follicle DEAE fractions. Lanes 1–3 are taken from DEAE fraction 45 (peak 2), and lanes 4–6 from DEAE fraction 55 (peak 3) from the elution profile shown in Figure 12.1B. Phosphorylation (P) and labeling with $8\text{-}N_3[^{32}P]cAMP$ in the presence (+) and absence (−) of 0.1-mM cAMP are indicated at the bottom of the figure as described in Methods.

free-RI and free-RII subunits, respectively (30, 35). DEAE fractions from the 3 peaks were photoaffinity-labeled with $8\text{-}N_3[^{32}P]cAMP$ to identify the R-subunits eluting in each peak.

Fractions from peak 1a contained one specifically labeled band, M_r 47,000, that was identified as RI (results not shown). Figure 12.2 shows the results of phosphorylation and photoaffinity labeling of fractions from peaks 2 and 3. Fractions from both peaks contained a band of apparent M_r 52,000 that specifically bound $8\text{-}N_3[^{32}P]cAMP$, was phosphorylated, and is apparently RII_{52}. It should be noted that the M_r of this band did not change appreciably upon phosphorylation. A second phosphorylated and photoaffinity-labeled band, M_r 56,000, was detected in peak 3 (Fig. 12.2, lanes 4–6). This higher M_r RII isoform, RII_{56}, appears to be present in a much lower concentration relative to RII_{52}, based on labeling intensity. Photoaffinity-labeled RI subunits were also present in these fractions, presumably due to the high levels of free RI in this tissue.

To confirm the presence of a type II holoenzyme as well as free RII in porcine follicle extracts, sucrose density gradient centrifugation was performed on DEAE fractions pooled from peaks 2 and 3. The resultant sedimentation profile (Fig. 12.3) showed a peak of A-kinase activity with $[^3H]cAMP$ binding activity that sedimented as a holoenzyme at 8.2S and a peak of $[^3H]cAMP$ binding activity that sedimented at approximately 5S as free-R subunit dimers. These sedimentation coefficients are consistent with reported values for holoenzyme and R-subunit dimers (3, 36–38). When the

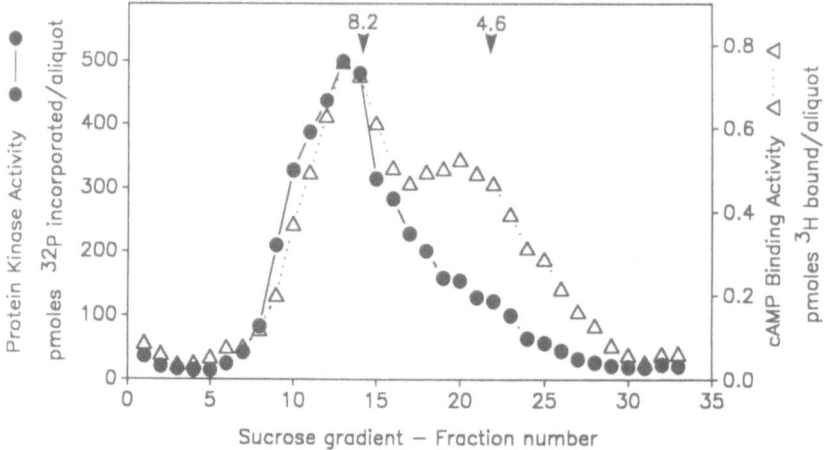

FIGURE 12.3. Sucrose gradient sedimentation analysis of porcine PO follicle DEAE peaks 2 and 3. Fractions 43–65 of a DEAE elution profile equivalent to that shown in Figure 12.1B were pooled and analyzed by sucrose density gradient centrifugation as described in Methods. Aliquots of fractions were assayed for [^{3}H]cAMP binding activity (open triangle) and A-kinase phosphorylation of Kemptide in the presence of 0.5-μM cAMP (solid circle). Sedimentation positions for phosphorylase b (8.2S) and hemoglobin (4.6S) are indicated by arrows.

areas under the 2 peaks were compared, [^{3}H]cAMP binding activity due to free R was approximately 30% lower than that due to holoenzyme. Photo-affinity labeling of fractions from the holoenzyme and free-R peaks confirmed that RII$_{52}$ was the major R-subunit in these fractions, and its concentration was notably greater in the holoenzyme peak relative to the free-R peak (results not shown).

A-kinases in porcine PO follicle soluble extracts exhibit several similarities to those of rat PO follicle soluble extracts when each are resolved on DEAE-cellulose. As in the rat, the predominant A-kinase in porcine PO follicles is a type II holoenzyme (indicated as peak 2). Both tissues also express free-RI and -RII subunits. The porcine type II kinase is comprised of RII$_{52}$ subunits, together with a minor amount of RII$_{56}$. However, the porcine type II A-kinase appears to be more acidic than the rat type II A-kinase, based on the co-elution of the rat type II holoenzyme (peak 2) with free-RI activity in contrast to the elution of the porcine type II holoenzyme (peak 2) following free RI (peak 1a).

An additional distinction between A-kinase subunits in rat and porcine follicles is that while porcine, like rat, PO follicles exhibited free RII$_{52}$, the level of RII$_{52}$ induction appears to be much lower in porcine follicles than in rat PO follicles. In porcine PO follicles, the level of [^{3}H]cAMP binding ac-

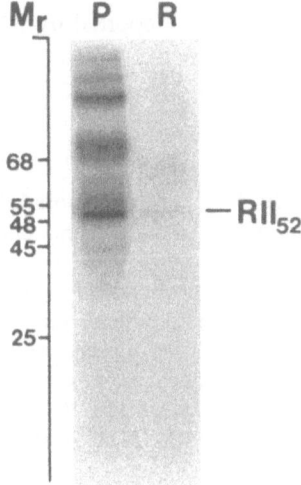

FIGURE 12.4. Comparison of phosphorylated RII_{52} in porcine and rat ovarian tissues. DEAE fractions from porcine and rat ovarian tissues were phosphorylated as described in Methods. The sample in lane P is a fraction from DEAE peak 2 of porcine corpora lutea (CL) preparation. We have determined that RII_{52} in peak 2 of CL is equivalent to RII_{52} in PO follicles. The sample in lane R is from rat immature ovary DEAE peak 2. Protein loaded in the 2 lanes is not equivalent.

tivity that sedimented as free R was approximately 30% lower than that which sedimented as holoenzyme when the areas of the 2 peaks are compared. In rat PO follicles, the free-RII [^{3}H]cAMP binding activity was several-fold greater than that attributable to holoenzyme when resolved on a sucrose density gradient (30).

The most prominent RII isoform in both rat and porcine PO follicles appears to be an RII_{52}. To compare the apparent RII_{52} subunits in rat and pig ovaries, aliquots of peak 2 DEAE fractions from the two species were phosphorylated and separated on the same SDS-polyacrylamide gel (Fig. 12.4). The porcine sample used was from a DEAE separation of corpora lutea (CL) soluble extracts; RII_{52} from CL is equivalent to that from PO follicles (DeManno, personal observation). As is evident in Figure 12.4, the 2 RII_{52} proteins indeed have the same apparent M_r.

In conclusion, the induction of RII_{52} in PO follicles is a phenomenon that is not limited to rat ovaries. Free RII_{52} is present in porcine PO follicles, but its level of expression is much lower than in the rat. The primary RII isoform in porcine PO follicles migrates with rat RII_{52} on SDS-PAGE and does not shift its M_r upon phosphorylation, suggesting that the porcine protein, like the rat protein, is likely an RIIβ.

Acknowledgments. This work was supported by NIH HD-21921 (M.H-D.) and NRSA HD-7244 (D.D.).

References

1. Hsueh AJW, Bicsak TA, Jia X-C, et al. Granulosa cells as hormone targets: the role of biologically active follicle-stimulating hormone in reproduction. Recent Prog Horm Res 1989;45:209-77.
2. Beebe SJ, Corbin JD. Cyclic nucleotide-dependent protein kinases. In: Boyer PD, ed. The enzymes. Orlando, FL: Academic Press, 1986;17:43-111.
3. Corbin JD, Kelly SL, Park CR. The distribution and dissociation of cyclic adenosine 3':5'-monophosphate-dependent protein kinases in adipose, cardiac, and other tissues. J Biol Chem 1975;250:218-25.
4. McKnight GS, Clegg CH, Uhler MD, et al. Analysis of the cAMP-dependent protein kinase system using molecular genetic approaches. Recent Prog Horm Res 1988;44:307-35.
5. Titani K, Sasagawa T, Ericsson LH, et al. Amino acid sequence of the regulatory subunit of bovine type I adenosine cyclic 3',5'-phosphate dependent protein kinase. Biochemistry 1984;23:4193-9.
6. Clegg CH, Cadd GG, McKnight GS. Genetic characterization of a brain-specific form of the type I regulatory subunit of cAMP-dependent protein kinase. Proc Natl Acad Sci USA 1988;85:3703-7.
7. Oyen O, Froysa A, Sandberg M, et al. Cellular localization and age-dependent changes in mRNA for cyclic adensoine 3',5'-monophosphate-dependent protein kinases in rat testis. Biol Reprod 1987;37:947-56.
8. Takio K, Smith SB, Krebs EG, Walsh KA, Titani K. Amino acid sequence of the regulatory subunit of bovine type II adenosine cyclic 3',5'-phosphate dependent protein kinase. Biochemistry 1984;23:4200-6.
9. Scott JD, Glaccum MB, Zoller MJ, et al. The molecular cloning of a type II regulatory subunit of the cAMP-dependent protein kinase from rat skeletal muscle and mouse brain. Proc Natl Acad Sci USA 1987;84:5192-6.
10. Jahnsen T, Hedin L, Kidd VJ, et al. Molecular cloning, cDNA structure, and regulation of the regulatory subunit of type II cAMP-dependent protein kinase from rat ovarian granulosa cells. J Biol Chem 1986;261:12352-61.
11. Jahsen T, Hedin L, Lohmann SM, Walter U, Richards JS. The neural type II regulatory subunit of cAMP-dependent protein kinase is present and regulated by hormones in the rat ovary. J Biol Chem 1986;261:6637-9.
12. Kurten RC, Navre M, Gaddy-Kurten D, et al. Induction of adenosine 3', 5'-monophosphate-dependent protein kinase subunits during adipogenesis in vitro. Endocrinology 1988;123:2408-18.
13. Erlichman J, Sarkar D, Fleischer N, Rubin CS. Identification of two subclasses of type II cAMP-dependent protein kinases. Neural-specific and non-neural protein kinases. J Biol Chem 1980;255:8179-84.
14. Hartl FT, Roskoski R, Jr. Cyclic adenosine 3':5'-monophosphate-dependent protein kinase. Comparison of type II enzymes from bovine brain, skeletal muscle and cardiac muscle. J Biol Chem 1983;258:3950-5.

15. Weldon SL, Mumby MC, Taylor SS. The regulatory subunit of neural cAMP-dependent protein kinase II represents a unique gene product. J Biol Chem 1985; 260:6440-8.

16. Stein JC, Rubin CS. Isolation and sequence of a tryptic peptide containing the autophosphorylation site of the regulatory subunit of bovine brain protein kinase II. J Biol Chem 1985;260:10991-5.

17. Schwartz DA, Rubin CS. Identification and differential expression of two forms of regulatory subunits (RII) of cAMP-dependent protein kinase II in Friend erythroleukemic cells. J Biol Chem 1985;260:6296-303.

18. Richards JS, Rolfes AI. Hormonal regulation of cyclic AMP binding to specific receptor proteins in rat ovarian follicles. J Biol Chem 1980;255:5481-9.

19. Ratoosh SL, Lifka J, Hedin L, Jahnsen T, Richards JS. Hormonal regulation of the synthesis and mRNA content of the regulatory subunit of cyclic AMP-dependent protein kinase type II in cultured rat ovarian granulosa cells. J Biol Chem 1987;262:7306-13.

20. Richards JS, Haddox M, Tash JS, Walter U, Lohmann S. Adenosine 3',5'-monophosphate-dependent protein kinase and granulosa cell responsiveness to gonadotropins. Endocrinology 1984;114:2190-8.

21. Richards JS, Kirchick HJ. Changes in content and phosphorylation of cytosol proteins in luteinizing ovarian follicles and corpora lutea. Biol Reprod 1984;30: 737-51.

22. Richards JS, Sehgal N, Tash JS. Changes in content and cAMP-dependent phosphorylation of specific proteins in granulosa cells of preantral and preovulatory ovarian follicles and in corpora lutea. J Biol Chem 1983;258:5227-32.

23. Darbon JM, Knecht M, Ranta T, Dufau ML, Catt KJ. Hormonal regulation of cyclic AMP-dependent protein kinase in cultured ovarian granulosa cells. Effects of follicle-stimulating hormone and gonadotropin-releasing hormone. J Biol Chem 1984;259:14778-82.

24. Ratoosh SL, Richards S. Regulation of the content and phosphorylation of RII by adenosine 3',5'-monophosphate, follicle-stimulating hormone, and estradiol in cultured granulosa cells. Endocrinology 1985;117:917-27.

25. Jahsen T, Lohmann SM, Walter U, Hedin L, Richards JS. Purification and characterization of hormone-regulated isoforms of the regulatory subunit of type II cAMP-dependent protein kinase from rat ovaries. J Biol Chem 1985;260: 15980-7.

26. Hedin L, McKnight GS, Lifka J, Durica JM, Richards JS. Tissue distribution and hormonal regulation of messenger ribonucleic acid for regulatory and catalytic subunits of adenosine 3',5'-monophosphate-dependent protein kinases during ovarian follicular development and luteinization in the rat. Endocrinology 1987; 120:1928-35.

27. Hunzicker-Dunn M, Maizels ET, Kern LC, Ekstrom RC, Constaninou AI. Separation of the complexes formed between the regulatory and catalytic subunits of cyclic adenosine monophosphate-dependent protein kinase and topoisomerase I activity in preovulatory follicle-enriched immature rat ovaries. Mol Cell Endocrinol 1989;3:780-9.

28. Lowry OW, Rosebrough NJ, Farr AL, Randall RJ. Protein measurement with the Folin phenol reagent. J Biol Chem 1951;193:265-75.

29. Hunzicker-Dunn M, Jungmann RA, Evely L, Hadawi GL, Maizels ET, West DE. Modulation of soluble ovarian adenosine 3',5'-monophosphate-dependent protein kinase activity during prepubertal development of the rat. Endocrinology 1984; 115;302-11.

30. Hunzicker-Dunn M. Lorenzini NA, Lynch LL, West DE. Coelution of the type II holoenzyme form of cAMP-dependent protein kinase with regulatory subunits of the type I form of cAMP-dependent protein kinase. J Biol Chem 1985;260: 13360-9.

31. Roskoski R, Jr. Assays of protein kinase. Methods in Enzymol 1983;99:3-6.

32. Corbin JD, Sugden PH, West L, Flockhart DA, Lincoln TM, McCarthy D. Studies on the properties and mode of action of the purified regulatory subunit of bovine heart adenosine 3':5'-monophosphate-dependent protein kinase. J Biol Chem 1978;253:3997-4003.

33. Hunzicker-Dunn M. Selective activation of rabbit ovarian protein kinase isozymes in rabbit ovarian follicles and corpora lutea. J Biol Chem 1981;256: 12185-93.

34. Rudolph SA, Krueger BK. Endogenous protein phosphorylation and dephospho-rylation. Adv Cyclic Nucleotide Protein Phosphorylation Res 1979;10:107-33.

35. Schwartz DA, Rubin CS. Regulation of cAMP-dependent protein kinase subunit levels in Friend erythroleukemic cells. J Biol Chem 1983;258:777-84.

36. Zoller MJ, Kerlavage AR, Taylor SS. Structural comparisons of cAMP-depen-dent protein-kinases I and II from porcine skeletal muscle. J Biol Chem 1979; 254:2408-12.

37. Erlichman J, Rubin CS, Rosen OM. Physical properties of a purified cyclic ad-enosine 3':5'-monophosphate-dependent protein kinase from bovine heart muscle. J Biol Chem 1973;248:7607-9.

38. Cobb CE, Beth AH, Corbin JD. Purification and characterization of an inactive form of cAMP-dependent protein kinase containing bound cAMP. J Biol Chem 1987;262:16566-74.

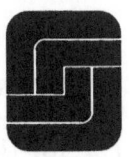

13

Regulation of Ovarian Inhibin and Activin Gene Expression by Gonadotropins

Robin E. Dodson, Lin Pei, Ok-Kyong Park, Joanna C. Dykema, and Kelly E. Mayo

Follicle stimulating hormone (FSH) plays a critical role in regulating ovarian function and is a key hormone in initiating follicular recruitment and promoting follicular maturation (1). Additionally, it influences differentiation by modulating steroidogenesis, inducing luteinizing hormone receptors and regulating the synthesis of ovarian hormones, such as inhibin and activin. Inhibin is an important regulator of FSH synthesis and secretion in rats (2), while activin appears to be a paracrine regulator of ovarian function (3, 4) that may also be involved in FSH regulation (5, 6). The study of how these two genes are regulated is important for understanding aspects of the reproductive cycle. This report focuses on the regulation of inhibin and activin gene expression in rat granulosa cells (GC) by gonadotropins.

The regulation of inhibin and activin expression is a complex issue since these hormones are structurally related but have functionally opposing effects, at least on FSH secretion. Inhibin is composed of one α-chain and one of 2 β-chains (β_A or β_B) that associate to form a 32-kD glycoprotein (7–10). Activin is a 28-kD dimer composed of 2 of the β-chains (5, 6). While inhibin suppresses FSH secretion from cultured pituitary cells, activin stimulates it (2). Inhibin and activin have both been identified in follicular fluid and are synthesized by the ovary. The identification of cells that produce inhibin has been facilitated by the availability of antibodies that recognize this protein. Inhibin has been shown to be localized to the GC of developing follicles (11–13), and these cells have also been shown to contain α-, β_A- and β_B-mRNAs by in situ hybridization (14–16). It is not clear at present if the same cells can also produce activin and if so, under what conditions.

FSH is an important regulator of inhibin expression both in vivo (17–20) and in vitro (11). In general, FSH acts to increase inhibin secretion and mRNA levels; however, there are exceptions to this. During much of the rat estrous cycle, FSH induces α- and β-mRNA levels in developing follicles (14, 16). However, the ovulatory surge of LH and FSH strongly suppresses expression of the two mRNA species (20, 21). While α- and β-mRNAs are regulated by FSH in the ovary, α- but not β_B-mRNA is regulated by gonadotropins in the testis (22, 23). The net effect of FSH on inhibin synthesis may depend on whether other hormones are present or absent, which tissue is being examined, and what stage of differentiation the follicles have reached.

The individual α- and β-genes appear to be regulated by different mechanisms since there are several conditions in which they are not coordinately expressed. Expression of α-mRNA has been reported in theca interstitial cells and in newly formed corpora lutea, as well as in GC; however, β-mRNA is found exclusively in GC of the ovary (15, 16). Expression of α-mRNA is also seen in follicles that do not express β (15, 16, 20, 21). In the male, α-gene expression occurs predominantly in Sertoli cells but is also found in Leydig cells, while β_B-expression is seen only in Sertoli cells (24). Beta mRNA expression has also been seen in tertiary follicles just prior to ovulation (16) and in small antral follicles of the monkey (25) at times when α-expression is not observed. In addition, comparison of the α-genes (26 and Pei, et al., submitted) and β_B-genes (26) reveals that the promoter regions have very different structures.

The inhibin α and β genes can be either co-expressed or independently expressed, and it is likely that the regulation of this expression pattern will prove to be complex. We describe here several examples that indicate the important role of FSH in regulating these genes, both in vitro and in vivo. We then briefly consider the use of GC to examine the expression and regulation of cloned and transfected α-inhibin genes.

Materials and Methods

In Situ Hybridization

Twenty-three-day-old female Sprague-Dawley rats (Harlan) were injected subcutaneously with pregnant mare's serum gonadotropin (PMSG) (10 IU) or vehicle alone. Rats were sacrificed 53 h after the final injection, and ovaries were processed for in situ hybridization analysis as described (15, 27) using ^{35}S-labeled riboprobes specific for the α- and β-cDNAs (14 and Dykema, unpublished).

Granulosa Cell Culture

Granulosa cells were cultured using the procedure described by Epstein-Almog and Orly (28). Ovaries were obtained from immature female Sprague-Dawley rats (23–27 days of age, Harlan). Granulosa cells were cultured in serum-free medium (50:50 Dulbecco's modified Eagles medium and Ham's F-12, 2-μg/mL insulin, 5-μg/mL transferrin, 40-ng/mL hydrocortisone and antibiotics) on fibronectin-coated plates (1.3 μg/cm^2) at a density of 2.2 to 2.6 × 10^7 cells per 100-mm plate. For transfections, cells were plated in medium containing 10% fetal bovine serum.

Transfections

Transfections were performed on day 5 of culture. Granulosa cells were transfected using either lipofectin reagent (BRL) or a modified calcium phosphate-mediated method. Lipofectin (30 μg) and DNA (10 μg) were added to 2 aliquots of serum-free medium, then mixed and added to cells (29, method B). After an 8-h incubation, the medium was aspirated, and medium containing serum and hormones was added. Alternatively, DNA (10 μg) was transfected using the method described by Chen and Okayama (30) in serum-containing medium. After incubation with the DNA for approximately 16 h, media was then removed, and fresh serum-containing medium with hormones was added. Granulosa cells were incubated an additional 48 h before assay. Media was analyzed by radioimmunoassay using an antibody specific for the inhibin α-chain (31).

Northern RNA Hybridization Analysis

RNA was extracted using the method of Chomczynski and Sacchi (32). RNA (20 μg) was electrophoresed on a 1% agarose formaldehyde denaturing gel and transferred to a nylon membrane. Hybridization was done under standard conditions using cDNA inserts as probes that were radiolabeled with ^{32}P-dCTP by random priming. Membranes were washed in 2X SSC and 0.1% SDS at 65°C, and hybridization products were visualized by autoradiography using Kodak XAR-5 film (~16 h).

Chloramphenicol Acetyl Transferase (CAT) and Luciferase Assays

Cell lysates were prepared by freezing and thawing cells in hypotonic buffer. CAT assays were performed as described by Gorman, et al. (33). Luciferase assays were performed using the method of Wood, et al. (34). Ten-second integrated light measurements were taken on a luminometer (Analytical Bioluminescence). Luciferase plasmids have been described (34, 35).

Results

FSH Regulation of Inhibin Gene Expression

FSH is an important regulator of inhibin expression in vivo, acting on the ovary to increase inhibin secretion and mRNA production (17–20). An example of

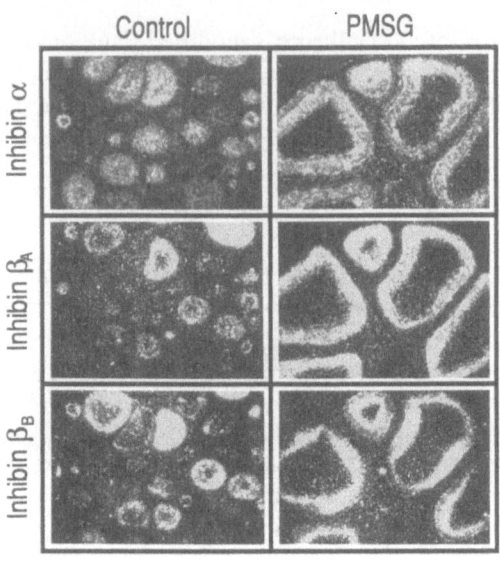

FIGURE 13.1. PMSG-induced inhibin gene expression in the ovary. Darkfield photomicrographs of ovaries from untreated (*left panels*) or PMSG-treated (*right panels*) immature rats following hybridization to inhibin α (inhibin α), β_A (inhibin β_A); or β_B (inhibin β_B) cDNA probes. Photomicrographs are from adjacent sections.

this, in which we examined the effect of PMSG exposure on the ovary of immature rats, is illustrated in Figure 13.1. Untreated control ovaries had numerous preantral and small antral follicles, many of which expressed inhibin α mRNA. Some, but not all of the follicles expressing α-mRNA also expressed β_A- and β_B-mRNA. PMSG exposure led to formation of large antral or preovulatory follicles, and most of these expressed all 3 mRNAs. PMSG stimulated follicular development and also appeared to increase the number of follicles expressing both the inhibin α and β mRNAs.

Since GC from immature rat ovaries express inhibin and respond to FSH, we next established an in vitro system of GC obtained from immature rats cultured in serum-free medium to study inhibin gene regulation. Similar GC culture systems have provided useful models for the study of inhibin biosynthesis (11, 36–40). Granulosa cells form monolayers in culture, and an example is shown in Figure 13.2, left panel. These cells also maintain their ability to respond to FSH, which is illustrated in Figure 13.2, right panel. Untreated GC appear elongated with groups of cells running parallel to one another. Addition of FSH (100 ng/mL for 24 h) caused the cells to round up. Effects on the morphology of GC by FSH have also been described in vivo (40).

Untreated **FSH-Treated**

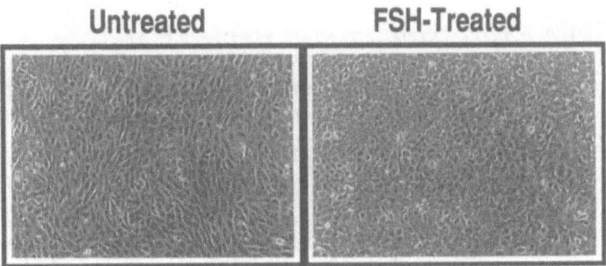

FIGURE 13.2. FSH alteration of the morphology of cultured GC. Granulosa cells are shown after 1 week in culture. Cells were untreated (*left panel*) or exposed to 100 ng/ mL FSH (*right panel*) for 24 h.

In addition to altering cellular morphology, FSH induced synthesis of inhibin protein and α-chain mRNA in a dose-dependent manner, as illustrated in Figure 13.3. Increasing doses of FSH were added to GC after 7 days in culture. After a 48-h exposure, inhibin release into the medium was measured by RIA, and α-mRNA content in the cells was assessed by Northern RNA hybridization analysis. Increasing doses of FSH led to elevated levels of α-mRNA and increased secretion of inhibin protein into the media.

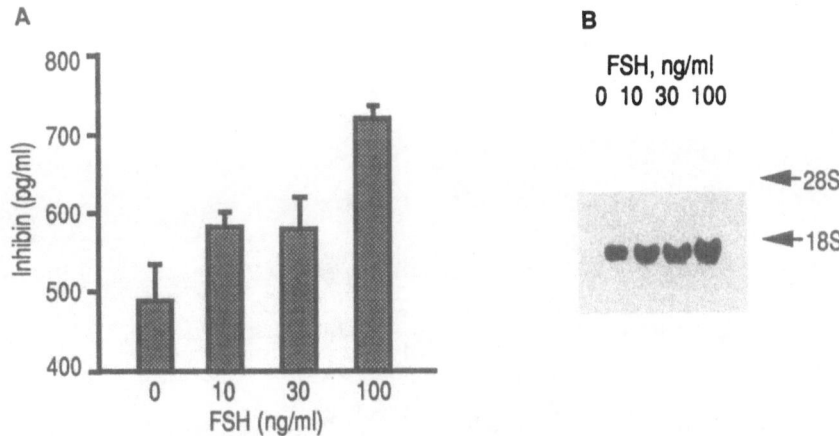

FIGURE 13.3. FSH-induced inhibin gene expression in cultured GC. *A*: Inhibin levels in medium as measured by RIA after 48 h of exposure to 0-, 10-, 30-, and 100-ng/mL FSH. *B*: Northern RNA hybridization analysis of total RNA (20 μg/lane), isolated from the same cultures as in (*A*), was probed with ^{32}P-labeled inhibin α-cDNA.

Inhibin Gene Expression in Transfected Cells

Besides providing a useful model for studying endogenous inhibin gene regulation, GC can also be used to identify regions of the inhibin α gene promoter that are important in controlling transcription of the gene. The strategy for identification of these DNA sequences is shown in Figure 13.4. The 5' flanking region of the α-inhibin gene was inserted upstream of a reporter gene, either luciferase or chloramphenicol acetyl transferase. These constructs were transfected into primary cultures of GC using either cationic liposomes or a modified calcium phosphate precipitation procedure. Cells were then incubated for an additional 48 h and cell lysates were assayed for the activity of the reporter gene. This approach has been successfully used to examine several aspects of inhibin promoter function.

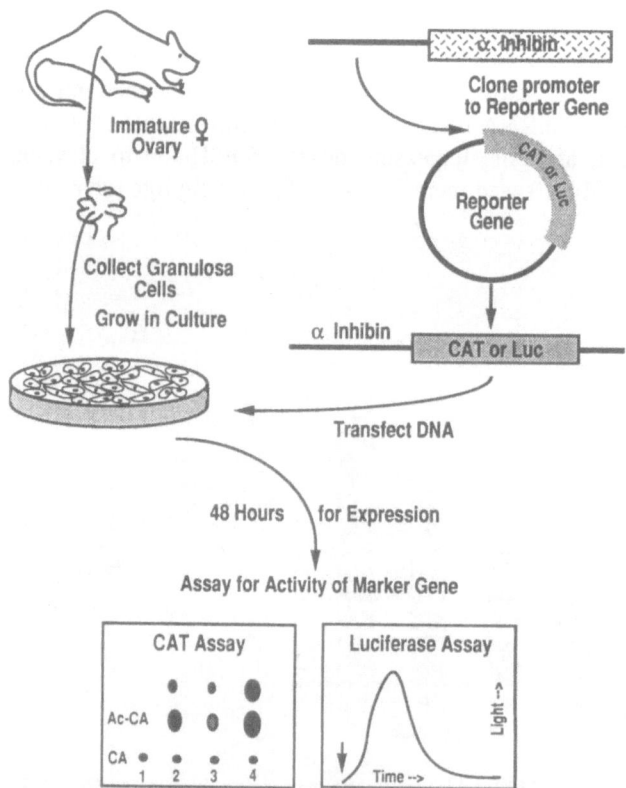

FIGURE 13.4. A GC transfection assay for studying inhibin gene expression. The 5' flanking region of the inhibin α gene was cloned upstream of either a CAT or luciferase reporter gene. Primary cultures of rat GC were transfected with these constructs, and after 48 h, cell lysates were prepared and assayed for CAT or luciferase activity.

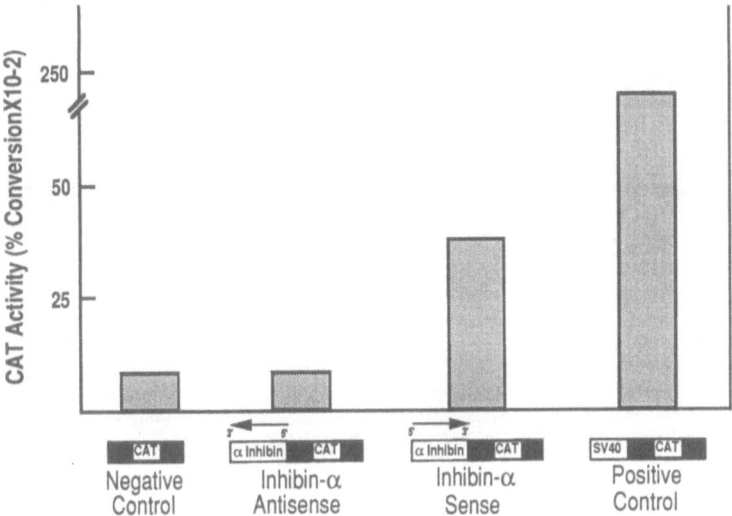

FIGURE 13.5. Activity of the α-inhibin gene promoter in GC. CAT activity is shown in cells transfected with the promoterless pUC-CAT construct (negative control) or with pSV2-CAT (positive control containing an SV40 promoter). Two constructs containing the α-inhibin promoter in the 3' to 5' orientation (inhibin-α antisense) or in the normal 5' to 3' orientation (inhibin-α sense) were also used for transfection.

We used the strategy outlined in Figure 13.4 to determine if the inhibin α gene promoter was functional in this system. A 2-kb portion of the 5' flanking region of the inhibin α gene was inserted in front of the CAT gene in either the 5' to 3' or 3' to 5' orientation. These constructs were transfected into GC using a liposome-mediated transfer procedure, and 48 h later, cell lysates were prepared and assayed for CAT activity. As illustrated in Figure 13.5, the 5' flanking region of the inhibin α gene could promote expression of the CAT gene. However in the 3' to 5' orientation, CAT activity was no different from cells transfected with the promoterless pUC-CAT construct.

We next determined whether the transfected inhibin α gene could respond to cAMP, the mediator of FSH action in ovarian GC (11). A 547-bp fragment of the 5' flanking region of the inhibin α promoter was fused to a luciferase reporter gene. This plasmid was transfected into GC using calcium phosphate-mediated transfer. These results are illustrated in Figure 13.6. Background luciferase activity was determined by transfection of a promoterless luciferase construct. Basal levels of luciferase expression from the inhibin α promoter were above background levels. Addition of forskolin, an agent that activates adenyl cyclase and elevates intracellular cAMP, led to an approximately 4-fold increase in luciferase activity. Therefore, this region of the inhibin α gene contains sequences able to mediate induction by cAMP.

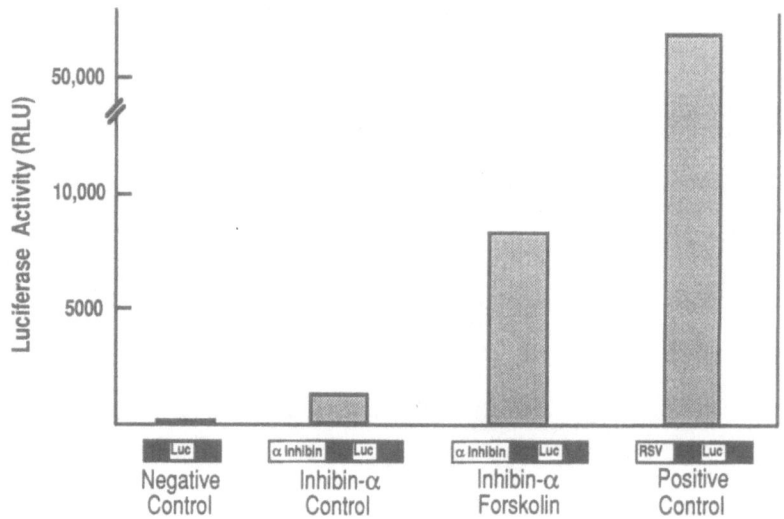

FIGURE 13.6. Forskolin regulation of the α-inhibin gene in transfected GC. Granulosa cells were transfected with either a promoterless luciferase construct (negative control), a luciferase gene containing the RSV-LTR (positive control), or a construct containing 547 bp of the 5' flanking region of the α-inhibin promoter inserted into a luciferase construct. Cells transfected with the inhibin α promoter were incubated in the absence (inhibin-α control) or presence of 10^{-5}M forskolin (inhibin-α forskolin). Luciferase activity is reported in relative light units (RLU).

Discussion

Gonadotropins are important regulators of inhibin and activin gene expression in the ovary. We have demonstrated that PMSG can increase α-, β_A-, and β_B-mRNA expression in the ovary of immature female rats. Inhibin and activin mRNAs were shown to be localized predominantly to GC of developing follicles. While some follicles express only the α-chain mRNA, many also express β_A- and β_B-mRNAs. These findings are in agreement with others (11, 14, 19). Meunier, et al. (18) have additionally shown that treatment with human chorionic gonadotropin (hCG) leads to decreased inhibin gene expression, mimicking the events occurring after the LH surge in adult cycling female rats.

An in vitro system of GC cultured in serum-free medium provides a useful model for the study of inhibin gene regulation. These cultures are enriched for the cell type that expresses inhibin, and the environment of the cells can be precisely controlled. In response to FSH, these cells synthesize inhibin mRNAs and protein in a dose-dependent manner. Granulosa cells in culture have been used by others to study inhibin regulation by hormones and growth factors (11, 37–39). To further our studies of inhibin regulation at the gene level, we have shown that these cells can be transfected using either lipofectin or calcium phosphate-mediated DNA transfer and that they express the exogenous DNA. This GC transfection system was used to examine the promoter activity of the 5' flanking region of the inhibin α gene. We demonstrated that the 5' flanking region of this gene can direct expression of a linked marker gene. We also showed that this region of the α-gene mediated cAMP responsiveness, consistent with the observation that the α-gene contains a cAMP response element (26 and Pei et al., submitted). This system should be useful to further study the expression and regulation of the α- and β-chain genes by hormones and growth factors.

Acknowledgments. Supported by grants from the NIH and NSF to K.E.M., a Lalor Foundation Fellowship to R.E.D., and an NIH Training Grant to J.C.D.

References

1. Dorrington J, Armstrong D. Effects of FSH on gonadal functions. Recent Prog Horm Res 1979;35:1-42.
2. De Jong FH. Inhibin. Physiol Rev 1988;68:555-607.
3. Hsueh AJW, Dahl KD, Vaughan J, et al. Heterodimers and homodimers of inhibin subunits have different paracrine action in the modulation of luteinizing hormone-stimulated androgen biosynthesis. Proc Natl Acad Sci USA 1987;84: 5082-6.
4. LaPolt PS, Soto D, Su J-G, et al. Activin stimulation of inhibin secretion and messenger RNA levels in cultured granulosa cells. Mol Cell Endocrinol 1989;3: 1666-73.
5. Ling N, Ying S-Y, Ueno N, et al. Pituitary FSH is released by a heterodimer of the β-subunits from the two forms of inhibin. Nature 1986;321:779-82.
6. Vale W, Rivier J, Vaughan J, et al. Purification and characterization of an FSH-releasing protein from porcine ovarian follicular fluid. Nature 1986;321:779-82.
7. Robertson DM, Foulds LM, Leversha L, et al. Isolation of inhibin from bovine follicular fluid. Biochem Biophys Res Commun 1985;126:220-6.
8. Miyamoto K, Hasegawa Y, Fukuda M, et al. Isolation of porcine follicular fluid inhibin of about 32 kDa. Biochem Biophys Res Commun 1985;129:396-403.
9. Ling N, Ying S-Y, Ueno N, Esch F, Denoroy L, Guillemin R. Isolation and partial characterization of a Mr 32,000 protein with inhibin activity from porcine ovarian follicular fluid. Proc Natl Acad Sci USA 1985;82:7217-21.
10. Rivier J, Spiess J, McClintock R, Vaughan J, Vale W. Purification and partial characterization of inhibin from porcine follicular fluid. Biochem Biophys Res Commun 1985;133:120-7.
11. Bicsak TA, Tucker EM, Cappel S, et al. Hormonal regulation of granulosa cell inhibin biosynthesis. Endocrinology 1986;119:2711-9.

12. Merchenthaler I, Culler MK, Petrusz P, Negro-Villar A. Immunocytochemical localization of inhibin in rat and human reproductive tissues. Mol Cell Endocrinol 1987;54:236-43.

13. Cuevas P, Ying S-Y, Ling N, Ueno N, Esch F, Guillemin R. Immunohistochemical detection of inhibin on the gonads. Biochem Biophys Res Commun 1987;142: 23-30.

14. Woodruff TK, Meunier H, Jones PBC, Hsueh AJW, Mayo KE. Rat inhibin: molecular cloning of α- and β-subunit complementary deoxyribonucleic acids and expression in the ovary. Mol Cell Endocrinol 1987;1:561-8.

15. Woodruff TK, D'Agostino J, Schwartz NB, Mayo KE. Dynamic changes in inhibin messenger RNAs in rat ovarian follicles during the reproductive cycle. Science 1988;239:1296-9.

16. Meunier H, Cajander SB, Roberts VJ, et al. Rapid changes in the expression of inhibin α-, β_A-, and β_B-subunits in ovarian cell types during the rat estrous cycle. Mol Cell Endocrinol 1988;2:1352-63.

17. Lee VWK, McMaster J, Quigg H, Findlay J, Leversha L. Ovarian and peripheral blood inhibin concentration increase with gonadotropin treatment in immature rats. Endocrinology 1981;108:2403-5.

18. Meunier H, Roberts VJ, Sawchenko PE, Cajander SB, Hseuh AJW, Vale W. Periovulatory changes in the expression of inhibin α-, β_A-, β_B-subunits in hormonally induced immature female rats. Mol Cell Endocrinol 1989;3:2062-9.

19. Davis SR, Burger HG, Robertson DM, Farnworth PG, Carson RS, Krozowski Z. Pregnant mare's serum gonadotropin stimulates inhibin subunit gene expression in the immature rat ovary: dose response characteristics and relationships to serum gonadotropins, inhibin and ovarian steroid content. Endocrinology 1988; 123:2399-407.

20. Rivier C, Roberts V, Vale W. Possible role of luteinizing hormone and follicle-stimulating hormone in modulating inhibin secretion and expression during the estrous cycle of the rat. Endocrinology 1989;125:876-82.

21. Woodruff TK, D'Agostino J, Schwartz NB, Mayo KE. Decreased inhibin gene expression in preovulatory follicles requires primary gonadotropin surges. Endocrinology 1989;124:2193-9.

22. Krummen LA, Toppari J, Kim WH, et al. Regulation of testicular inhibin subunit messenger ribonucleic acid levels in vivo: effects of hypophysectomy and selective follicle-stimulating hormone replacement. Endocrinology 1989;125:1630.

23. Feng Z-M, Bardin CW, Chen C-LC. Characterization and regulation of testicular inhibin β-subunit mRNA. Mol Cell Endocrinol 1989;3:939-48.

24. Bardin CW, Morris PL, Shaha C, et al. Inhibin structure and function in the testis. Ann NY Acad Sci 1989;565:10-23.

25. Schwall RH, Mason AJ, Wilcox JM, Bassett SC, Zeleznik AJ. Localization of inhibin activin subunit messenger RNAs within the primate ovary. Mol Cell Endocrinol 1990;4:75-9.

26. Feng Z-M, Li Y-P, Chen C-LC. Analysis of the 5'-flanking regions of rat inhibin α- and β_B-subunit genes suggests two different regulatory mechanisms. Mol Cell Endocrinol 1989;3:1914-25.

27. Suhr ST, Rahal JO, Mayo KM. Mouse growth hormone-releasing hormone:

precursor structure and expression in brain and placenta. Mol Cell Endocrinol 1989;3:1693-1700.

28. Epstein-Almog R, Orly J. Inhibition of hormone-induced steroidogenesis during cell proliferation in serum-free cultures of rat granulosa cells. Endocrinology 1985; 116:2103-12.

29. Felgner PL, Holm M. Cationic liposome-mediated transfection. Focus 1989; 11:21-5.

30. Chen C, Okayama H. High-efficiency transformation of mammalian cells by plasmid DNA. Mol Cell Biol 1987;7:2745-52.

31. Ackland JF, D'Agostino J, Ringstrom SJ, Hostetler JP, Mann BG, Schwartz NB. Circulating radioimmunoassayable inhibin during periods of transient follicle-stimulating hormone rise: secondary surge and unilateral ovariectomy. Biol Reprod 1990;43:347-52.

32. Chomczynski P, Sacchi N. Single step method of RNA isolation by acid guanidium thiocyanate phenol-chloroform extraction. Anal Biochem 1987;162:156-9.

33. Gorman CM, Moffat LF, Howard BH. Recombinant genomes which express chloramphenicol acetyltransferase in mammalian cells. Mol Cell Biol 1982;2: 1044-51.

34. Wood WM, Kao MY, Gordon DF, Ridgway EC. Thyroid hormone regulates the mouse thyrotropin β-subunit gene promoter in transfected primary thyrotrophs. J Biol Chem 1989;264:14840-7.

35. Maxwell IH, Harrison GS, Wood WM, Maxwell F. A DNA cassette containing a trimerized SV40 polyadenylation signal which efficiently blocks spurious plasmid-initiated transcription. BioTechniques 1989;7:276-80.

36. Bicsak TA, Cajander SB, Vale W, Hsueh AJW. Inhibin: studies of stored and secreted forms by biosynthetic labeling and immunodetection in cultured rat granulosa cells. Endocrinology 1988;122:741-8.

37. Suzuki T, Miyamoto K, Hasegawa Y, et al. Regulation of inhibin production by rat granulosa cells. Mol Cell Endocrinol 1987;54:185-95.

38. Zhang Z, Lee VWK, Carson RS, Burger HG. Selective control of rat granulosa cell inhibin production by FSH and LH in vitro. Mol Cell Endocrinol 1988;56: 35-40.

39. LaPolt PS, Piquette GN, Soto D, Sincich C, Hseuh AJW. Regulation of inhibin subunit messenger ribonucleic acid levels by gonadotropin, growth factors and gonadotropin-releasing hormone in cultured rat granulosa cells. Endocrinology 1990;127:823-31.

40. Amsterdam A, Rotmensch S. Structure-function relationships during granulosa cell differentiation. Endocr Rev 1987;8:309-337.

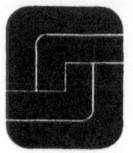

14

Gonadotropin Regulation of Apolipoprotein E Production by Steroidogenic Cells

J.R. Schreiber, K.L. Wyne, L.M. Olson, D.M. Driscoll, M.W. Beckmann, V.M. Schmit, and G.S. Getz

Apolipoprotein E (apo E) is a 34-kD protein that is found in association with various lipoproteins, including chylomycron remnants, very low density lipoproteins (VLDL), and certain subclasses of high-density lipoprotein (HDLc) (1, 2). Apo E plays an important role in cholesterol metabolism and thus has been the subject of much investigation. First, it functions as a ligand for the receptor-mediated uptake of plasma lipoproteins by the B/E (LDL) receptor of peripheral cells and the E-receptor on hepatocytes (3). Second, it serves as the ligand for the recently described LDL receptor-related protein (LRP) of hepatic and peripheral cells (4). Third, apo E can serve as a distributor of lipids between cells in tissue and as a mediator of reverse transport of cholesterol from peripheral cells back to the liver (2), especially in species lacking the cholesterol ester transfer protein. Apo E is synthesized predominantly in the liver, but unlike the other apoproteins, it is also produced in most extrahepatic tissues, including brain, spleen, and the steroidogenic organs (adrenal, testis, and ovary) (5, 6). In individual extrahepatic tissues, apo E could serve some or all the functions mentioned previously. The steroidogenic tissues have a great demand for cholesterol as the substrate for steroid hormone production. A role for apo E as a tissue distributor of lipids would likely be identified in them.

We have studied the regulation of the production of apo E in cultured rat ovarian granulosa cells (GC). This well-examined model has several characteristics that make it attractive. First, these cells mature in vitro in response to the gonadotropin FSH with the development of LH and prolactin receptors, the synthesis of enzymes necessary for steroidogenesis, and the production of numerous secretory proteins (7). Second, these cells are cultured in serum-free (i.e., lipoprotein-free) medium, making them dependent on endogenous cholesterol synthesis for steroidogenesis (7). Inhibition of cholesterol synthesis would severely restrict the availability of cholesterol and potential regulatory sterol products. Third, rat GC can utilize both LDL and HDL cholesterol for cellular needs, including steroidogenesis (8). Cell cholesterol can therefore be restricted or provided, and the availability of cell cholesterol can be easily ascertained by measuring progestin production. This ability to manipulate cell cholesterol is important for the study of apo E since it has been shown in macrophages that apo E production is positively correlated with cell cholesterol content (9).

In our studies, we set out to answer the following questions. First, do rat ovarian GC synthesize and secrete apo E? Second, is apo E production regulated by the gonadotropin FSH? Third, if FSH has an effect, is it mediated by A-kinase? Fourth, does cell cholesterol availability affect apo E production? Fifth, is the regulation of apo E production transcriptionally regulated? Sixth, is apo E production unique to the rat ovarian GC? Seventh, what role does locally produced apo E play in the ovary?

Materials and Methods

Cell Culture

Rat ovarian GC were isolated from ovaries obtained from 23-day-old hypophysectomized diethylstilbestrol treated Sprague-Dawley female rats (Johnson Laboratories, Chicago, IL) and cultured in McCoy's 5A medium as previously described (10). Cell media contained 2-mM L-glutamine, 100-U/mL penicillin, 100-µg/mL streptomycin, 10^{-7}M androstenedione, plus additives noted in the text and figure legends.

Human ovarian GC were aspirated from preovulatory (PO) follicles of women undergoing ovum retrieval for in vitro fertilization. Women were treated with urinary gonadotropin (Pergonal or Metrodin, Serono, Randolph, MA) at a daily I.M. dose of 150–300 IU starting day 2 of the menstrual cycle. Exogenous gonadotropins were continued until serum estradiol was >500-pg/mL and at least 2 follicles were >16 mm in diameter by ultrasound. After ova were removed, GC were isolated from the follicular aspirates by centrifugation (room temperature, 7 min, 500 × g). GC were separated from erythrocytes and polymorphonuclear leukocytes by centrifugation over 3-mL Ficoll as previously described (11). To remove contaminating monocytes/macrophages, the GC preparation was suspended in 3-mL incubation medium and incubated in plastic tissue culture dishes for 1 h at 37°C (95% humidified air, 5% CO_2). The nonadherent GC were cultured for 24 h in incubation medium (DMEM + 4-mM L-glutamine, 100-U/mL penicillin, and 100-µg/mL streptomycin) plus 20%-v/v human male serum. After 24 h, the cells were cultured in serum-free medium plus additives as described in the figure legend.

Measurement of Secreted Apo E

During the last hours of culture, GC were incubated with 50–100-μCi/mL [^{35}S]methionine. The media were removed, and ^{35}S-labeled apo E secretion was quantitated by representative immunoprecipitation (12). In brief, a monospecific apo E antibody was added to the media; the immune complex was precipitated by the addition of protein A bearing *S. aureus* and electrophoresed on SDS-PAGE. The ^{35}S-apo E bands on autoradiograms were quantitated.

Measurement of Cellular Content of Apo E mRNA

Total cellular RNA was isolated from the GC at the end of the culture period by the guanidine thiocyanate/cesium chloride procedure of Chirgwin, et al. (13). Slot blots were hybridized by specific ^{32}P-cDNA probe as previously described (14), and the autoradiograms were quantitated.

Measurement of Secreted Progestins

Rat GC secretion of 5α-dihydroprogesterone (DHP) and estrogen (E) and human GC secretion of progesterone (P) were measured by specific radioimmunoassay (RIA)(8) of aliquots of media removed prior to the addition of the [^{35}S]methionine.

Results

Rat Ovarian GC

Preliminary experiments demonstrated that cultured rat ovarian GC synthesized and secreted a protein with characteristics that identified it as apo E. It was immunoprecipitated with a monospecific apo E antibody, migrated on SDS-PAGE as does authentic apo E, and had a pattern of limited proteolytic cleavage (Cleveland digest [15]) that was the same as authentic apo E (12).

To characterize the regulation of apo E synthesis and secretion, we tested whether FSH had an effect on GC apo E production. As shown in Figure 14.1, FSH alone stimulated a 1-fold increase in apo E secretion. To test whether the FSH effect was mediated via adenylate cyclase activation and A-kinase stimulation, we examined the effects of the phosphodiesterase inhibitor isobutylmethylxanthine (IBMX) and dibutyryl cAMP (Bt$_2$cAMP). Both cause elevated levels of cellular cAMP and activate A-kinase. As shown in Figure 14.1, IBMX augmented the FSH effect, and Bt$_2$cAMP stimulated apo E synthesis significantly. Therefore, FSH stimulates apo E production via the cAMP:A-kinase pathway.

To determine whether the cAMP:A-kinase effect is transcriptionally regulated, we tested the effect of cholera toxin (CT), an adenylate cyclase activa-

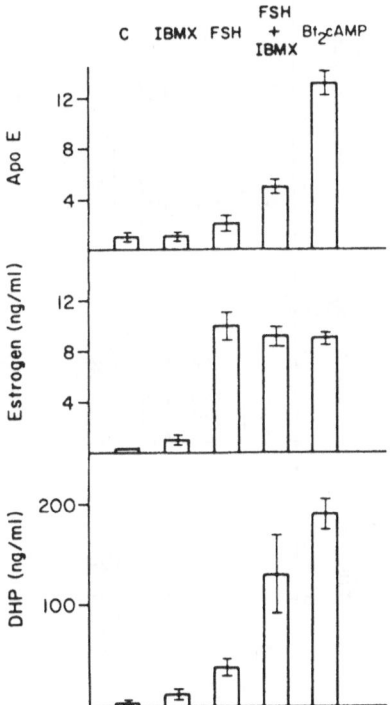

FIGURE 14.1. Effects of FSH and cAMP on apo E secretion and steroidogenesis by cultured rat ovarian GC. Granulosa cells were cultured for 48 h in serum-free medium (control = C), 0.2-mM IBMX, 50-ng/mL FSH, IBMX + FSH, or 5-mg/mL Bt$_2$cAMP. An aliquot of medium was assayed for DHP and E by specific RIA, and the cells were labeled for 16 h with [^{35}S]methionine. ^{35}S-apo E was measured as described in Materials and Methods. (1 apo E secretion unit = amount secreted in control cultures.) Results are mean ± SD; n = 4. Reprinted with permission from Driscoll, Schreiber, Schmit, and Getz (12).

tor, on cellular content of apo E mRNA (14). As shown in Figure 14.2, an increasing concentration of CT stimulated a step-wise increase in apo E secretion, cell content of apo E mRNA, and DHP production. The data indicate that the A-kinase stimulation of apo E production is at least partially at the transcriptional level. An examination of the time course of the CT effect supports this conclusion. As shown in Figure 14.3, CT stimulated an increase in apo E mRNA after 16 h of culture, a peak at 32 h, and a decline at 48 h and beyond. The effect on apo E secretion has the same pattern, except that the effect on mRNA precedes the effect on apo E protein synthesis.

The regulation of the apo E gene is complex (16), and studies of other apo E-producing cells, such as macrophages, indicate that apo E production is

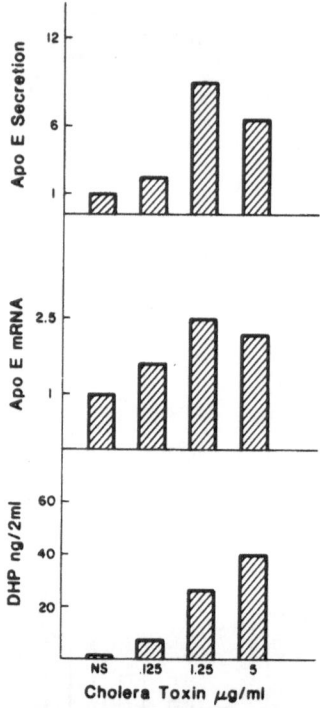

FIGURE 14.2. Effect of cholera toxin (CT) on apo E secretion, apo E mRNA content, and DHP production of rat GC. Granulosa cells were cultured in serum-free medium without (nonstimulated = NS) or with the indicated concentration of CT. After 24 h, an aliquot of medium was assayed for DHP by RIA; then cells were labeled for 8 h with [^{35}S]methionine. Medium ^{35}S-apo E and cellular apo E mRNA content were assayed as described. (1 apo E mRNA or apo E secretion unit = amount in NS culture.) Results are the average of 2 experiments. Reprinted with permission from Wyne, Schreiber, Larsen, and Getz (14).

up-regulated by an increasing cell content of cholesterol (9). We tested the effect of cell cholesterol content on GC apo E production. As shown on Figure 14.4, Bt$_2$ cAMP stimulated apo E secretion 6-fold, mevinolin (an inhibitor of cholesterol synthesis) blocked the cAMP effect, and mevalono-lactone (which overcomes the mevinolin block) reversed the mevinolin effect on apo E secretion (17). Since these cells were cultured in serum-free medium and, thus, were dependent on endogenously synthesized cholesterol, the data indicate that decreased available cell cholesterol down-regulated the apo E production. The effects of mevinolin and mevalonolactone on steroidogenesis support this interpretation since mevinolin blocked DHP production and mevalonolactone restored it by providing the cell with the material

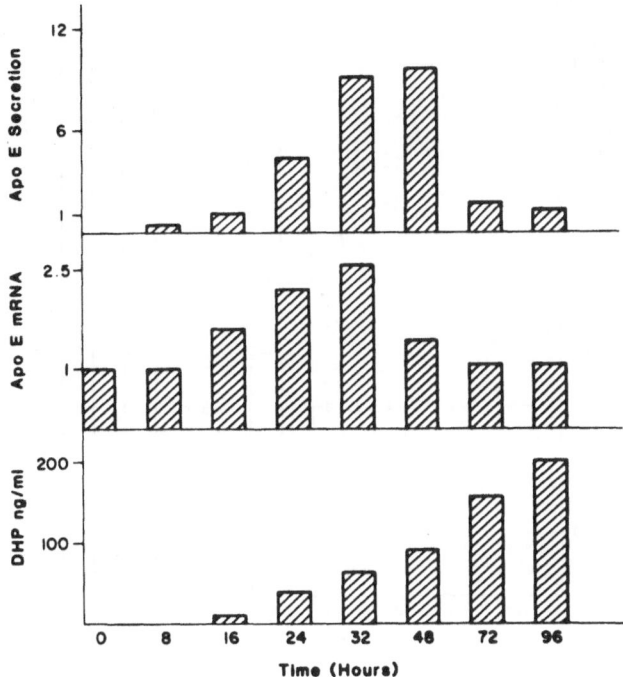

FIGURE 14.3. Cholera toxin time course. Granulosa cells were cultured for the time indicated in serum-free medium plus 1.25-μg/mL CT. Eight hours prior to indicated time, an aliquot of medium was removed for DHP assay. Apo E secretion and apo E mRNA were assayed as described in Figure 14.1, and results were normalized to the 32-h nonstimulated control, which was set equal to 1. Values are mean of 2 experiments. Reprinted with permission from Wyne, Schreiber, Larsen, and Getz (14).

needed to produce cholesterol substrate for steroidogenesis. Changes in apo E mRNA content parallel the apo E secretion changes, suggesting that the regulation is at least partially at the level of gene expression.

To examine the role of cholesterol further, we tested the effect of HDL, an effective provider of cholesterol to the rat GC, on apo E synthesis. As shown in Figure 14.5, HDL stimulated a significant increase in apo E secretion over that of CT alone. To test which component of HDL was responsible for this stimulation, we examined the effect of 2 synthetic particles. Particle 1 contained apo A-1 + phospholipid, while particle 2 contained A-1 + phospholipid + cholesterol. As shown in Figure 14.5, particle 2 stimulated apo E more effectively than did particle 1. These data indicate that HDL cholesterol is a likely candidate as the mediator of the HDL effect on apo E production. In further studies, we determined that increased secretion of apo E due to

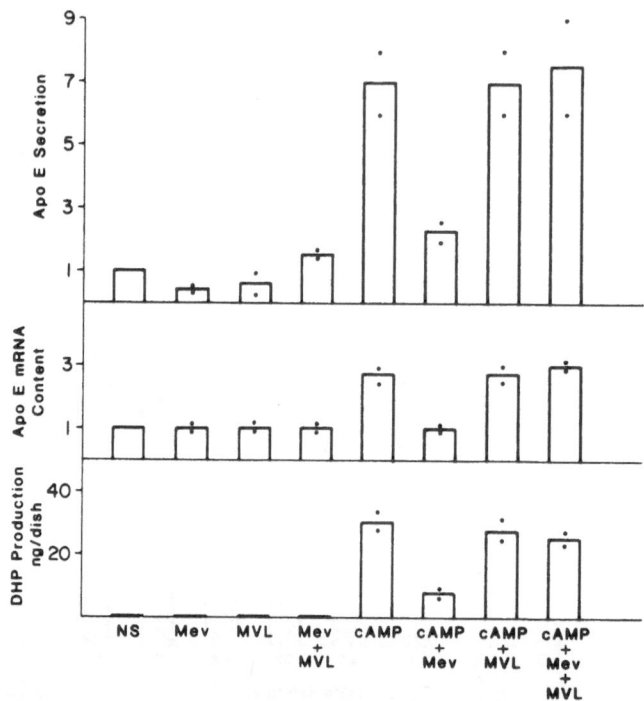

FIGURE 14.4. Effect of limited cellular cholesterol on steroidogenesis, apo E secretion, and apo E mRNA content of rat GC. Granulosa cells were cultured for 32 h in serum-free medium (nonstimulated = NS), 10^{-6}M mevinolin (Mev), 10-mM mevalonolactone (MVL), 5-mg/mL Bt$_2$cAMP (cAMP), or the indicated combination. At 28 h, an aliquot of medium was removed for DHP RIA, and the cells were cultured with [^{35}S]methionine. ^{35}S-apo E secretion and apo E mRNA content were measured as described, and values were normalized to the 32-h NS control, which was set equal to 1. Reprinted with permission from Wyne, Schreiber, Larsen, and Getz (17).

added HDL was not accompanied by a change in cellular apo E mRNA content, suggesting that the HDL effect is posttranscriptional.

Human Ovarian GC

To learn the general applicability of the rat GC apo E studies to other steroidogenic cells, we examined the effect of cAMP stimulation and cholesterol manipulation on human GC apo E synthesis. In preliminary experiments, we determined that cultured human GC also produced a ^{35}S-labeled protein identified as apo E. It was immunoprecipitated by a monospecific apo E antibody, migrated to the same position as authentic apo E on SDS-

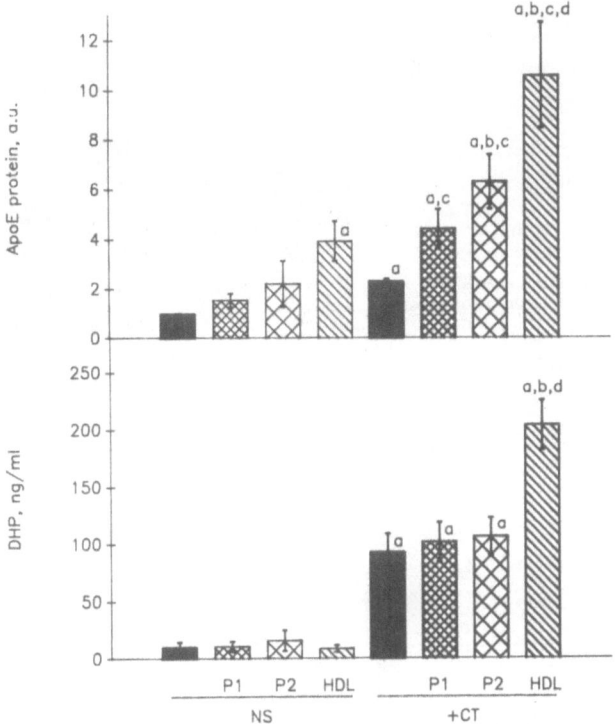

FIGURE 14.5. Effect of lipoprotein cholesterol on steroidogenesis and apo E secretion by rat GC. Granulosa cells were cultured for 32 h in serum-free medium alone or with particle 1 (P1 = 10.4-µg protein/mL, no cholesterol), particle 2 (P2 = 10.4-µg protein/mL + 4.1-µg unesterified cholesterol/mL), or HDL (100-µg protein/mL + 4.1-µg unesterified cholesterol/mL + 29.3-µg esterified cholesterol/mL) with and without CT (1.25 µg/mL). DHP and apo E secretion were measured as described in the legend to Figure 14.4. Values are mean ± SEM. Different letters mean significant difference (P < 0.05). From Olsen et al., VIII Ovarian Workshop, Maryville, TN, Serono Symposia USA, 1990.

PAGE, and had a partial proteolytic digest pattern (Cleveland digest [15]), the same as authentic apo E. Apo E mRNA was identified by binding of a ^{32}P-cDNA probe by Northern analysis (18). As shown in Figure 14.6, human chorionic gonadotropin (hCG), which binds to specific surface receptors and stimulates cAMP production, caused the expected increase in progesterone production and a 50% decrease in apo E secretion. Aminoglutethimide, which blocks cholesterol metabolism to progestin (17), and LDL, which provides cholesterol to the cell, both stimulated apo E secretion and reversed the hCG effect. As with the rat cells, the human ovarian GC apo E production is regulated by both A-kinase and cell cholesterol. In further studies, the cell

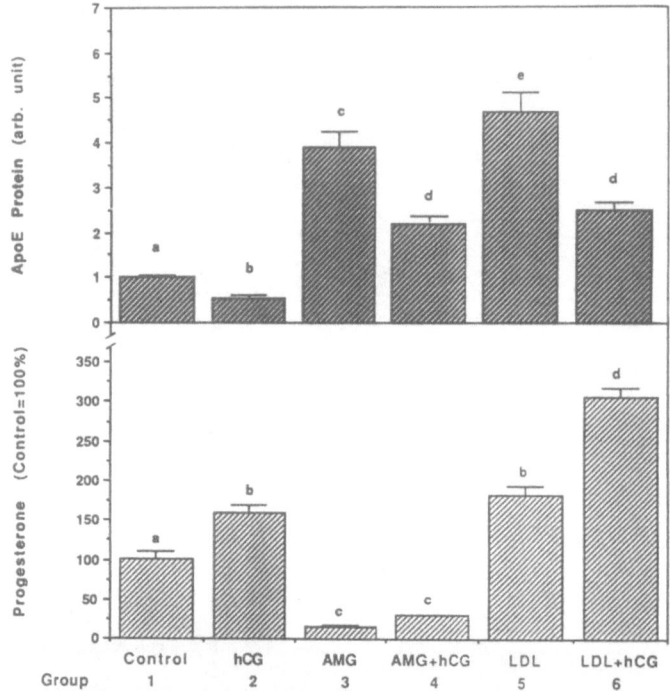

FIGURE 14.6. Regulation of apo E secretion and steroidogenesis by human ovarian GC. Human GC were incubated in medium + 20% human male serum for 24 h. The medium was replaced with serum-free medium ± aminoglutethimide (AMG = 100 µg/mL) or LDL (100 µg/mL) as noted in the figure. At 48 h of culture, hCG (1 IU/mL) was added to the indicated groups. At 68 h of culture, aliquots of media were removed for progesterone (P) analysis by RIA, and 100-µCi/mL of [^{35}S]methionine was added. At 72 h, the media were assayed for ^{35}S-apo E, with the values normalized so that control = 1. Values are mean ± SEM. Different letters mean significant difference (P < 0.05).

content of apo E mRNA changed in parallel with apo E secretion, indicating that the regulation is probably at least partially at the transcriptional level.

Discussion

Apo E has been detected in numerous organs throughout the body, making it unique among the apolipoproteins (5, 6). Our studies have added to this list with the demonstration that steroidogenic cells in human and rat ovaries secrete apo E (12). In both rat and human, apo E production is under A-kinase and cholesterol control. Rat preantral GC contain specific FSH receptors (7). FSH and other agents that increase cellular cAMP and activate A-kinase stimulate apo E secretion (12).

This effect of A-kinase stimulation on apo E secretion is time dependent, with a marked increase during the first 48 h of culture followed by a marked decrease over the next 48 h (Fig. 14.3). In the rat, which has a 4-day estrous cycle, day 2 corresponds to the time of ovulation. This reasoning can reconcile the rat and human results. The preovulatory human GC possess LH/hCG receptors (11) that were induced by the in vivo administration of gonadotropins. The hCG stimulates the cAMP:A-kinase system, which results in an increase in steroidogenesis and a decrease in apo E and apo E mRNA. The fall in human apo E production after hCG can be considered analogous to the fall in rat apo E secretion during the last 2 days of A-kinase stimulation. In any case, cAMP:A-kinase stimulation has effects on both rat and human GC apo E synthesis that are mediated at least partially at the transcriptional level, based upon the above described experiments as well as on transfection experiments to be reported elsewhere.

In both rat and human cells, cholesterol or a cholesterol product has regulatory effects. Restricting cholesterol to the cell causes decreased apo E secretion, while increased cholesterol causes increased apo E secretion. These data are in agreement with the results of studies of macrophages in which it has been shown that increased cell cholesterol levels lead to increased apo E production (9). However, in each of these cells, the mechanisms accounting for the cholesterol effects appear to differ somewhat from cell to cell. Thus, in human ovarian GC, exogenous cholesterol provided as lipoprotein influences apo E production and its message in similar fashion. This is not the case in primary ovarian GC, where a posttranscriptional influence of lipoprotein is evident.

The regulation of the apo E gene has been shown to be exceedingly complex. Smith, et al. (16) have shown that the apo E gene is regulated by multiple positive and negative elements. It is thus not surprising that the interplay between A-kinase stimulators and a modification of cholesterol availability can have competing effects on apo E expression. In studies of genes in which cholesterol, or a cholesterol metabolite, regulates gene expression, an octanucleotide, termed *sterol regulatory element* (SRE), has been identified in the 5' promotor region (19). Inspection of the published sequences of both the rat and human apo E genes reveals that this octanucleotide is located in the first and second intron in the human gene and in the third intron in the rat gene (20, 21). Closely related sequences are in several other gene locations. Whether these sequences are involved in apo E gene regulation awaits further study. Steroidogenic cells are exceedingly good models for studying this issue. Cholesterol synthesis and utilization can be stimulated so that the flow of cholesterol increases, and the ability to raise and lower available cell cholesterol is easily accomplished.

The role of apo E in the ovary is unknown, but several possibilities exist. As has been suggested for other tissue, apo E could be secreted in order to mediate excess cholesterol movement from peripheral cells back to the liver—that is, reverse cholesterol transport (1, 2). However, this is unlikely to be the case for steroidogenic tissue, such as the ovary, because of its need for cholesterol as substrate for steroidogenesis. However, apo E could be important for the redistribution of cholesterol and/or other lipids within the tissue. This could be particularly important for the avascular ovarian follicle. Cells requiring cholesterol would express LDL receptors, which avidly mediate the uptake of apo E-containing particles (2). Apo E particles could also be taken up by the recently described LRP-mediated pathway (4). A model for such tissue redistribution has been described at the site of nerve injury, where macrophage-produced apo E particles containing cholesterol are taken up locally by regenerating nerves that need the cholesterol for membrane synthesis (2).

There could also be functions for apo E that are unrelated to lipid transport. Apo E could have paracrine-like activity, whereby one ovarian cell could influence another. Data suggesting such a function were published by Dyer and Curtiss (22), who demonstrated that apo E-containing lipoproteins inhibit theca cell androgen production, converting them to progesterone producers. A possible regulatory role for apo E in the human ovary is suggested by the finding that apo E in human ovarian follicular fluid falls dramatically as serum estrogen is rising and ovulation approaches (23). Apo E could thus serve several functions in the ovary, and the regulation of the apo E gene in steroidogenic cells can serve as a model for its regulation in other tissues.

Acknowledgments. The research projects reported in this paper were supported by the NIH, grant HL-15062.

References

1. Getz GS, Mazzone T, Soltys P, Bates SR. Atherosclerosis and apoprotein E. Arch Pathol Lab Med 1988;112:1048-55.
2. Mahley RW. Apoprotein E. Science 1988;240:622-30.
3. Sherrill BC, Innerarity TL, Mahley RW. Rapid hepatic clearance of canine lipoproteins containing only apo E by a high affinity receptor. J Biol Chem 1980; 255:1804-7.
4. Kowal RC, Herz J, Goldstein JL, Esser J, Brown MS. Low density lipoprotein receptor related-protein mediates uptake of cholesterol esters derived from apoprotein E-enriched lipoproteins. Proc Natl Acad Sci USA 1989;86:5810-4.
5. Reue KL, Quon DH, et al. Cloning and regulation of mRNA for mouse apo E. J Biol Chem 1984;259:2100-7.

6. Driscoll DM, Getz GS. Extrahepatic synthesis of apolipoprotein E. J Lipid Res 1984;25:1368-79.
7. Hsueh AJ, Adashi EY, Jones PC, Welsh TH. Hormonal regulation of the differentiation of cultured granulosa cells. Endocr Rev 1984;5:76-127.
8. Schreiber J, Hsueh AJ, Weinstein D, Erickson G. Plasma lipoproteins stimulate progestin production by rat ovarian granulosa cells cultured in serum-free medium. J Steroid Biochem 1980;13:1009-14.
9. Mazzone T, Gump H, Diller P, Getz GS. Macrophage free cholesterol content regulates apo E production. J Biol Chem 1987;262:11657-62.
10. Erickson G, Hsueh AJ. Stimulation of aromatase activity by FSH in rat granulosa cells in vivo and in vitro. Endocrinology 1978;102:1275-82.
11. Golos TG, Soto EA, Tureck RW, Strauss JF III. Human chorionic gonadotropin and 8-bromo cAMP stimulate ^{125}I-LDL uptake and metabolism by luteinized human granulosa cells in culture. J Clin Endocrinol Metab 1985;61:633-8.
12. Driscoll DM, Schreiber JR, Schmit V, Getz GS. Regulation of apo E synthesis in rat ovarian granulosa cells. J Biol Chem 1985;260:9031-8.
13. Chirgwin JM, Przybyla A, MacDonald R, Rutter W. Isolation of biologically active ribonucleic acid from sources enriched in ribonuclease. Biochemistry 1978; 18:5294-9.
14. Wyne K, Schreiber J, Larsen A, Getz GS. Regulation of apo E biosynthesis by cAMP and phorbol ester in rat ovarian granulosa cells. J Biol Chem 1989;264: 981-9.
15. Cleveland DW, Fischer SG, Kirschner MW, Laemmli UK. Peptide mapping by limited proteolysis in SDS and analysis by gel electrophoresis. J Biol Chem 1977; 252:1102-6.
16. Smith JD, Melian A, Leff T, Breslow J. Expression of the human apo E gene is regulated by multiple positive and negative elements. J Biol Chem 1988;263: 8300-8.
17. Wyne KL, Schreiber JR, Larsen A, Getz GS. Rat granulosa cell apolipoprotein E secretion: regulation by cell cholesterol. J Biol Chem 1989;264:16530-6.
18. Alwine JC, Kemp DJ, Stark GR. Method for detection of specific RNA's in agarose gels by transfer to diabenzyloxymethyl paper and hybridization with DNA probes. Proc Natl Acad Sci USA 1977;74:5350-4.
19. Osborne TF, Gil G, Goldstein JL, Brown MS. Operator constitutive mutation of HMG CoA reductase promoter abolishes protein binding to SRE. J Biol Chem 1988;263:3380-7.
20. Fung WP, Howlett GJ, Schreiber G. Structure and expression of the rat apo E gene. J Biol Chem 1986;261:13777-83.
21. Reardon CA, Paik YK, Chang DJ, et al. Cloning and expression of the human apo E gene. In: Segrest JP, Albers JJ, eds. Methods in enzymology: plasma lipoproteins, part A. New York: Academic Press, 1986:811-23.
22. Dyer CA, Curtiss LK. Apo E-rich HDL's inhibit ovarian androgen synthesis. J Biol Chem 1988;263:10965-73.
23. Brown SA, Hay RV, Schreiber JR. Relationship between serum estrogen and level of apo E in human ovarian follicular fluid. Fertil Steril 1989;51:639-43.

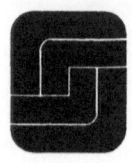

15

Insulin-Like Growth Factors and Their Binding Proteins: Ovarian Modulators of FSH Action

JAMES M. HAMMOND, JUDITH S. MONDSCHEIN, SUSAN E. SAMARAS, RANDALL W. GRIMES, JOHN K. LEIGHTON, SANDRA F. CANNING, AND DANIEL R. HAGEN

The focus of this chapter is the role of the ovarian insulin-like growth factor (IGF) system as an amplification mechanism for FSH action in the ovarian follicle. Recent data from our own laboratory will be emphasized, although numerous investigators have made important contributions to this area. Collectively, these efforts have established the ovarian IGF system as one of the most persuasive and best documented of the putative ovarian paracrine/autocrine systems. For the purpose of discussion, it is convenient to divide the IGF system into its intracellular transduction mechanism and its extracellular components (Fig. 15.1), each of which is affected by FSH. The current emphasis in our laboratory is on the extracellular components of the IGF system—locally secreted IGFs and their binding proteins—and this emphasis will be reflected in this paper. However, a brief summary of the actions of IGFs on ovarian cells is appropriate.

Each of the 3 insulin-related peptides—insulin, IGF-I, and IGF-II—have demonstrated effects on ovarian cells (reviewed in 1–3). However, IGF-I has been found to be the most potent in the majority of instances (3, 4), and the type I (IGF-I) receptor appears to be the most important binding site involved in IGF signal transduction (5). Further, these binding sites are induced by FSH (6) as well as by estrogens (7), which may be secreted under FSH control. In serum-free culture, particularly in the presence of other growth factors, insulin and the IGFs are potent stimulators of granulosa cell (GC) replication (8, 9). However, in the presence of gonadotropins, the dominant effect of the IGFs is a synergistic enhancement of gonadotropin-dependent steroidogenesis. These cytodifferentiative effects are the best-studied ovarian actions of the IGFs and entail amplification of multiple steps in the

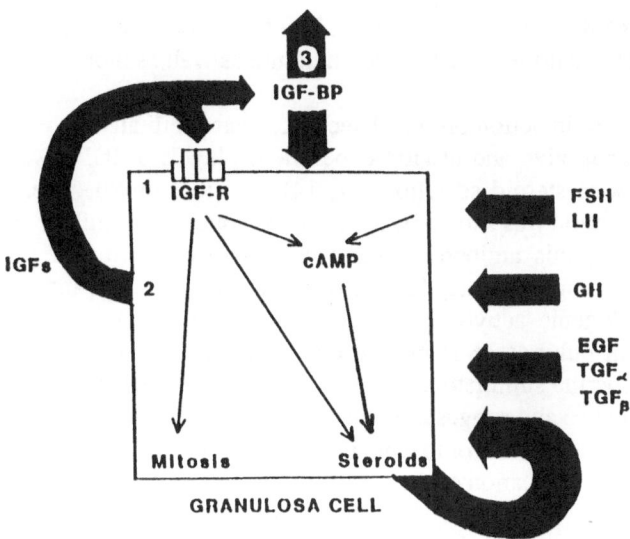

FIGURE 15.1. Components of the ovarian IGF system. *1*: IGF signal transduction system. *2*: Locally secreted IGFs. *3*: IGF binding proteins. As shown, each of these components is regulated by the hormonal signals of the reproductive cycle and modulated locally by gonadal steroids and other ovarian growth factors. In this paper, the FSH-IGF interaction is emphasized. See text for details.

cAMP-dependent steroidogenic cascade (reviewed in 1, 3). These data provide strong support for the concept of IGFs as an FSH-amplifying mechanism.

Ovarian IGF Secretion

Data from a number of investigative strategies have now shown conclusively that the IGFs are synthesized and secreted in the ovary. Our own studies have emphasized immunoassays for IGF-I and/or IGF-II in porcine follicular fluid (FF) and media conditioned by porcine ovarian cells in vitro. More recently, these analyses have been supported by measurement of mRNA for the IGFs.

Our studies have indicated high concentrations of immunoactive IGF-I in pFF and an increase in levels when large follicles were compared to small follicles or serum (10). In vitro, we found that GC from immature follicles secreted immunoreactive IGF-I for at least 10 days in culture (10). More recent studies with GC from more mature follicles have indicated enhanced secretion of IGF-I and a greater degree of hormone responsivity (11). Of most direct relevance to the concept of the IGFs as amplifiers or mediators of FSH action, we found that PMSG treatment of swine in vivo resulted in a doubling of IGF-I levels in pFF (12). In vitro, FSH (as well as LH) enhanced IGF levels in cultures of GC from immature as well as more mature follicles (11, 13).

Gonadotropin action on IGF-I secretion was facilitated by estradiol (13). In both our in vivo and in vitro experiments, levels of IGF-I were found to correlate with steroid secretion (12, 14). A direct link between IGF-I and steroid secretion was shown by the use of a monoclonal antibody to IGF-I. In GC cultures, this antibody blunted the FSH stimulation of progesterone secretion by approximately 50% (15). In addition, the same antibody blocked the steroidogenic activity of preovulatory (PO) pFF when that fluid was assessed in cultures of immature GC (15). These experiments indicate a direct, autocrine stimulatory action of the IGFs on FSH-dependent steroidogenesis in vitro and suggest that the IGFs are an important component of the autocrine/paracrine steroidogenic milieu in the PO follicle.

As another indication of the biosynthetic capacity of the porcine ovary for IGF-I, we have assessed the mRNA for this peptide in whole ovarian homogenates as a function of the porcine cycle, in dissected ovarian components, and in frozen sections of porcine ovary (Samaras and Hammond, unpublished observations). IGF-I mRNA was readily detectable by both Northern analysis and in situ hybridization techniques. Northern analysis indicated multiple transcripts that seem similar or identical to those found in other porcine tissues.

Changes in levels of ovarian IGF-I mRNA during the cycle were modest when such assessments were based on whole ovarian homogenates. However, comparative studies on dissected ovarian components indicated a substantial enrichment of IGF-I message in GC from medium-sized and larger follicles, as well as significant expression of IGF-I mRNA in the functioning corpus luteum. With in situ hybridization, we found that IGF-I mRNA was expressed in the membrane GC of a small population of early antral follicles in ovaries from immature and luteal phase animals. Expression was enhanced in the GC of PO follicles and persisted in the functioning corpus luteum. Collectively, these observations suggest that expression of IGF-I mRNA is a property of growing follicles and persists throughout their life span. We hypothesize that such expression could enhance the FSH responsivity of such follicles and further their growth and development for ovulation.

A topic of ongoing interest is the relative importance of IGF-I and IGF-II for ovarian physiology. Our original studies using receptor assays for IGF-II (10, 16) suggested that both IGF-I and IGF-II were present in the porcine ovary, and this hypothesis has now been confirmed and extended by analysis with specific RIAs (17, 18) and Northern analysis (Samaras et al., unpublished). We found that IGF-I and IGF-II were approximately equally abundant in pFF (17, 18). Cultures of immature GC secreted little if any IGF-II

(17), but cultures from more highly differentiated follicles secreted both peptides (Mondschein et al., unpublished). mRNA for IGF-II was detectable in the porcine ovary. In contrast to that for IGF-I, it appeared to be selectively enriched in the theca layer (Samaras et al., unpublished).

The hormonal regulation of IGF-II secretion in the porcine ovary has not been defined as completely as has that of IGF-I, but the regulation of the two peptides is clearly different. In particular, our studies in vivo and in vitro indicated that IGF-II concentrations were not increased by PMSG or FSH treatment; in fact, they were somewhat diminished (18, unpublished). This situation may differ from that in the human. In that species, IGF-II, the predominant or exclusive GC IGF, appeared to be gonadotropin responsive (19, 20). Whether these intriguing discrepancies actually resulted from species differences, differences in techniques, or in the physiological preparations examined has not been conclusively determined. Thus, additional studies will be required to fully define the role of IGF-II in ovarian physiology in general and in gonadotropin action in particular.

IGF Binding Proteins (IGFBPs)

While developing and validating assays for IGFs in ovarian samples and conditioned media, we found that IGFBPs were abundant in these samples (10, 21); in some samples, they appeared to be in substantial excess of the IGFs themselves (12, 14). More recently, we and other laboratories have defined the nature and regulation of the ovarian IGFBPs to a considerably greater extent. Emerging from these studies is a picture of a family of abundant ovarian secretory proteins, including at least 4 discrete gene products that may exert major effects on the ovarian IGF system. In addition, they may have some physiological actions through other mechanisms.

The cDNAs for 3 IGFBPs have been cloned and sequenced, and a nomenclature suggested (IGFBP-1, IGFBP-2, and IGFBP-3) (22). In addition, a fourth, smaller, protein has been purified, and partial sequence data suggest that it is an additional gene product (23). By common usage, this IGFBP is called IGFBP-4, although a formal designation has not been agreed upon. In addition to serving as carrier proteins for the IGFs in the circulation, these proteins can influence local cellular function in either a positive or negative fashion (reviewed in 24). To date, positive effects of the IGFBPs have not been demonstrated in the ovary. However, a number of negative actions on gonadotropin-dependent differentiation as well as on GC replication have been reported (25). In the main, these effects were mimicked by a monoclonal antibody to IGF-I (25), indicating that sequestration of locally produced IGFs might be an important mode of action. However, some qualitative and quantitative differences between the effects of IGFBPs and antibodies led Biczak et al. to postulate that additional mechanisms might be involved (25).

Each of the aforementioned IGFBPs is expressed in the ovary (26–29). However, the dominant forms encountered depend on the physiological circumstances and the techniques employed. IGFBP-1 was the first ovarian IGFBP described (26), and its regulation has been examined in some detail with human ovarian cells (30). In the pig ovary, our studies have suggested that IGFBP-3 and IGFBP-2 are the predominant forms (Figs. 15.2 and 15.3). However, smaller forms corresponding to the molecular weights of IGFBP-1 and IGFBP-4 are present under some circumstances (28, 29). We have achieved presumptive identification of IGFBP-2 and IGFBP-3 by immuno-precipitation studies (28, 29) and by demonstrating mRNA for these forms in

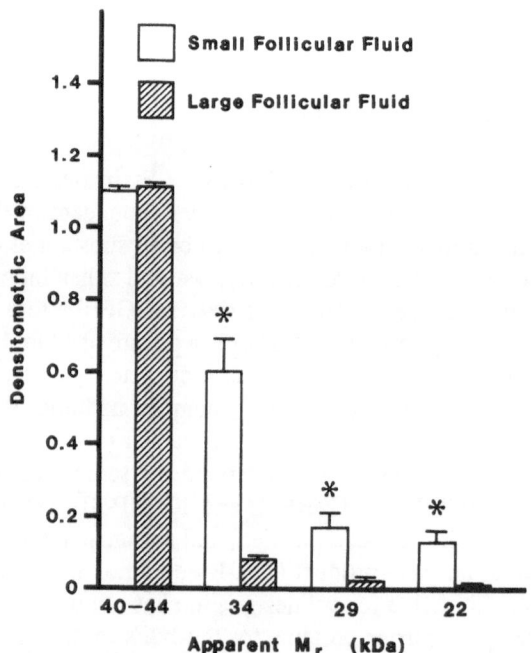

FIGURE 15.2. IGFBP complement of pFF. Four batches of "small" pFF (from 1- to 3-mm follicles) were compared with 4 batches of "large" pFF (from 8- to 10-mm follicles) on 10% polyacrylamide gels that were blotted and probed with ^{125}I-IGF-II (ligand blotting) as described in reference 29. The resulting autoradiographs were scanned densitometrically, and results were presented as mean ± SEM. The 40- to 44-kD bands were identified as IGFBP-3 and the 34-kD band as IGFBP-2 by immunoprecipitation. The 29- and 22-kD bands migrate with IGFBP-1 and IGFBP-4 respectively. (*Small follicles > large; $P < 0.01$.)

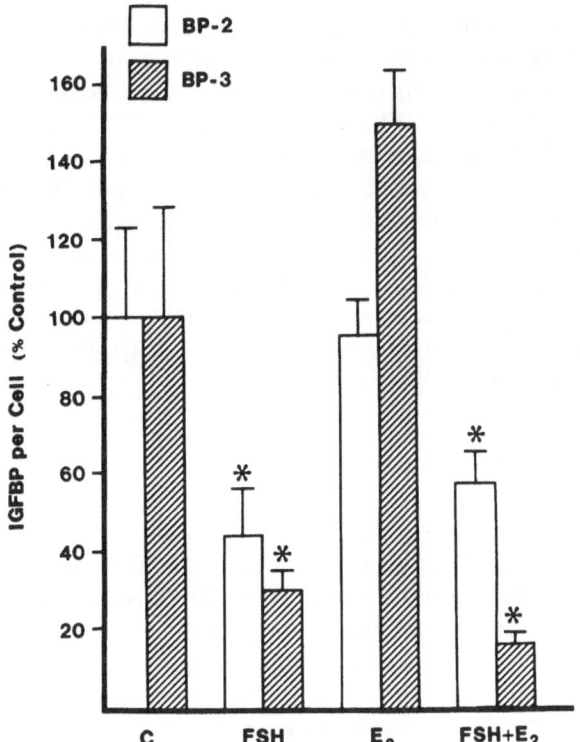

FIGURE 15.3. Effect of FSH and/or estradiol (E_2) on IGFBP production by porcine GC. Granulosa cells from 3- to 5-mm follicles were cultured for 3 days in serum-free medium in the presence or absence (C) of the hormones indicated. The media were analyzed as indicated in Figure 15.2 and the results from 3 to 5 experiments were pooled. (*$P < 0.05$ vs. C.)

the porcine ovary (Samaras et al., unpublished). However, comparable data have not as yet been generated for IGFBP-1 and IGFBP-4. Antibodies and probes to human IGFBP-1 do not recognize this form in pig ovary (28), and antibodies and probes to IGFBP-4 have not yet been employed.

A particular interest of our laboratory has been the physiological regulation of the IGFBPs in ovarian pFF and in ovarian cells in vitro. Using ligand blotting, we found that the complement of IGFBPs in pFF from small and large ovarian follicles was quantitatively and qualitatively different. Small follicles contained about twice the total IGFBP activity of large follicles in general and contained higher concentrations of the lower molecular weight forms in particular (29) (Fig. 15.2). In animals treated with PMSG to induce follicular development, a significant diminution in IGFBP activity was noted

(18). Thus, it appears that gonadotropin-induced follicular enlargement is associated with a diminution in IGFBP activity in vivo.

This phenomenon has also been examined in vitro. We found that cultured GC secreted each of the IGFBP forms detected in pFF. However, the amount and type of IGFBP secreted varied with the follicle of origin of the cultured cells, the duration of culture, and the hormones and growth factors to which the cells were exposed in vitro (28). Of particular relevance to the theme of this symposium was the inhibitory effect of FSH on the secretion of IGFBP-2 and IGFBP-3 (28) (Fig. 15.3). In addition, secretion of IGFBP-3 was inhibited by transforming growth factor β (TGFβ) while growth hormone, epidermal growth factor, insulin, and IGF-I increased IGFBP secretion (28, 31, unpublished observations).

Summary and Conclusions

The central theme developed in this paper has been the role of the IGF system as a local amplification mechanism for FSH action. While compelling proof of the operation of this mechanism in vivo remains elusive, numerous in vivo data and an even greater number of in vitro observations provide support for this hypothesis. The interactions of FSH with this system are numerous and interlocking: (1) FSH induction of IGF receptors, (2) synergistic interaction of FSH with IGFs on the cAMP-dependent steroidogenic cascade, (3) FSH induction of IGF secretion, and (4) FSH inhibition of the production of inhibitory IGFBPs. Collectively, these observations suggest a finely tuned, integrated, and mutually reinforcing autocrine/paracrine network in the ovarian follicle. The development of such a system could markedly enhance FSH action in follicles selected for further growth, development, and ovulation.

Acknowledgments. Work on this project was supported by grants from the NIH (HD-24536) and from the Competitive Grants Program, USDA. The authors gratefully acknowledge the provision of antibodies and probes by Drs. J. Van Wyk, M. Rechler, G. Veomette, T. Etherton, N. Ling, and F. Simmens. In addition, we appreciate the technical support of Mrs. Sheila Smith and Ms. Judith Pearn and the secretarial assistance of Mrs. Carrie Leitzell and Ms. Lisa Doster.

References

1. Adashi EY, Resnick CE, D'Ercole AA, Svoboda ME, Van Wyk JJ. Insulin-like growth factors as intraovarian regulators of granulosa cell growth and function. Endocr Rev 1985;6:400-20.
2. Hammond JM, Hsu C-J, Mondschein JS, Canning SF. Paracrine and autocrine

functions of growth factors in the ovarian follicle. J Anim Sci 1988;66(suppl 2): 21-31.

3. Hammond JM, Mondschein JS, Samaras SE, Canning SF. The ovarian insulin-like growth factors, a local amplification mechanism for steroidogenesis and hormone action. J Steroid Biochem (suppl) (in press).

4. Baranao JLS, Hammond JM. Comparative effects of insulin and insulin-like growth factors on DNA synthesis and differentiation of porcine granulosa cells. Biochem Biophys Res Commun 1984;124:484-90.

5. Adashi EY, Resnick CE, Rosenfeld RG. Insulin-like growth factor-I (IGF-I) and IGF-II hormonal action in cultured rat granulosa cells: mediation via type I but not type II receptors. Endocrinology 1990;126:216-33.

6. Adashi EY, Resnick CE, Svoboda ME, Van Wyk JJ. Follicle-stimulating hormone enhances somatomedin C binding to cultured rat granulosa cells. J Biol Chem 1986;261:3923-6.

7. Veldhuis JD, Rogers RF, Furlanetto RW, Azumi P, Juchter D, Garmey J. Synergistic actions of estradiol and the insulin-like growth factor somatomedin-C on swine ovarian (granulosa) cells. Endocrinology 1986;119:530-8.

8. Hammond JM, English HF. Regulation of deoxyribonucleic acid synthesis in cultured porcine granulosa cells by growth factors and hormones. Endocrinology 1987;120:1039-46.

9. Hammond JM, Mondschein JS, Canning SF. Insulin-like growth factors (IGFs) as autocrine/paracrine regulators in the porcine ovarian follicle. In: Hirshfield AN, ed. Growth factors and the ovary. New York: Plenum Press, 1989:107-20.

10. Hammond JM, Baranao JLS, Skaleris D, Knight AB, Romanus JA, Rechler MM. Production of insulin-like growth factors by ovarian granulosa cells. Endocrinology 1985;117:2553-5.

11. Hammond JM, Smith SA, Mondschein JS. FSH enhances insulin-like growth factor (IGF)-I and attenuates IGF binding protein (BP)-3 production in porcine granulosa cell (GC) from medium sized follicles [Abstract 31]. VIII Ovarian Workshop, Serono Symposia, USA. Maryville, TN, 1990.

12. Hammond JM, Hsu C-J, Klindt J, Tsang BK, Downey BR. Gonadotropins increase concentrations of immunoreactive insulin-like growth factor-I in porcine follicular fluid in vivo. Biol Reprod 1988;38:304-8.

13. Hsu C-J, Hammond JM. Gonadotropins and estradiol stimulate immunoreactive insulin-like growth factor-I production by porcine granulosa cells in vitro. Endocrinology 1987;120:198-207.

14. Hsu C-J, Hammond JM. Concomitant effects of growth hormone on secretion of insulin-like growth factor-I and progesterone by cultured porcine granulosa cells. Endocrinology 1987;121:1343-8.

15. Mondschein JS, Canning SF, Miller DQ, Hammond JM. Insulin-like growth factors (IGFs) as autocrine/paracrine regulators of granulosa cell differentiation and growth: studies with a neutralizing monoclonal antibody to IGF-I. Biol Reprod 1989;40:79-85.

16. Hammond JM, Yoshida K, Veldhuis JD, Rechler MM, Knight AB. Intrafollicular role of somatomedins: comparison with effects of insulin. In: Greenwald GS, Terranova P, eds. Factors regulating ovarian function. New York: Raven Press, 1983:197-201.

17. Mondschein JS, Hammond JM, Canning SF. Profiles of immunoreactive (i) insulin-like growth factors (IGFs) -I and -II in porcine follicular fluid (FF) and granulosa cell conditioned medium (GCCM) [Abstract 429]. Biol Reprod 1988; 38(suppl 1):191.

18. Samaras SE, Mondschein JS, Bryan K, Hagen D, Hammond JM. Growth hormone effects on ovarian function in gilts: changes in insulin-like growth factors and their binding proteins [Abstract 256]. Biol Reprod 1990;42(suppl 1):126.

19. Ramasharma K, Li CH. Human pituitary and placental hormones control insulin-like growth factor II secretion in human granulosa cells. Proc Natl Acad Sci 1987;84:2643-7.

20. Voutilainen R, Miller WL. Coordinate tropic hormone regulation of mRNAs for insulin-like growth factor II and the cholesterol side-chain-cleavage enzyme $P450_{ssc}$, in human steroidogenic tissues. Proc Natl Acad Sci 1987;84:1590-4.

21. Hammond JM, Veldhuis JD, Seale TW, Rechler MM. Intraovarian regulation of granulosa-cell replication. In: Channing CP, Segal SJ, eds. Intraovarian control mechanisms. New York: Plenum, 1983:341-56.

22. Ballard FJ, Baxter RC, Binoux M, et al. Report on the nomenclature of the IGF binding proteins. J Clin Endocrinol Metab 1990;70:817-8.

23. Mohan S, Bautista CM, Wergedal J, Baylink DJ. Isolation of an inhibitory insulin-like growth factor (IGF) binding protein from bone cell-conditioned medium: a potential local regulator of IGF action. Proc Natl Acad Sci USA 1989; 86:8338-42.

24. Baxter RC, Martin JL. Binding proteins for the insulin-like growth factors: structure, regulation and function. Prog Growth Factor Res 1989;1:49-68.

25. Bicsak TA, Motoyuki S, Malkowski M, Ling N. Insulin-like growth factor-binding protein (IGFBP) inhibition of granulosa cell function: effect on cyclic adenosine 3',5'-monophosphate, deoxyribonucleic acid synthesis, and comparison with the effect of an IGF-I antibody. Endocrinology 1990;126:2184-9.

26. Seppala M, Wahlstrom T, Koskimies AI, et al. Human preovulatory follicular fluid, luteinized cells of hyperstimulated preovulatory follicles, and corpus luteum contain placental protein 12. J Clin Endocrinol Metab 1984;58:505-10.

27. Shimasaki S, Shimonaka M, Ui M, Inouye S, Shibata F, Ling N. Structural characterization of a follicle-stimulating hormone action inhibitor in porcine ovarian follicular fluid. Its identification as the insulin-like growth factor-binding protein. J Biol Chem 1990;265:2198-2202.

28. Mondschein JS, Smith SA, Hammond JM. Production of insulin-like growth factor binding proteins (IGFBPs) by porcine granulosa cells: identification of IGFBP-2 and -3 and regulation by hormones and growth factors. Endocrinology 1990;127 (in press).

29. Mondschein JS, Etherton TD, Hammond JM. Characterization of insulin-like growth factor binding proteins of porcine ovarian follicular fluid. Biol Reprod 1991 (in press).

30. Jalkanen J, Suikkari A-M, Koistenen R, et al. Regulation of insulin-like growth factor binding protein-1 production in human granulosa-luteal cells. J Clin Endocrinol Metab 1989;69:1174-9.

31. Hammond JM, Mondschein JS, Samaras SE, Smith SA, Hagen DR. The ovarian insulin-like growth factor system. J Reprod Fertil 1991;43(suppl) (in press).

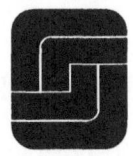

16

Regulation of the LH/CG Receptor by Gonadotropins

Deborah L. Segaloff, JoAnne S. Richards,
Mario Ascoli, and Haiyun Wang

The induction of the lutropin/choriogonadotropin receptor (LH/CG-R) by follicle-stimulating hormone (FSH) is one of the hallmarks of the differentiating granulosa cell (GC) (1–3). The mechanisms underlying the induction and regulation of the LH/CG-R, however, are for the most part not well understood. Utilizing cultured GC, many different laboratories have characterized the FSH-dependent induction of LH/CG-R as defined by hCG binding activity. From these experiments, it has been possible to make the following conclusions. (1) The induction of the LH/CG-R by FSH is mediated by the FSH-induced increase in intracellular cAMP (4–7). Thus, other agents that increase intracellular cAMP, such as cholera toxin, forskolin, or exogenously added cAMP derivatives, are capable of mimicking the induction of the LH/CG-R. (2) The dose-response curve for the induction of the LH/CG-R by FSH or agents that increase cAMP is bell shaped, such that at high concentrations of hormone or cAMP, the induction is submaximal (5, 8, 9). (3) The time course of this induction process is relatively slow, with increased hCG binding activity in cells cultured with FSH observed only 24 h after the incubation has been initiated. Maximal binding is typically observed at 72–96 h (5, 8–10). (4) The induction and the maintenance of the LH/CG-R in GC requires the continual presence of FSH. If FSH is removed at any time, the levels of LH/CG-R return to basal within 24 h (4). Thus, the induction process does not involve a "committed step," but is a continuous process. (5) The FSH-dependent increase in cell-surface LH/CG-R in GC is not due to the mobilization of an intracellular pool of preformed receptors to the cell surface (11). (6) The FSH-dependent increase in LH/CG-R can be prevented when protein synthesis is inhibited (11).

Taken altogether, these data had suggested that the induction of the LH/CG-R in GC was a result of de novo synthesis of the receptor protein. With the cloning of the LH/CG-R cDNA (12–14) it is now possible to begin to address this question directly.

LH/CG-R mRNA Expression in Differentiating Rat GC

In order to better understand the mechanisms underlying the FSH-dependent induction of the LH/CG-R, we analyzed the content of LH/CG-R mRNA during the differentiation of rat GC (15). In all the experiments described herein, a cDNA probe corresponding to nucleotides 1–622 of the rat luteal LH/CG-R cDNA was used (12). This partial cDNA encodes for the initial two-thirds of the extracellular domain of the receptor.

It is known that rat corpora lutea, preovulatory (PO) theca cells, and PO GC express LH/CG-R, as determined by hCG binding activity. When Northern blots are prepared from these tissues and probed with the afore-mentioned cDNA for the LH/CG-R, multiple mRNA transcripts are observed, the most prominent ones being 6.7, 4.3, 2.6, and 1.2 kb in length. The relative abundance of LH/CG-R mRNA appears greatest in the corpora lutea.

To examine whether the induction of the LH/CG-R in GC is associated with an increase in LH/CG-R mRNA, Northern blots were prepared using RNA from immature GC taken from small antral follicles and mature GC obtained from PO follicles. Indeed, there is a striking absence of all LH/CG-R mRNA in the immature GC. These data show that the induction of the LH/CG-R is associated with a coordinate increase in all LH/CG-R mRNA species, suggesting that there is an increase in the transcription of the LH/CG-R gene and/or an increase in the stability of the LH/CG-R mRNA during the differentiation of the GC.

In rat GC, it is well known that the induction of the LH/CG-R is dependent upon both FSH and estrogen (E). To examine the role that each of these hormones plays in the induction of LH/CG-R mRNA, hypo-physectomized rats were untreated or were injected with estradiol alone, with FSH alone, or with a combination of estradiol and FSH. GC were isolated, and LH/CG-R mRNA content was analyzed by Northern blots and quantitated by solution hybridization. In the absence of any hormone treatment, there was little or no LH/CG-R mRNA present. Interestingly, neither FSH alone nor estradiol alone had any effect on the levels of LH/CG-R mRNA. Only the synergistic actions of the two hormones together caused an increase in the steady state levels of LH/CG-R mRNA. The amount of LH/CG-R mRNA induced by E plus FSH was comparable to that observed in GC of PO follicles of intact rats.

A widely used in vitro system for studying the induction of the LH/CG-R in GC is to isolate GC from E-primed immature rats and culture them with FSH. The levels of LH/CG-R mRNA were thus examined in this experimental system. Cells from immature rats primed with estradiol were cultured with no additions, with FSH alone, or with FSH plus estradiol. Having been pretreated with estradiol, the cells incubated with FSH showed elevated levels of both LH/CG mRNA and hCG binding activity. The further addition of estradiol (in addition to FSH) to the cultures had no augmenting effect. The same experiment was also performed with cells isolated from immature rats that had not been primed with estradiol. When FSH alone was added to cultures of these cells, there was a modest increase in LH/CG-R mRNA content. This was augmented by the further addition of estradiol. We conclude that the ability of FSH to increase LH/CG-R mRNA levels in GC from the immature rat is most likely due to the prior exposure of the ovary in those rats to low levels of E.

As mentioned above, the appearance of hCG binding activity in FSH-treated cultures of GC is generally not apparent until approximately 24 h after the addition of FSH. To examine the time course of LH/CG-R mRNA induction, GC were isolated from estradiol-primed rats and cultured in the presence of FSH. At 12-, 24-, and 48-h time points, the RNA was isolated and analyzed by Northern blots. No apparent increase in LH/CG-R mRNA was observed until 24 h after FSH addition, in accordance with the appearance of hCG binding activity. The long time required before LH/CG-R mRNA is induced by FSH and estradiol suggests that these hormones may be inducing the synthesis of one or more proteins that in turn are required for increased LH/CG-R gene transcription and/or LH/CG-R mRNA stability.

It has previously been shown that the removal of FSH from cultures of GC results in the disappearance of LH/CG-R (4). To examine whether this decrease is associated with a loss of LH/CG-R mRNA, PO follicles were isolated from rat ovaries and used immediately for RNA extraction or were incubated in vitro for 6 h with no hormone additions and used for RNA extraction. By Northern analysis, it is apparent that in follicles incubated 6 h with no hormone additions, all LH/CG-R mRNA transcripts have decreased to barely detectable levels. These data suggest that the LH/CG-R mRNA in rat GC is indeed turning over rapidly.

Down-Regulation of the LH/CG-R

Once the LH/CG-R has been induced in GC, it can be down-regulated by high concentrations of hCG or LH (1, 16–19). We examined whether the LH/CG-induced loss of LH/CG-R in GC is associated with a loss of LH/CG-R mRNA by injecting rats with a high dose of hCG, isolating the GC from PO follicles 2, 4, and 6 h later, and quantitating the LH/CG-R mRNA content in them by solution hybridization. There is a rapid loss of LH/CG-R mRNA such that 2 and 6 h after hCG administration, the levels of LH/CG-R mRNA have decreased to approximately 70% and 20% of control values, respectively.

The LH/CG-induced down-regulation of the LH/CG-R mRNA in GC in vivo can be reproduced in vitro. Thus, when GC from E-primed rats are isolated and cultured with FSH (50 ng/mL) and estradiol (10 nM) for 48 h and then are challenged for 6 h (in the continued presence of FSH and estradiol) with either no additions, forskolin (10 µM), cycloheximide (10 µg/mL), LH (500 ng/mL), or LH plus cycloheximide, the LH/CG-R mRNA contents were determined to be 9.5, 1.3, 22.5, 2.3, and 18.9 pg/µg of total RNA, respectively. These data suggest that the down-regulation of the LH/CG-R by LH is mediated by cAMP, which in turn induces the synthesis of a protein(s) that suppresses LH/CG-R gene transcription and/or decreases LH/CG-R mRNA stability.

Another model system that can be used to examine the LH/CG-induced down-regulation of the LH/CG-R is the MA-10 cell line, a clone of murine Leydig tumor cells that constitutively express LH/CG-R (20, 21). In a separate study (22), we examined the mechanisms involved in the LH/CG-induced down-regulation of LH/CG-R in MA-10 cells.

When MA-10 cells are incubated with either hCG or oLH, as shown previously (23, 24), there is a rapid loss of LH/CG-R, such that within 3 h, receptors are decreased to about 10% of control levels. This down-regulation is not due to occupancy of the receptors by hormone, but is a true loss of numbers of receptors. In the same experiments, LH/CG-R mRNA content was quantitated by solution hybridization. After 3 h with hCG or oLH, there was no decrease in LH/CG-R mRNA. Note that at this time point, most of the cell-surface receptors have disappeared. Beginning at about 8 h after hormone addition, one observes a loss of LH/CG-R mRNA, such that by 16 h, the content of LH/CG-R mRNA is decreased to about 50% of control.

Since hCG and oLH stimulate cAMP accumulation and since 8-Br-cAMP is known to down-regulate the LH/CG-R in a similar murine Leydig tumor cell line (25), the MA-10 cells were incubated with 8-Br-cAMP for increasing lengths of time and then assayed for LH/CG-R mRNA content and hCG binding activity. The addition of 8-Br-cAMP to the MA-10 cells causes a loss of LH/CG-R mRNA such that the time course and extent of this decrease is comparable to that observed with the LH/CG-treated cells. Unlike the LH/CG-treated cells, however, the loss of hCG binding activity occurs after, not prior to, the loss of LH/CG-R mRNA.

The conclusion that the loss of LH/CG-R mRNA is mediated by cAMP is further supported by the observations that deglycosylated hCG does not decrease LH/CG-R mRNA and that neither hCG nor 8-Br-cAMP decrease LH/CG-R mRNA in a line of MA-10 cells that express a cAMP-resistant phenotype (26). The LH/CG-induced loss of LH/CG-R in MA-10 cells, however, is not due primarily to the cAMP-induced decrease in LH/CG-R mRNA. This conclusion is supported by the experiment described above, where the majority of receptor loss induced by LH/CG precedes LH/CG-R mRNA loss, as well as by the observations that (1) deglycosylated hCG down-regulates the LH/CG-R despite not having any effects on LH/CG-R mRNA levels, and (2) hCG, but not 8-Br-cAMP, down-regulates the LH/CG-R in the cAMP-resistant subclone of MA-10 cells where neither decreases LH/CG-R mRNA content.

Thus, in MA-10 cells there appear to be two distinct mechanisms involved in the LH/CG-induced down-regulation of the LH/CG-R. In the initial phase, the loss of receptors occurs in a cAMP-independent manner and is not associated with any changes in LH/CG-R mRNA. This phase is most probably due to the previously documented LH/CG-induced increase in the rate of degradation of the LH/CG-R (23) as a result of receptor-mediated internalization and degradation of the hormone-receptor complex (27–29). There is a second phase (beginning after about 4 h of hormone addition) in which there is a cAMP-dependent loss of LH/CG-R mRNA. In the MA-10 cells, the increased degradation of the receptor is quantitatively the prime cause of LH/CG-induced down-regulation of the receptor.

It seems reasonable to assume that the LH/CG-induced down-regulation in all LH/CG-R-bearing cells would be composed of these two mechanisms (i.e., a cAMP-independent increase in the rate of degradation of the receptor as a result of receptor-mediated endocytosis and degradation of the hormone-receptor complex and a cAMP-dependent decrease in the levels of LH/CG-R mRNA). However, the relative quantitative contributions of each may vary between cell types and/or species. For instance, as discussed above, the LH/CG-induced loss of LH/CG-R mRNA in rat ovarian GC occurs much more rapidly than in MA-10 cells. Thus, the cAMP-dependent loss of LH/CG-R mRNA may contribute far more to the down-regulation of the LH/CG-R in rat GC than in MA-10 cells.

In addition to providing information regarding the mechanisms involved in the LH/CG-induced down-regulation of the LH/CG-R, these data also provide information that now allows us to better understand the FSH-dependent induction of the LH/CG-R in GC. In particular, we now know that high concentrations of cAMP act to decrease levels of LH/CG-R mRNA, presumably by decreasing the rate of LH/CG-R gene transcription and/or by decreasing the stability of LH/CG-R mRNA. Thus, the observation that high concentrations of FSH (cAMP) induce submaximal levels of LH/CG-R in GC can now be explained by the finding that high concentrations of cAMP decrease LH/CG-R mRNA content.

Summary

In summary, the induction, maintenance, and regulation of the LH/CG-R in GC is a complex phenomenon in which FSH is a central player. The concentrations of FSH and the context within which it is presented to the GC are critical. Thus, in the rat ovary, the synergistic actions of estradiol and low concentrations of FSH (via cAMP) induce the receptor by increasing the levels of LH/CG-R mRNA. However, high concentrations of cAMP induce the synthesis of a protein(s) that acts to decrease the content of LH/CG-R mRNA. Whether these stimulatory and inhibitory actions are exerted at the level of gene transcription and/or mRNA stability and the precise mechanisms by which these actions occur are under investigation.

References

1. Richards JS, Ireland JJ, Rao MC, Bernath GA, Midgley AR, Jr. Ovarian follicular development in the rat: hormone receptor regulation by estradiol, follicle stimulating hormone and luteinizing hormone. Endocrinology 1976;99:1562-70.
2. Uilenbroek JTJ, Richards JS. Ovarian follicular development during the rat estrous cycle: gonadotropin receptors and follicular responsiveness. Biol Reprod 1979;20:1159-65.
3. Richards JS, Kersey KA. Changes in theca and granulosa cell function in antral follicles developing during pregnancy in the rat: gonadotropin receptors, cyclic AMP, and estradiol-17β. Biol Reprod 1989;21:1185-1201.
4. Segaloff DL, Limbird LE. Luteinizing hormone receptor appearance in cultured porcine granulosa cells requires continual presence of follicle-stimulating hormone. Proc Natl Acad Sci USA 1983;80:5631-5.
5. Knecht M, Catt KJ. Induction of luteinizing hormone receptors by adensoine 3',5'-monophosphate in cultured granulosa cells. Endocrinology 1982;111:1192-1200.
6. Nimrod A. The induction of ovarian LH-receptors by FSH is mediated by cyclic AMP. FEBS Lett 1981;131:31-3.
7. Erickson GF, Wang C, Casper R, Mattson G, Hofeditz C. Studies on the mechanism of LH receptor control by FSH. Mol Cell Endocrinol 1982;27:17-30.
8. Segaloff DL, May J, Schomberg DW, Limbird L. A model system for the biochemical study of luteinizing hormone/chorionic gonadotropin receptor synthesis. Acta Biochim Biophys Hung 1984;804:31-6.
9. Sanders MM, Midgley AR, Jr. Rat granulosa cells differentiation: an in vitro model. Endocrinology 1982;111:614-24.
10. Erickson GF, Wang C, Hsueh AJW. FSH induction of functional LH receptors in granulosa cells cultured in a chemically defined medium. Nature 1979;279:336-8.
11. Segaloff DL, Limbird LE. The cAMP-dependent induction of LH receptors in primary cultures of porcine granulosa cells is not due to the expression of an intracellular pool of LH receptors. Endocrinology 1983;113:825-7.
12. McFarland KC, Sprengel R, Phillips HS, et al. Lutropin-choriogonadotropin receptor: an unusual member of the G protein-coupled receptor family. Science 1989;245:494-9.
13. Segaloff DL, Sprengel R, Nikolics K, Ascoli M. The structure of the lutropin/choriogonadotropin receptor. Recent Prog Horm Res 1990;46:261-303.
14. Loosfelt H, Misrahi M, Atger M, et al. Cloning and sequencing of porcine LH-hCG receptor cDNA: variants lacking transmembrane domain. Science 1989; 245:525-8.
15. Segaloff DL, Wang H, Richards JS. Hormonal regulation of LH/CG receptor

mRNA in rat ovarian cells during follicular development and luteinization. Mol Endocrinol (in press).

16. Channing CP, Dammerman S. Characteristics of gonadotropin receptors of porcine granulosa cells during follicle maturation. Endocrinology 1973;114:1114-23.

17. Jonassen JA, Richards JS. Granulosa cell desensitization: effects of gonadotropins on antral and preantral follicles. Endocrinology 1981;106:1786-94.

18. Rao MC, Richards JS, Midgely AR, Jr, Reichert LE, Jr. Regulation of gonadotropin receptors by luteinizing hormone in granulosa cells. Endocrinology 1977; 101:512-23.

19. Schwall RH, Erickson GF. A new in vitro model system for the study of luteinizing hormone receptor down-regulation. J Biol Chem 1983;258:3442-5.

20. Ascoli M. Functions and regulation of cell surface receptors in cultured Leydig tumor cells. In: Conn PM, ed. The receptors. Boca Raton, FL: Academic Press, 1985:368-400.

21. Ascoli M. Characterization of several clonal lines of cultured Leydig tumor cells: gonadotropin receptors and steroidogenic responses. Endocrinology 1981;108: 88-95.

22. Wang H, Segaloff DL, Ascoli M. Two distinct pathways for the lutropin/ choriogonadotropin (LH/CG)-induced down-regulation of the LH/CG receptor: receptor-mediated endocytosis and a cAMP-dependent reduction in receptor mRNA. J Biol Chem (in press).

23. Lloyd CE, Ascoli M. On the mechanisms involved in the regulation of the cell surface receptors for human choriogonadotropin and mouse epidermal growth factor in cultured Leydig tumor cells. J Cell Biol 1983;96:521-6.

24. Freeman DA, Ascoli M. Desensitization to gonadotropins in cultured Leydig tumor cells involves loss of gonadotropin receptors and decreased capacity for steroidogenesis. Proc Natl Acad Sci USA 1981;78:6309-13.

25. Rebois RV, Fishman PH. Down-regulation of gonadotropin receptors in a murine Leydig tumor cell line. J Biol Chem 1984;259:3096-101.

26. Wang H, Ascoli M. Reduced gonadotropin responses in a novel clonal strain of Leydig tumor cells established by transfection of MA-10 cells with a mutant gene of the type I regulatory subunit of the cAMP-dependent protein kinase. Mol Cell Endocrinol 1990;4:80-90.

27. Ascoli M. Internalization and degradation of receptor-bound human choriogonadotropin in Leydig tumor cells. Fate of the hormone subunits. J Biol Chem 1982;257:13306-11.

28. Ascoli M. Lysosomal accumulation of the hormone-receptor complex during receptor-mediated endocytosis of human choriogonadotropin. J Cell Biol 1984; 99:1242-50.

29. Ascoli M, Segaloff DL. On the fates of receptor-bound human ovine luteinizing hormone and human choriogonadotropin in cultured Leydig tumor cells. Demonstration of similar rates of internalization. Endocrinology 1987;120:1161-72.

17

Recombinant FSH and Regulation of Ovulation

A. Brenda Galway, Philip S. LaPolt, Irving Boime,
and Aaron J.W. Hsueh

FSH Structure

The pituitary glycoprotein hormone FSH consists of two dissimilar, non-covalently linked polypeptide chains. The α-subunit is common to all three pituitary glycoprotein hormones (FSH, LH, and TSH) and the placental-derived chorionic gonadotropin (CG). The unique β-subunit confers each molecule with its biological specificity. Although all subunits of the gonadotropins are believed to be derived from a common ancestral gene, each subunit is encoded for by a separate gene. The gene structure of the α- and β-subunits is well conserved, with the FSHβ subunit gene structure identified in 3 exons separated by 2 introns. The FSHβ gene is unique among the glycoprotein hormones in possessing a 3'-untranslated region of approximately 1 kb. The importance of this long 3' tract is unknown, but is potentially involved in mRNA stability.

FSH molecules from all species contain carbohydrate units covalently linked to the polypeptide chain. Human FSH has 4 N-linked carbohydrate chains, at positions 52 and 78 on the α-subunit and at positions 7 and 24 of the β-subunit (1). Numerous studies suggest that these oligosaccharides are important in determining the metabolic half-life of FSH in the circulation and, therefore, govern the in vivo biological action of this hormone. In addition, chemical and enzymatic deglycosylation of gonadotropins yields molecules with potential antagonistic properties. Several studies have shown that the anterior pituitary contains a spectrum of FSH isoforms with different isoelectric properties, bioactivities, and circulating half-lives (2), presumably due to a microheterogeneity of the carbohydrate side chains.

TABLE 17.1. FSH-induced genes in GC.

1. Steroidogenic enzymes
   Cytochrome P450 cholesterol side-chain cleavage
   Cytochrome P450 aromatase
   3β-hydroxysteroid dehydrogenease (HSD) and 17β-HSD

2. Hormones and their receptors
   LH, FSH, and PRL receptors
   β₂-adrenergic receptor
   Inhibin (α, β_A, β_B) and follistatin (activin-binding protein)

3. Differentiation-related genes
   Tissue-type plasminogen activator (tPA)
   Prostaglandin synthase
   Gap junction proteins and microvillus proteins

4. Signal transduction genes
   Protein kinase A regulatory subunit II (RII)
   Phosphodiesterase

5. Others
   Renin

FSH Action in the Ovary

Pituitary FSH is essential for ovarian follicular development, whereas LH is primarily responsible for ovulation and transformation of follicles into the corpus luteum. During follicular growth up to the preovulatory (PO) stage, numerous genes are activated and inactivated in the developing oocyte and surrounding granulosa cells (GC). In the ovary, FSH receptors (FSH-R) are found exclusively on the GC where, upon binding, FSH induces a number of genes whose products are essential for normal GC differentiation (Table 17.1). In the rapidly proliferating GC, FSH induces the steroidogenic enzymes necessary to produce estrogen (E), which then acts as an amplifier of many gene products necessary for ongoing follicular development. Numerous steroid and polypeptide hormone receptors subsequently appear, thereby allowing the growing follicle(s) the means to selectively prepare for ovulation (3). Furthermore, growth factors produced locally can modulate this process through specific receptors. FSH also induces the gene for tissue-type plasminogen activator (tPA), a protease that leads to digestion of the follicular wall at the time of ovulation (4, 5). The precise role of FSH in the postovulatory period remains to be elucidated, although there exists potential for its involvement in maintenance of the corpus luteum as well as in follicular growth for the next cycle (6).

Recombinant Human FSH

Expression of FSH in Eukaryotic Cells

The semipurified human menopausal gonadotropins used to stimulate follicular maturation in anovulatory women contain a mixture of urinary FSH and LH (7), and the purified pituitary FSH preparations currently available also contain small residual quantities of LH (8). As the effects of the LH contamination upon successful follicular maturation remain unknown, it would be advantageous to have a source of homogeneous FSH that is not contaminated by LH and could be standardized with respect to mass and bioactivity. The enhanced expression of isolated genes in mammalian cell lines has provided the unique opportunity to obtain a large quantity of relatively homogeneous preparations of gonadotropins for physiological studies. Recently, Keene and Boime have isolated the human FSH gene and expressed the α- and β-genes in a Chinese hamster ovary (CHO) cell line (9). Cotransfection of the common α- and β-genes into eukaryotic cell lines results in the expression of FSH dimers. The secreted recombinant FSH (wild-type, FSH-WT) has been shown to be biologically active in vitro (9).

In ovarian GC, FSH specifically stimulates the aromatase enzyme, allowing production of estrogen (E) from the androgen precursor androstenedione. Therefore, to determine if the recombinant human FSH was biologically active, we examined its ability to stimulate steroidogenesis in an in vitro GC aromatase bioassay (10) and found it to be comparable to the pituitary FSH standard, LER-907. We further analyzed the charge heterogeneity of the recombinant human FSH molecule based on its migration in a chromatofocusing column (PBE-94) with a pH gradient from 7.0 to 3.5. When compared to a highly purified pituitary FSH preparation (NIADDK-hFSH-I-3), the recombinant FSH eluted with an almost identical pH range (5–3.6), suggesting the presence of a relatively uniform molecule (9). Using this transfected cell line, coupled with the chromatofocusing method and other traditional isolation protocols, one would expect the availability of large quantities of purified bioactive FSH for various future clinical and experimental studies.

Studies Using Glycosylation-Deficient FSH

The oligosaccharide side chains of FSH terminate in sialic acid, thus accounting for its relatively acidic elution range following chromatofocusing (9). The terminal sialic acids prolong the biological half-life and, thus, in vivo bioactivity of FSH (11). While glycosylation of FSH is not critical for receptor binding, it is important in the coupling of the receptor to adenyl cyclase and the subsequent stimulation of steroidogenesis (12). Although there is agreement on the importance of oligosaccharides in the biological action of FSH in vitro and in vivo, earlier studies have relied on either chemical or enzymatic methods to remove carbohydrate side chains of glycoproteins. These procedures may result in incomplete deglycosylation and/or conformational changes in the polypeptide backbone (13). Moreover, several studies have demonstrated that N-linked oligosaccharides on gonadotropins are heterogeneous and may have site-specific roles (14). Since the structure of the oligosaccharides may affect biological activity, the availability of homogeneous oligosaccharide structure is critical for structure-function studies of FSH.

Gene transfer techniques, together with mutant cell lines defective in one or more steps of the oligosaccharide-processing pathway, provide an alternative approach to the use of chemical or enzymatic methods for modifying the carbohydrate side chains of FSH. We transfected the FSH genes into two glycosylation-deficient cell lines and studied the in vitro and in vivo activity of these recombinant FSH variants with altered carbohydrate side chains. These include CHO cells deficient in cytidine monophosphate (CMP)-sialic acid transport into the Golgi (ST– or 1021 cells), resulting in sialic acid-deficient glycoproteins (15) or CHO cells deficient in the glycosylation enzyme N-acetylglucosamine transferase-I (NAGT– or 15 cells), resulting in the synthesis of glycoproteins with Asn-linked $(GlcNAc)_2$-$(mannose)_5$ oligosaccharides (16). The cells were transfected with the common α and FSHβ genes to allow their expression.

Determination of in vitro bioactivity, using the GC aromatase bioassay, indicates that both FSH variants (ST– and NAGT–) are as active as FSH secreted by the wild-type cells (FSH-WT) and purified pituitary FSH (17). Also, the normal (WT) and variant forms of FSH (ST– and NAGT–) are equipotent in a radioligand receptor assay using rat testis membranes (17). However, both the variant FSH molecules (ST– and NAGT–) are more basic than the FSH-WT, as determined using a chromatofocusing column (pI: FSH-WT, 3.6–5.0; NAGT– FSH > 7.0; and ST– FSH $\approx$ 6.0 and > 7.0). Unexpectedly, injection of immature E-treated rats with FSH-WT induced high aromatase activity in their GC, whereas treatment with either one of the FSH variants was ineffective. The lack of in vivo activity of the FSH variants was correlated with rapid clearance of these molecules in serum (17).

Although the FSH isoforms studied here are derived from CHO cell lines with transfected genes, alteration in the hormonal milieu bathing the anterior pituitary gland, as occurs during different physiological states, may also lead to changes in the endogenous isoforms of FSH secreted. Evidence also exists for sex- and age-related variations in sialic acid content of FSH, further emphasizing that alteration in the degree of hormone glycosylation may be of physiologic significance.

Furthermore, treatment of hypogonadal postmenopausal women with a

GnRH antagonist results in the formation of circulating antagonistic isoforms of FSH that display lower molecular weights and more basic isoelectric points (pH 8.9–9.2) than native FSH (18), reinforcing the notion that glycosylation is important in determining in vitro bioactivity. Our studies using mutant cell lines of CHO cells that produce partially glycosylated FSH (17) confirms that specific oligosaccharide structure is important in FSH function. Future use of these and other mutant CHO cells, combined with site-directed mutagenesis of the transfected FSH genes, should reveal the exact carbohydrate structures responsible for in vitro and in vivo bioactivities of FSH.

FSH Induction of Ovulation

Role of tPA in Ovulation

Numerous structural and biochemical changes occur around the time of the release of a mature oocyte from the PO follicle. The extracellular matrix components of the follicle wall are broken down, and this process is thought to be mediated through the action of proteolytic enzymes. One group of such proteases that are present in the ovary are plasminogen activators (PAs). These enzymes, normally considered to be important for vascular fibrinolysis, catalyze the limited cleavage of the inactive zymogen, plasminogen, to form the active enzyme, plasmin. Plasmin has trypsin-like activity, and may also be involved in the activation of another zymogen, procollagenase (19). The generation of active collagenase, in turn, leads to the breakdown of collagen fibers present in the connective tissues surrounding the ovulating follicle.

In vitro studies in rat GC have shown that tPA activity is stimulated by the gonadotropins (FSH and LH), GnRH and the growth factors, epidermal growth factor (EGF), and basic fibroblast growth factors (bFGF) (20–22). As the gonadotropins, GnRH and growth factors utilize different pathways of tPA gene activation (protein kinase A, protein kinase C, and tyrosine kinases, respectively), it is apparent that complex mechanisms are involved in the regulation of tPA genes during ovulation. In vivo studies have also shown that ovarian tPA activity rises in a manner temporally correlated with the ovulation process. Maximal tPA levels occur several hours before ovulation induced by LH, hCG, or GnRH, suggesting a more direct role of tPA in follicular rupture (23, 24). Furthermore, intrabursal injection of serine protease inhibitors or antibodies to tPA inhibits ovulation (25, 26), lending more support to an essential role of tPA in ovulation.

FSH in Ovulation

The pituitary glycoprotein hormones LH and FSH are independently secreted and as such, account for the different phases of the reproductive cycle. FSH secretion during the follicular phase is essential for follicle growth, thereby nourishing the developing oocyte in preparation for ovulation. LH, in turn, is responsible for maintaining progesterone production by the corpus luteum until the placenta is capable of independent function. Although a simultaneous surge of both LH and FSH precedes follicular rupture in most mammals (27, 28), it is the larger surge of LH that is believed to be essential for ovulation. Despite several studies using highly purified FSH preparations, suggesting that FSH has inherent ovulatory activity (29–31), the relative contribution of FSH to triggering ovulation has been unclear because of the unavailability of FSH preparations that are entirely free of LH contamination.

We utilized the LH-free recombinant FSH (FSH-WT) to assess the ovulation-inducing potential of FSH alone (5). When immature E-treated hypophysectomized rats were treated with PMSG to induce follicular maturation and injected 52 h later with either hCG or recombinant FSH, a dose-dependent increase in ovulation rate was stimulated by FSH (Fig. 17.1, left panel). Ovulation induced by either FSH or hCG was associated with a periovulated increase in the ovarian tPA activity and message levels of this enzyme, indicating that FSH shares similar mechanisms of follicle rupture with the other ovulatory hormones, such as LH/hCG and GnRH.

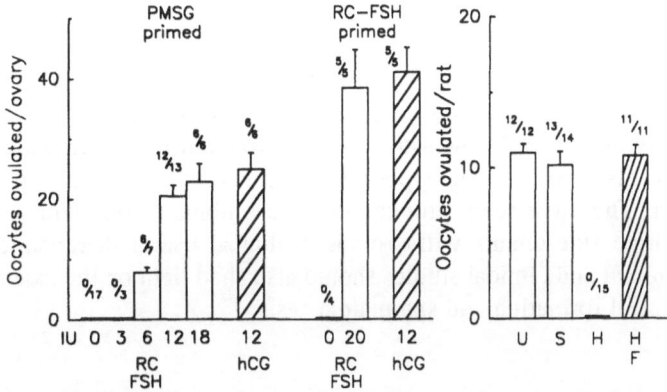

FIGURE 17.1. Ovulation induction in hypophysectomized rats by recombinant FSH. Estrogen-implanted hypophysectomized immature rats (*left panel*) either received a single injection of 15-IU PMSG subcutaneously (PMSG-primed) or were implanted with a minipump releasing RCFSH (4 IU/day; RCFSH-primed) to induce follicle growth. Fifty-two h later, they were injected with saline, hCG (12 IU), or RCFSH (3–20 IU). Ovulation was determined 24 h later. The fractions above each bar on the graph indicate the ratio of successful ovulating rats to total numbers studied in each group. Adult cyclic rats (*right panel*) were hypophysectomized on proestrous morning and injected IP with either saline alone (H) or 7.8-IU RCFSH (HF). Unoperated control rats (U) and sham-operated rats (S) were also studied. Rats were sacrificed the next morning, and ovulation was determined. Results are expressed as mean ± SEM.

Because PMSG has inherent LH-like activity in rats, we also implanted hypophysectomized rats with a minipump (sc) that released FSH (FSH-WT) to induce follicle growth. Fifty-two hours after insertion of the minipump, a single sc injection of a surge dose of FSH was administered, and ovulation was successfully induced (Fig. 17.1). To test if FSH can also induce ovulation in adult animals, rats were hypophysectomized on proestrous morning and treated with increasing doses of FSH (IP) (Fig. 17.1, right panel). Again, ovulation was successfully induced.

These studies indicate that LH-free recombinant FSH is capable of inducing ovulation in hypophysectomized immature and adult rats and is associated with increases in ovarian tPA gene expression (5). Thus, FSH may be involved in follicular rupture in addition to its role in follicle recruitment and maturation. The PO surges of both LH and FSH may represent a protective mechanism to ensure an optimal ovulatory stimulus. This finding may also serve to provide a basis for formulating new ovulation induction protocols.

Conclusion

The use of recombinant FSH molecules secreted by transfected eukaryotic cells allows detailed analysis of the immunoreactivity and receptor binding ability, as well as the in vitro and in vivo bioactivity, of normal and variant FSH. Structure-function analysis of FSH with different carbohydrate side-chain structures demonstrates the important role of terminal sugars in the in vivo processing of FSH. The availability of FSH molecules without contaminating LH also provides the opportunity to study the specific role of FSH in ovulation. The large-scale production of recombinant FSH with unaltered carbohydrate side chains will provide a clinical useful therapeutic agent. Future animal and clinical studies should also shed light on the exact role of FSH in luteal formation and spermatogenesis.

References

1. Shome B, Parlow AF. Human follicle-stimulating hormone: first proposal for the amino acid sequence of the hormone-specific, α-subunit (hFSH)..J Clin Endocrinol Metab 1974;39:203-5.
2. Chappel SC, Ulloa-Aquirre A, Coutifaris C. Biosynthesis and secretion of follicle-stimulating hormone. Endocr Rev 1983;4:179-211.
3. Hsueh AJW, Bicsak TA, Jia XC, et al. Granulosa cells as hormone targets: the role of biologically active follicle-stimulating hormone in reproduction. Recent Prog Horm Res 1989;45:209-77.
4. Ny T, Bjersing L, Hsueh AJW, Loskutoff DJ. Cultured granulosa cells produce two plasminogen activators and an antiactivator, each regulated differently by gonadotropin. Endocrinology 1985;116:1666-8.

5. Galway AB, LaPolt PS, Tsafriri A, Dargan CM, Boime I, Hsueh AJW. Recombinant FSH induced ovulation and tissue plasminogen activator expression in hypophysectomized rats. Endocrinology 1990.
6. Schwartz NB. The role of FSH and LH and their antibodies on follicular growth and on ovulation. Biol Reprod 1974;10:236-72.
7. Laufer N, DeCherney AJ, Haseltine FP, et al. The use of high dose human menopausal gonadotropins in in vitro fertilization programs. Fertil Steril 1983; 40:734-41.
8. Jones GS, Acosta AA, Garcia JE, Bernardus RE, Rosenwak Z. The effect of follicle stimulating hormone without additional luteinizing hormone on follicle stimulation and oocyte development in normal ovulatory women. Fertil Steril 1985;43:696-702.
9. Keene JL, Matzuk MM, Otani T, et al. Expression of biologically active human follitropin in Chinese hamster ovary cells. J Biol Chem 1989;264:4769-75.
10. Jia XC, Hsueh AJW. Granulosa cell aromatase bioassay (GAB) for follicle stimulating hormone: validation and application of the method. Endocrinology 1986;119:1578-87.
11. Morell AG, Gregoriadis G, Scheinberg IH. The role of sialic acid in determining the survival of glycoproteins in the circulation. J Biol Chem 1971;245:1461-7.
12. Sairam MR, Bhargave GN. A role of glycosylation of the α-subunit in transduction of biological signal in glycoprotein hormones. Science 1985;229:65.
13. Sairam MR. Protein glycosylation and receptor-ligand interactions. In: Conn PM, ed. The receptors. New York: Academic Press, 1985;2:307-40.
14. Matzuk MM, Spangler MM, Camel M, Suganuma N, Boime I. Mutagenesis and chimeric genes define determinants in the α-subunits of human chorionic gonadotropin and lutropin for secretion and assembly. Biol Reprod 1989.
15. Briles EB, Li E, Kornfeld S. Isolation of wheat germ agglutimin-resistant clones of Chinese hamster ovary cells deficient in membrane sialic acid and galactose. J Biol Chem 1977;252:1107-16.
16. Gottlieb C, Skinner SAM, Kornfeld S. Isolation of a clone of Chinese hamster ovary cells deficient in plant lectin-binding sites. Proc Natl Acad Sci USA 1974; 71:1078-82.
17. Galway AB, Hsueh AJW, Keene JL, Yamoto M, Fauser BCJM, Boime I. In vitro and in vivo bioactivity of recombinant human follicle-stimulating hormone and deglycosylated variants secreted by transfected eukaryotic cell lines. Endocrinology 1990;127:93-100.
18. Dahl KD, Bicsak TA, Hsueh AJH. Naturally occurring antihormones: secretion of FSH antagonists by women treated with a GnRH analog. Science 1988;239: 72-4.
19. Werb Z, Mainardi CL, Vater CA, Harris ED. Endogenous activation of latent collagenase by rheumatoid synovial cells. New Engl J Med 1977;296:1017-23.
20. Ny T, Bjersing L, Hsueh AJW. Loskutoff OJ. Cultured granulosa cells produce two plasminogen activators and an antiactivator, each regulated differently by gonadotropins. Endocrinology 1985;116:1666-8.
21. Galway AB, Oikawa M, Ny T, Hsueh AJW. Epidermal growth factor stimulates tissue plasminogen activator activity and messenger ribonucleic acid levels in cultured rat granulosa cells: mediation by pathways independent of protein kinases-A and -C. Endocrinology 1989;125:126-35.

22. LaPolt PS, Yamoto M, Veljkovic M, et al. Basic fibroblast growth factor induction of oocyte maturation and granulosa cell tissue plasminogen activator gene expression. Endocrinology 1990.

23. Liu YX, Cajander SB, Ny T, Kristensen D, Hsueh AJW. Gonadotropin regulation of tissue-type plasminogen activator activity in granulosa and theca-interstitial cells during the periovulatory period. Mol Cell Endocrinol 1987;54; 221-9.

24. Hsueh AJW, Liu YX, Cajander S, et al. Gonadotropin-releasing hormone induces ovulation in hypophysectomized rats: studies on ovarian tissue-type plasminogen activator activity, messenger ribonucleic acid content and cellular localization. Endocrinology 1988;122:1486-95.

25. Reich R, Miskin R, Tsafriri A. Follicular plasminogen activator: involvement in ovulation. Endocrinology 1985;116:516-21.

26. Tsafriri A, Bicsak TA, Cajander SB, Ny T, Hsueh AJW. Suppression of ovulation rate by antibodies to tissue-type plasminogen activator and α_2-antiplasmin. Endocrinology 1981;124:415-21.

27. McClintock JA, Schwartz NB. Changes in pituitary and plasma follicle stimulating hormone concentrations during the rat estrous cycle. Endocrinology 1968;83: 433-41.

28. Yamaji T, Peckham WD, Alkinson LE, Dierschke DJ, Knobil E. Radioimmunoassay of rhesus monkey follicle-stimulating hormone (Rh FSH). Endocrinology 1973;92:1652-9.

29. Nuti LC, McShan WH, Meyer RK. Effect of ovine FSH and LH on serum steroids and ovulation in hypophysectomized immature female rats. Endocrinology 1974;95:682-9.

30. Greenwald GS, Papkoff H. Induction of ovulation in the hypophysectomized proestrous hamster by purified FSH or LH (40992). Proc Soc Exp Biol Med 1980;165:391-3.

31. Armstrong DT, Opavsky MA. Superovulation of immature rats by continuous infusion of follicle-stimulating hormone. Biol Reprod 1988;39:511-8.

Part IV

Molecular Mechanisms of
FSH Action in the Testis

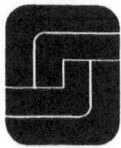

18

FSH Actions on Sertoli Cell Secretions in Stationary and Superfused Cultures

Anna Steinberger, Andrzej Janecki, and Andrzej Jakubowiak

It is commonly accepted that FSH is essential for the initiation of spermatogenesis in the sexually maturing rat (1) and that Sertoli cells (Sc) are the primary site of FSH action in the testis (2, 3). The testicular development during puberty is accompanied by dramatic changes in Sc responsiveness to FSH (4, 5), the formation of the blood-testis barrier (6), and the appearance of first postmeiotic germ cells in the seminiferous epithelium (7). There is increasing evidence suggesting that all of these events are interrelated, but the precise role of FSH during the maturational process is still not very clear. The functional and morphological complexity of the testis make it difficult to study FSH actions in vivo. Thus, much of our knowledge on the regulation of Sc functions has been derived from experiments conducted in vitro with Sc cultures. Two culture techniques have been employed recently for this purpose: the superfusion culture system (8) and the two-compartment culture system (9). The superfusion system is particularly well suited for defining the kinetics of Sc secretions and their responses to FSH, whereas the two-compartment system can be used to investigate the regulation of Sc vectorial secretions and the development of the blood-testis barrier. Our results concerning FSH actions on Sc secretions and the formation of Sc tight junctions are summarized below.

Kinetics of Sertoli Cell Secretions in Response to FSH in Superfused Cultures

It is commonly accepted that the initial phase of Sc response to FSH involves cAMP formation, activation of cAMP-dependent protein kinases, and phosphorylation of proteins (10–12). Although many aspects of more distal steps in the signaling cascade have been determined (13), it remains unclear by what mechanisms exposure to FSH leads to increased Sc secretions or how

Sc maintain increased secretion rates in the continuous presence of FSH (14). We have utilized superfused rat Sc cultures for determining the effects of FSH on the dynamics of inhibin and transferrin (Trf) secretion and correlated the data with changes in α-inhibin subunit mRNA levels and cAMP output. The methods used to isolate and culture Sc from 18-day-old rats have been described previously (9).

It is well established that the early effects of FSH on signal transduction (stimulation of adenyl cyclase, cAMP formation, and metabolism) occur within minutes, whereas increased secretion of proteins is significantly delayed (10, 15). In our culture system, significant increases in the secretion of Trf (Fig. 18.1A) and inhibin (Fig. 18.1B) were noted after 5–6 h of FSH exposure (14, 16). Maximal secretion rates were observed after 8–12 h of FSH exposure and, in the continuous presence of FSH, remained elevated for at least 24 h. The delay in accelerated secretion suggests that protein synthesis and/or transcription of RNA may be involved in this process. A significant increase in amino acids incorporation was, in fact, observed shortly after Sc

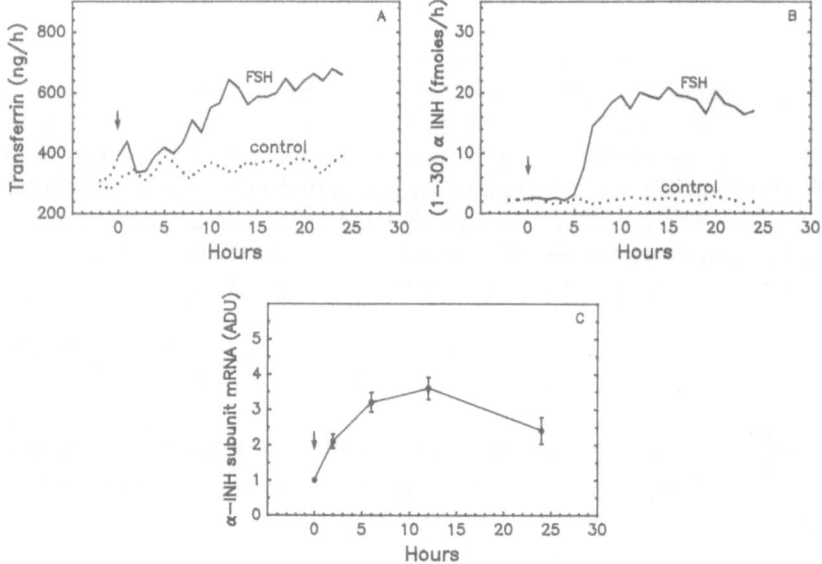

FIGURE 18.1. Effects of FSH on the time courses of immunoactive transferrin (A) and inhibin [(1–30) α-INH] secretion (B), and the expression of inhibin α-subunit mRNA (C) in Sc cultures. Three-day Sc cultures (1.5 × 10⁷ cells/chamber) were exposed to FSH (100 ng/mL), as indicated by the solid lines. The secretion dynamics were determined in superfused cultures, and representative patterns are shown in A and B. Levels of α-inhibin mRNA (C) were determined in static cultures by Northern blot analysis using an α-inhibin cDNA probe (kindly provided by Dr. A. Singh, Genentech, Inc., CA). The relative amounts are expressed in arbitrary densitometric units (ADU) and represent mean ± SD from 2 independent experiments. The arrows indicate the time of FSH addition.

exposure to FSH (10). Moreover, inhibition of protein synthesis by cyclo-heximide decreased the secretion of Sc products within 0.5–1 h (14).

Such close coupling of protein synthesis with secretory activity indicates that the regulation of Sc secretions by FSH may occur in the steps preceding protein synthesis. The results of our studies (Fig. 18.1C), as well as reports of other investigators, indicate that the addition of FSH to Sc cultures increases mRNA levels for α-inhibin (17) and Trf (18) within 1.5–2 h. This suggests that regulation of α-inhibin subunit and Trf mRNA by FSH may be at the transcriptional level, although other mechanisms cannot be excluded at this time (19). Also, it remains to be determined what processes take place between the increase of mRNA and protein secretion. In our experiments, there was a 3- to 4-h interval between the increase of mRNA for α-inhibin and increased inhibin secretion (Fig. 18.1B and 18.1C). Others reported even a longer time interval and suggested that posttranslational modifications of inhibin may need to occur before its release from the cell (17).

Interestingly, at the time when Sc responded to FSH with increased protein secretion, their cAMP responsiveness was drastically diminished (Fig. 18.2A). After several hours of continuous (Fig. 18.2A) or intermittent (Fig. 18.2B) exposure to FSH, the Sc became refractory to FSH stimulation in terms of cAMP release, whereas the secretion of inhibin and Trf remained

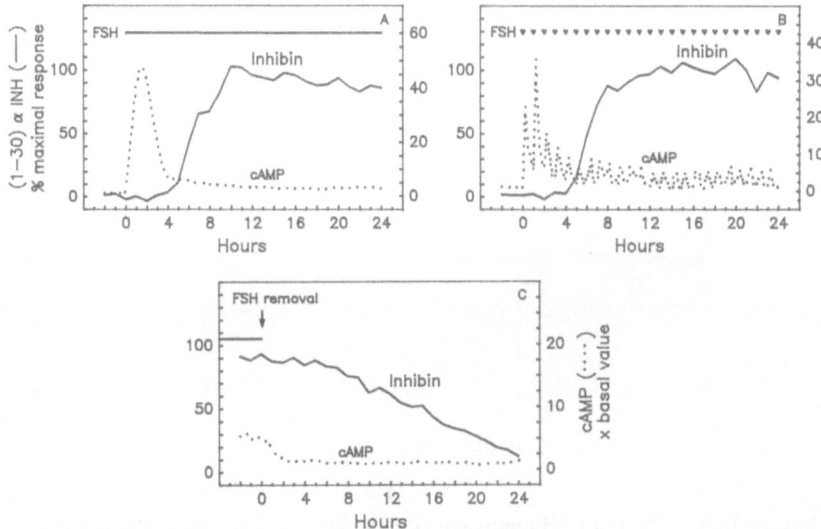

FIGURE 18.2. Comparison of inhibin (solid lines) and cAMP (dotted lines) time courses in superfused Sc cultures during exposure to FSH (100 ng/mL) and after FSH removal. A: Continuous exposure to FSH, as indicated by the horizontal bar. B: Pulsatile FSH stimulation (5 min/h). C: After 12-h exposure to FSH, the cultures were superfused with medium without FSH. The values for inhibin are expressed as percent of maximal response to FSH and the values for cAMP in multiples of baseline value.

elevated for at least 24 h in the continuous presence of FSH (Figs. 18.1A and 18.1B; Fig. 18.2A). It should be noted that although the cAMP levels declined sharply after the initial increase, they remained above the baseline values for at least 24 h (Figs. 18.2A and 18.2B). The declining pattern of cAMP responses in cultures exposed to FSH pulses (5 min/h) was surprising (Fig. 18.2B). FSH stimulation, either intermittently or continuously, resulted in similar total secretion of inhibin (Figs. 18.2A and 18.2B) and Trf (14).

When FSH was removed after several hours of exposure, the levels of Trf and inhibin slowly declined, reaching basal values after approximately 24–30 h (Figs. 18.3A and 18.3B). The decrease of inhibin secretion was preceded by a decline of α-inhibin subunit mRNA (Fig. 18.3C) and cAMP output (Fig. 18.2C). There are at least two mechanisms by which FSH could maintain increased Sc secretion. First, mediators of FSH action other than cAMP, or other pathways, may be involved in the regulation of Sc secretion, particularly at times when the cAMP pathway becomes desensitized. The recent observation that the FSH receptor itself may function as a calcium channel (20), together with earlier observations on the role of Ca^{++} in the regulation of the Sc function (10, 21), leaves such a possibility open. The

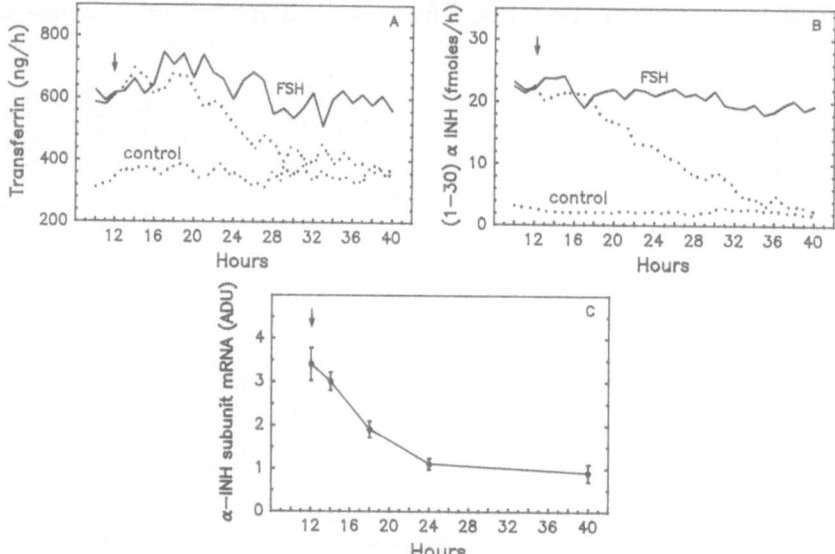

FIGURE 18.3. Effect of FSH removal on the secretion of Trf and inhibin in superfused cultures and on the expression of α-inhibin subunit mRNA in stationary Sc cultures (C). After 3 days of incubation in basal conditions, the Sc were exposed to FSH (100 ng/mL). After 12-h exposure, FSH was removed from some cultures, as indicated by the arrows. Representative secretory patterns for Trf and immunoactive inhibin are shown in A and B, respectively. The values for α-inhibin mRNA represent mean ± SD from 2 independent experiments.

roles of purine nucleotides and adenosine receptor system (22) and phosphoinositide pathway (23, 24) should also be considered.

Alternatively, the cAMP pathway may play a role not only in the initial steps of FSH stimulation, but also in maintaining the increased secretion. Observations that derivatives of cAMP can mimic FSH action in many respects (13, 25, 26) support this concept. Also, our observation that cAMP values remained above the baseline in desensitized Sc suggests that cAMP may mediate the long-term effects of FSH. It should be noted that full desensitization of the adenyl cyclase system was not achieved with high doses of FSH (27). Additional studies are clearly needed to clarify the mechanism(s) responsible for the continuous FSH stimulation of Sc secretions.

Based on results available to date, it appears that Sc secretory activity can be maintained for long time periods at a relatively high level despite the continuous presence of FSH. This may explain why relatively steady circulating levels of FSH in the male rat do not cause desensitization of Sc secretions. Moreover, hormones other than FSH and other factors could also directly or indirectly influence the dynamics of Sc responses to FSH.

Effects of FSH on the Vectorial Secretion of Trf, ABP, and Inhibin by Immature Rat Sc In Vitro

In the rat, changes in Sc responsiveness to FSH during puberty are accompanied by changes in the polarity of Sc secretions. Although experiments in vivo were limited to the secretion of androgen binding protein (ABP) and inhibin (11, 28), it is possible that other, if not all, Sc secretions follow a similar pattern. Since endocrine and paracrine interactions in the maturing testis are extremely complex, we investigated the regulation of vectorial Sc secretions utilizing the previously described two-compartment culture system (9, 29). In the initial experiments, we explored the effects of FSH on the total (basal plus apical) and polarized secretion of Trf, ABP, and inhibin by immature rat Sc. The culture system was carefully controlled, since such factors as binding of basolaterally secreted products by the supporting filter, differences in pH between the two compartments, and surface characteristics of the cell supports can significantly affect the results (30, 31). Most probably, methodological differences contributed to the discrepancies in results reported by various laboratories.

When Sc from 18-day-old rats were cultured in the two-compartment system, Trf, ABP, and inhibin were secreted bidirectionally (Fig. 18.4). The ratio of the amounts secreted into the basal and apical compartments (BC:AC ratio) for Trf and inhibin was 1.4–1.8. In case of ABP, however, the BC:AC ratio was 0.6–0.8. Virtually identical data were obtained when the Sc were cultured in the superfused two-compartment culture system (8). In the pres-

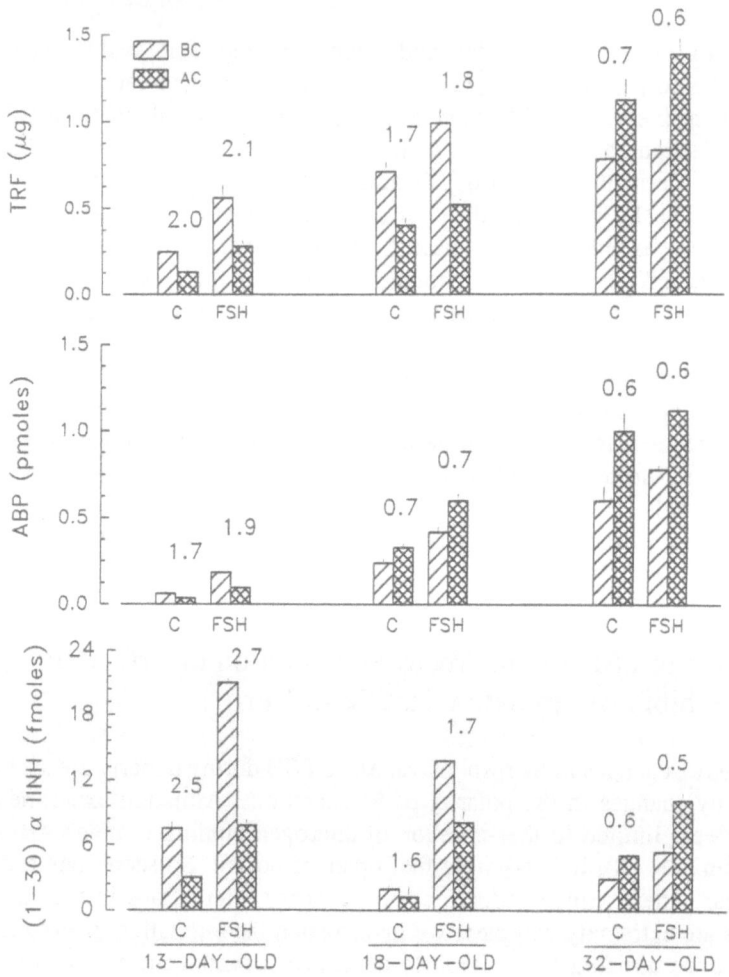

FIGURE 18.4. Vectorial secretion of Trf, ABP, and immunoactive inhibin [(1–30) α INH] by Sc from 13-, 18-, and 32-day-old rats. Cultures (1.2×10^6 cells/cm^2) were maintained on Matrigel-coated Nucleopore filters in the two-compartment culture system, either in control medium (C) or medium containing FSH (200 ng/mL). The media were replenished at 1- to 20-day intervals. The glycoproteins in the basal (BC) and apical (AC) compartments were measured separately in 7-day cultures. The bars represent the amounts secreted into each compartment by 10^6 cells during a 48-h period. Mean ± SD from triplicate cultures. Numbers above the bars indicate the BC:AC ratio.

ence of a maximally stimulating dose of FSH (200 ng/mL), the total secretion of all three glycoproteins was increased. The stimulation of Trf and ABP was relatively small 150%–180% of control), whereas the secretion of immunoactive inhibin increased 5- to 9-fold. Interestingly, FSH did not significantly affect the polarity of secretion of either protein.

However, stimulation with FSH resulted in a much smaller increase of inhibin bioactivity (B) relative to its immunoactivity (I), causing the B:I ratio to decline from 3.0 in control to 1.0 in FSH-stimulated cultures (31). The reason for this change, reported also by others, is unclear. Recently, Risbridger and colleagues (32) identified in Sc-conditioned medium a peptide (M_r 27,000) with high inhibin immunoactivity and low bioactivity that was stimulated by FSH. Secretion of this peptide may be responsible for the decreased B:I ratio of inhibin in our cultures.

The secretion of inhibin in vitro differed significantly from that of Trf and ABP at different animal ages. The results obtained with cultures of Sc from 13-, 18-, and 32-day-old rats are summarized in Figure 18.4. Basal and FSH-stimulated secretion of both Trf and ABP increased with animal age, as also reported by others (33, 34). In contrast, the secretion of inhibin appeared to decrease with age, the effect being more pronounced in FSH-stimulated cultures. The responsiveness to FSH decreased sharply with age for all three glycoproteins. These data suggest that FSH, while stimulating the total secretion of these glycoproteins, does not directly regulate the polarity of Sc secretions. It should be pointed out, however, that these results were obtained from relatively pure cultures of Sc, and the absence of specific germ cell population(s) may have influenced the effects of FSH on Sc secretions. The results of our experiments (described below) indicate that certain types of germ cells may play a role in the regulation of vectorial protein secretion in immature rat Sc.

Modulating Effects of Germ Cells on the Vectorial Secretion of ABP, Trf, and Inhibin

An increasing body of information (mostly indirect) suggests that the polarity of Sc secretions changes dramatically during sexual maturation. For example, inhibin is secreted predominantly basolaterally in immature animals, whereas in adults, virtually all inhibin is secreted apically into the adluminal compartment of the seminiferous tubule (28, 35, 36). A similar pattern was observed for ABP secretion (37, 38). Moreover, the polarity of both glycoproteins in vivo was shown to be altered in situations where the number of certain germ cell types was depleted (36, 39–41).

We explored the role of pachytene spermatocytes in the regulation of vectorial ABP secretion more directly utilizing Sc cocultures in the two-compartment system. The Sc were isolated from 14-day-old rats, and enriched populations of pachytene spermatocytes (>85% pure, obtained from 26-day-old rats) were plated directly on top of confluent Sc monolayers. The results are summarized in Figure 18.5. In the absence of FSH, the pachytene spermatocytes did not affect the polarity of ABP secretion. However, in the presence of FSH, the ABP BC:AC ratio was significantly decreased (from

1.8–2.1 in Sc-only groups to 0.8–0.5 in cocultures). The changes in ratio resulted from both increased apical and decreased basolateral secretion. The polarity of Trf secretion was not altered by the germ cells in either the presence or absence of FSH (not shown).

In other experiments, residual germ cells (predominantly spermatocytes and some early spermatids) initially present in Sc monolayers from 32-day-old animals were eliminated by hypotonic treatment (42). Removal of the germ cells significantly increased the BC:AC ratio of ABP, the effect being FSH independent (Fig. 18.5). The polarity of Trf secretion was not affected. These results suggest that certain germ cells may, indeed, modulate the polarity of ABP secretion, as was observed in vivo following germ cell depletion. Since the polarity changes in vivo were observed 30 days after hypophysectomy, the lack of FSH as a direct cause seems improbable.

Our results also indicate that FSH may be essential for the effects of pachytene spermatocytes on ABP secretion in 14-day-old rats but be less critical in older animals. The lack of FSH effect in Sc monolayers from

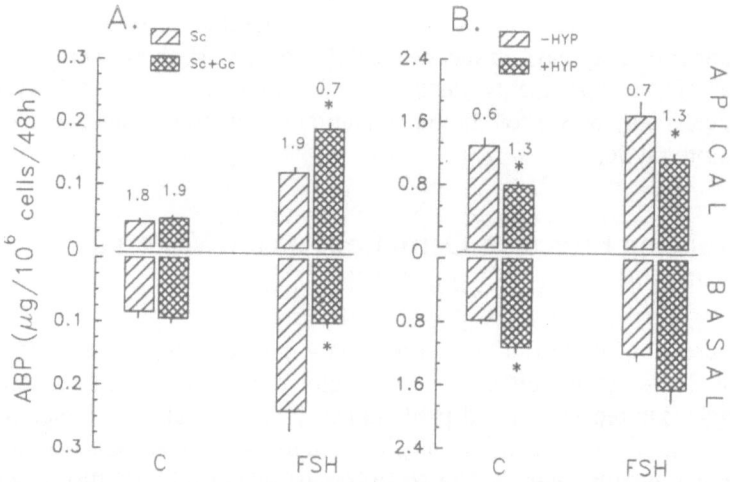

FIGURE 18.5. Effect of germ cells on the vectorial secretion of ABP. A: Sc from 14-day-old rats were cocultured for 48 h with enriched populations of pachytene spermatocytes (Sc + Gc). The pachytene spermatocytes (>85% pure) were plated (8×10^5 cells/cm^2) on top of 2-day-old confluent Sc monolayers. B: Three-day cultures of Sc from 32-day-old animals were subjected to hypotonic treatment (+HYP) to remove contaminating germ clels and were reincubated for an additional 48h. All cultures were maintained either in control medium (C) or medium containing FSH (200 ng/mL). The ABP that accumulated in the media during the last 48 h was measured separately in the basal and apical compartments. The values are mean ± SD from triplicate cultures. Numbers above the bars indicate the BC:AC ratio. Asterisks indicate a significant difference ($P < 0.01$) from corresponding untreated groups.

32-day-old rats supports this hypothesis but could be also due to the well-documented declining responsiveness of Sc to FSH with age (4, 10).

Cells other than pachytene spermatocytes can also modulate Sc secretions in vitro. Coculture of enriched populations (65%) of round spermatids with Sc from 14-day-old rats reversed the BC:AC ratio of immunoactive inhibin from 1.6–1.8 to 0.8–0.6. This effect was enhanced in the presence of FSh and was more pronounced than that observed in cocultures with pachytene spermatocytes. Moreover, coculture with round spermatids resulted in greater increases of mRNA for the α-subunit of inhibin, compared to cocultures with pachytene spermatocytes (data not shown). These results are in agreement with recent data from Sc cultures on plastic reported by Pineau et al. (43). Results of the coculture experiments suggest that the regulation of vectorial Sc secretions may involve populations of germ cells, FSH, and probably many other endocrine and paracrine factors.

Effect of FSH on the Electrical Resistance of Sc Monolayers

The blood-testis barrier in the rat is formed at 14–16 days of life and matures over the next 2–3 weeks (44, 45). The main structural component of the barrier is at the level of specialized tight (occluding) junctions formed between the basolateral aspects of neighboring Sc. Functionally, the selective transport of products from the circulation across the blood-testis barrier and the vectorial secretory activity of the Sc aid to maintain the unique intratubular milieu, which is believed to be essential for normal spermatogenesis. However, little is known about the mechanisms that regulate the formation, maturation, and maintenance of the tight junctions.

The two-compartment culture system provides an excellent model for the study of these events in vitro, although there was no sensitive, reliable method for monitoring the tight junction status in culture until recently. The [^{3}H]inulin permeability test commonly used for this purpose (29, 46, 47) had several disadvantages, the major one being low precision and radioactive contamination of the cultures, which prevented repeated measurements of the same monolayer. Recently, a new Millipore ERS device became available that we utilized to measure changes in electrical resistance of Sc monolayers. When appropriately standardized, this method provides a reliable estimation of the tight junction status under different culture conditions. It is generally accepted that electrical resistances 80–120 ohms/cm^2 or higher indicate the presence of tight junctions (48–50), whereas the resistance of cell monolayers known to lack tight junctions (e.g., peritubular myoid cells or testicular fibroblasts) is usually in the range of 25–40 ohms/cm^2.

The results of our study on the hormonal regulation of tight-junction formation in vitro by Sc from 18-day-old rats are summarized in Figure 18.6.

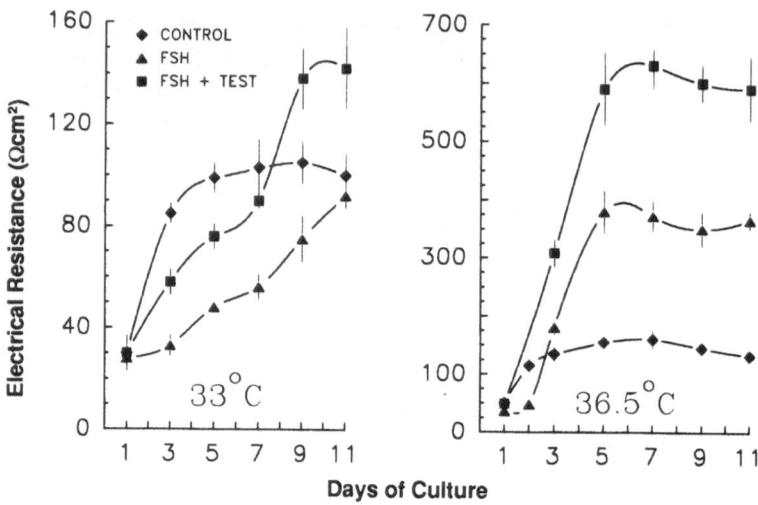

FIGURE 18.6. Effects of hormones and incubation temperature on the electrical resistance of Sc monolayers. Sc from 18-day-old rats were cultured on Matrigel-coated Nucleopore filters either in control medium (C), medium containing FSH (200/ng/ml) or medium containing FSH (200 ng/ml) plus testosterone (10^{-6}M). The cultures were incubated at 33°C or 36.5°C. Electrical resistance was measured at indicated times after equalizing the medium temperature at 26°C. The results are expressed as ohms per cm^2 (Ω/cm^2) and represent mean ± SD of triplicate cultures.

In monolayers maintained at 33°C in control medium, the resistance gradually increased, reaching a plateau at 90–130 ohms/cm^2. The initial increase of electrical resistance was accompanied by a decreasing permeability to [^{3}H]inulin; however, the inulin flux was maximally restricted at resistance values of 80–100 ohms/cm^2. A further increase in resistance, believed to reflect "maturation" of the tight junctions, was not accompanied by an additional decrease of [^{3}H]inulin flux (31). These results suggest that resistance values of 80–100 ohms/cm^2 correspond to the formation of one continuous strand of tight junctions that maximally restricts the passage of [^{3}H]inulin. Higher resistances, most probably, reflect an increasing number and "debranching" of strands that cannot be monitored by [^{3}H]inulin permeability (45, 49). In the presence of FSH (200 ng/mL), the resistance increased gradually but remained significantly below control values for up to 9 culture days. The simultaneous presence of testosterone (10^{-6}M) and FSH (200 ng/mL) minimized the inhibitory effect of FSH, and after 7 days of culture, the resistance values were increased above those of controls.

In searching for optimal conditions for the development and "maturation" of tight junctions in vitro, we found that incubation temperature was a critical factor. Although the electrical resistance in control cultures at 36.5°C only slightly exceeded that noted at 33°C (~100 ohms/cm^2), the addition of FSH increased the resistance up to 350–500 ohms/cm^2 after 3–4 culture days. Testosterone amplified the effect of FSH, raising the resistance into the range of 550–800 ohms/cm^2. It is important to emphasize that these changes did not result from differences in cell viability or cell number. The reason for the inhibitory effect of FSH at 33°C is not clear at the present time, but the effect of temperature may not be surprising since intratesticular temperature in the rat at 14–20 days of age is approximately 36°–36.5°C (51). It seems, therefore, that the combined effects of FSh and testosterone may be of importance in the initiation and "maturation" of the blood-testis barrier in the mammalian testis.

Acknowledgments. This work was supported by NIH grant HD-17802 (A.S.). The authors thank Mr. Clinton John-Phillip for excellent technical assistance and Ms. Mary Gilliland for typing the manuscript. The authors also gratefully acknowledge NIDDK and NHPP, University of Maryland School of Medicine, for providing the ovine FSH used in these studies.

References

1. Steinberger E. Hormonal control of mammalian spermatogenesis. Physiol Rev 1971;51:1-21.
2. Dorrington JH, Armstrong DT. Follicle-stimulating hormone stimulates estradiol-17β synthesis in cultured Sertoli cells. Proc Natl Acad Sci USA 1975;72: 2677-81.
3. Steinberger A, Heindel JJ, Lindsey JN, Elkington JSH, Sanborn BM, Steinberger E. Isolation and culture of FSH responsive Sertoli cells. Endocr Res 1975;2: 261-72.
4. Steinberger A, Walther J, Heindel JJ, Sanborn BM, Tsai YH, Steinberger E. Hormone interactions in the Sertoli cells. In Vitro 1979;15:23-31.
5. Sanborn BM, Wagle JR, Steinberger A, Greer-Emmert D. Maturation and hormonal influences on Sertoli cell function. Endocrinology 1986;118:1700-9.
6. Vitale R, Fawcett DW, Dym M. The normal development of the blood-testis barrier and the effects of clomiphene and estrogen treatment. Anat Rec 1973; 176:333-44.
7. Russell LD, Alger LE, Nequin LG. Hormonal control of pubertal spermatogenesis. Endocrinology 1987;120:1615-32.
8. Janecki A, Jakubowiak A, Steinberger A. Study of the dynamics of Sertoli cell secretion in a new superfusion, two-compartment culture system. In Vitro 1987; 23:492-500.
9. Janecki A, Steinberger A. Polarized Sertoli cell functions in a new two-compartment culture system. J Androl 1986;7:69-71.
10. Means AR, Dedman JR, Tash JS, Tindall DJ, van Sickle M, Welsh MJ. Regula-

tion of the testis Sertoli cell by follicle stimulating hormone. Annu Rev Physiol 1980;42:59-70.

11. Bardin CW, Cheng CY, Musto NA, Gunsalus GL. The Sertoli cell. In: Knobil E, Neill J, eds. The physiology of reproduction. New York: Raven Press, 1988: 933-73.

12. Reichert LE, Jr, Dattatreyamurty B. The follicle-stimulating hormone (FSH) receptor in testis: interaction with FSH, mechanism of signal transduction, and properties of the purified receptor. Biol Reprod 1989;40:13-26.

13. Oyen O, Eskild W, Jahnsen T, Hansson V. FSH, cAMP and gene regulation in testis. In: Serio M, ed. Perspectives in andrology. New York: Serono Symposia Publications from Raven Press, 1989:259-69.

14. Jakubowiak A, Janecki A, Steinberger A. Transferrin secretion in response to different modes of FSH stimulation and cycloheximide in superfused Sertoli cell cultures. J Androl 1988;9:390-6.

15. Sanborn BM, Caston LA, Buzek SW, Ussuf KK. Hormonal regulation of Sertoli cell function. In: Mahesh VB, Dhindsa DS, Anderson E, Kalra SP, eds. Regulation of ovarian and testicular function. 1987:561-88.

16. Jakubowiak A, Janecki A, Steinberger A. Kinetics of inhibin secretion in static and superfused Sertoli cell cultures in response to follicle-stimulating hormone. Biol Reprod 1990.

17. Toebosch AMW, Robertson DM, Klaij IA, de Jong FH, Grootegoed JA. Effects of FSH and testosterone on highly purified rat Sertoli cells: inhibin α-subunit mRNA expression and inhibin secretion are enhanced by FSH but not by testosterone. J Endocrinol 1989;122:757-62.

18. Huggenvik JI, Idzerda RL, Haywood L, Lee DC, McKnight GS, Griswold MD. Transferrin messenger ribonucleic acid: molecular cloning and hormonal regulation in rat Sertoli cells. Endocrinology 1987;120:332-40.

19. Klaij IA, Toebosch AMW, Themmen APN, Shimasaki S, de Jong FH, Grootegoed JA. Regulation of inhibin α- β_B-subunit mRNA levels in rat Sertoli cells. Mol Cell Endocrinol 1990;68:45-52.

20. Grasso P, Reichert LE, Jr. Follicle-stimulating hormone receptor mediated uptake of $^{45}Ca^{2+}$ by cultured Sertoli cells does not require activation of cholera toxin- or pertussis toxin-sensitive guanine nucleotide binding proteins or adenylate cyclase. Endocrinology 1990;127:949-56.

21. Grasso P, Reichert LE, Jr. Follicle-stimulating hormone receptor-mediated uptake of $^{45}Ca^{2+}$ by proteoliposomes and cultured rat Sertoli cells: evidence for involvement of voltage-activated and voltage-independent calcium channels. Endocrinology 1990;125:3029-36.

22. Conti M, Boitani C, Demanno D, Migliaccio S, Monaco L, Szymeczek C. Characterization and function of adenosine receptors in the testis. Ann NY Acad Sci 1989;564:39-47.

23. Quirk SM, Reichert LE, Jr. Regulation of the phosphoinositide pathway in cultured Sertoli cells from immature rats: effects of follicle-stimulating hormone and fluoride. Endocrinology 1988;123:230-7.

24. Monaco L, Adamo S, Conti M. Follicle-stimulating hormone modulation of phosphoinositide turnover in the immature rat Sertoli cell in culture. Endocrinology 1988;123:2032-9.

25. de Jong FH, Grootenhuis AJ, Klaij IA, et al. Regulation of inhibin production in rat Sertoli cells. In: Serio M, ed. Perspectives in andrology. New York: Serono Symposia Publications from Raven Press, 1989:235-42.
26. Skinner MK, Schlitz SM, Anthony CT. Regulation of Sertoli cell differentiated function: testicular transferrin and androgen-binding protein expression. Endocrinology 1989;124:3015-24.
27. Le Gac F, Attramadal H, Jahnsen T, Hansson V. Studies on the mechanism of follicle-stimulating hormone-induced desensitization of Sertoli cell adenyl cyclase in vitro. Biol Reprod 1985;32:916-24.
28. Maddocks S, Sharpe RM. The effects of sexual maturation and altered steroid synthesis on the production and route of secretion of inhibin-alpha from the rat testis. Endocrinology 1990;126:1541-50.
29. Janecki A, Steinberger A. Bipolar secretion of androgen-binding protein and transferrin by Sertoli cells cultured in a two-compartment culture chamber. Endocrinology 1987;120:291-8.
30. Janecki A, Steinberger A. Experimental pitfalls in evaluating vectorial protein secretion in vitro: Sertoli cell secretion of androgen binding protein and transferrin in two-compartment culture chamgers. In Vitro 1988;24:518-24.
31. Janecki A, Jakubowiak A, Steinberger A. Vectorial secretion of inhibin by immature rat Sertoli cells in vitro: reexamination of the previous results. Endocrinology 1990;127.
32. Risbridger GP, Hancock A, Robertson DM, Hodgson Y, de Kretser DM. Follitropin (FSH) stimulation of inhibin biological and immunological activities by seminiferous tubules and Sertoli cell cultures from immature rats. Mol Cell Endocrinol 1989;67:1-9.
33. Perez-Infante V, Bardin CW, Gunsalus GL, Musto NA, Rich KA, Mather JP. Differential regulation of testicular transferrin and androgen-binding protein secretion in primary cultures of rat Sertoli cells. Endocrinology 1986;118:383-92.
34. Rich KA, Bardin CW, Gunsalus GL, Mather JP. Age-dependent pattern of androgen-binding protein secretion from rat Sertoli cells in primary culture. Endocrinology 1983;113:2284-93.
35. Maddocks S, Sharpe RM. The route of secretion of inhibin from the rat testis. J Endocrinol 1989;120:R5-8.
36. Maddocks S, Sharpe RM. Assessment of contribution of Leydig cells to the secretion of inhibin by the rat testis. Mol Cell Endocrinol 1989;67:113-8.
37. Gunsalus GL, Musto NA, Bardin CW. Bidirectional release of Sertoli cell product, androgen binding protein, into the blood and seminiferous tubule. In: Steinberger A, Steinberger E, eds. Testicular development, structure and function. New York: Raven Press, 1980:291-7.
38. Mather JP, Gunsalus GL, Musto NA, et al. The hormonal and cellular control of Sertoli cell secretion. J Steroid Biochem 1983;19:41-51.
39. Musto NA, Bardin CW. Decreased levels of androgen binding protein in reproductive tract of the restricted (Hre) rat. Steroids 1976;28:1-11.
40. Morris ID, Bardin CW, Musto NA, Thau RB, Gunsalus GL. Evidence suggesting that germ cells influence the bidirectional secretion of androgen binding protein by the seminiferous epithelium demonstrated by selective impairment of spermatogenesis with busulphan. Int J Androl 1987;10:691-700.

41. Sharpe RM, Bartlett JM. Changes in the secretion of ABP into testicular interstitial fluid with age and in situations of impaired spermatogenesis. Int J Androl 1987;10:701-10.

42. Galdieri M, Ziparo E, Palombi F, Russo MA, Stefanini M. Pure Sertoli cell cultures: a new model for the study of somatic-germ cell interactions. J Androl 1981;2:249-54.

43. Pineau C, Sharpe RM, Saudners PTK, Gerrard N, Jegou B. Regulation of Sertoli cell inhibin production and of inhibin alpha-subunit mRNA levels by specific germ cell types. Mol Cell Endocrinol 1990;72:13-22.

44. Setchell BP, Pollanen P, Zupp JL. Development of the blood-testis barrier and changes in vascular permeability at puberty in rats. Int J Androl 1988;11:225-33.

45. Russell LD, Peterson RN. Sertoli cell junctions: morphological and functional correlates. Int Rev Cytol 1985;94:177-211.

46. Ailenberg M, Tung PS, Pelletier M, Fritz IB. Modulation of Sertoli cell functions in the two-chamber assembly by peritubular cells and extracellular matrix. Endocrinology 1988;122:2604-12.

47. Djakiew D, Hadley MA, Byers SW, Dym MK. Transferrin-mediated transcellular transport of 59Fe across confluent epithelial sheets of Sertoli cells grown in bicameral cell culture chambers. J Androl 1986;7:355-66.

48. Gumbiner B. Structure, biochemistry, and assembly of epithelial tight junctions. Am J Physiol 1987;253:C747-58.

49. Madara JL, Dharmsathaphorn K. Occluding junction structure-function relationships in a cultured epithelial monolayer. J Cell Biol 1985;101:2124-33.

50. Cereijido M, Meza I, Martinez-Palomo A. Occluding junctions in cultured epithelial monolayers. Am J Physiol 1981;240:C96-102.

51. Bergh A. Early morphological changes in the abdominal testes in immature unilaterally cryptorchid rats. Int J Androl 1983;6:73-90.

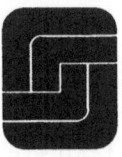

19

Cell-Cell Interactions that Influence FSH Regulation of Testis Function

JOHN N. NORTON, CATHERINE TANANIS ANTHONY,
AND MICHAEL K. SKINNER

Follicle stimulating hormone (FSH) is a gonadotropin secreted from the pituitary that influences the function and differentiation of the testicular Sertoli cell (Sc). This influence of FSH on Sc is mediated through activation of adenylate cyclase, followed by elevation of cAMP levels, stimulation of cAMP-dependent protein kinase, and regulation of gene expression (1–5). FSH promotes and regulates Sc function and differentiation throughout pubertal development; however, the role of FSH in the adult animal is unclear and remains to be fully elucidated.

Under endocrine, paracrine, and/or autocrine regulation, several testicular somatic cells influence testis function and the maintenance of spermatogenesis. Although FSH is an endocrine agent, FSH is speculated to promote paracrine interactions in the testis. For example, spent media from FSH-stimulated Sc has been shown to stimulate testosterone secretion from Leydig cells (6). In addition, local cell-cell interactions may also influence the actions of FSH on Sc. The focus of this chapter is a review of testicular cell-cell interactions that influence FSH actions, with emphasis on peritubular cell-Sc communication and the paracrine factor PModS.

Cell-Cell Interactions and FSH Action

Leydig Cell-Sc Interactions

Leydig cells are responsible for androgen production (7) that subsequently acts on the seminiferous tubule and maintains the process of spermatogenesis (8). Sc contain and express the androgen receptor gene (9); however, in vitro studies have demonstrated that androgens alone have less of an effect on Sc function than FSH (10). Androgens have generally been shown to have little influence on the actions of FSH on Sc. The role androgens have in the regulation of Sc functions requires further investigation. A nonsteroidal Leydig cell product that may influence Sc function is the proopiomelanocortin (POMC)-derived peptides. Adrenocorticotropin (ACTH) and α-melanocyte stimulating hormone (α-MSH) elevate cAMP levels in Sc (11, 12), but functional effects are small. Leydig cells also produce β-endorphin (β-END), which may interact with receptors on Sc to decrease cAMP levels in FSH-stimulated Sc (13). The POMC peptides, however, require high concentrations to elicit responses in Sc cultures, and the effects are less dramatic than those seen with FSH. Further investigation of regulatory agents, such as the POMC-derived β-END is needed to elucidate the importance of Leydig cell products and their potential influence on the regulation of FSH actions on Sc.

Germinal Cell-Sc Interactions

Several important interactions exist between germinal cells and Sc. Co-culture of these cells has been shown to influence several functional parameters of Sc, such as increased androgen binding protein (ABP) production and inhibition of estradiol production (14, 15). Similar effects on Sc functions have been observed with germinal cell-conditioned medium (16). Secretory products of germinal cells may be important for regulation of FSH action on Sc. For example, nerve growth factor (NGF) has been demonstrated to be produced by germinal cells (17), and Sc express the NGF receptor (NGF-R) gene under androgen influence (18). Further investigation of germinal cell-Sc interactions requires the identification and characterization of germinal cell regulatory agents, such as NGF, that may influence FSH actions on Sc.

Peritubular Cell-Sc Interactions

Growth factors are postulated to mediate numerous regulatory interactions between peritubular cells and Sc. For example, both cell types produce TGFα and TGFβ (19, 20). Receptors for TGFα are speculated to be present on Sc (21), and lactate production by Sc may be influenced by TGFβ (22); thus, growth factors such as TGFα and TGFβ may influence FSH regulation of Sc functions. An additional interaction between these cell types is mediated through a nonmitogenic paracrine factor, PModS. This protein is produced by peritubular cells under androgen stimulation (23) and has been shown to influence Sc function in vitro to a greater extent than any individual regulatory agent previously examined, including FSH (24, 25). PModS has been purified into two potentially related forms with $M_r \approx 56,000$ and $M_r \approx 59,000$ (24), and both forms of PModS have equivalent biological activities in vitro (24, 25).

Interactions Between PModS and FSH

The effects of FSH on Sc are dependent upon the stage of pubertal development. Utilizing transferrin (Trf) secretion as a marker of Sc function, the effects of PModS on Sc function and differentiation were investigated at various stages of pubertal development. PModS alone was found to increase Trf secretion from Sc isolated and cultured from 10-day-old rats (prepubertal). Simultaneous treatment with FSH greatly enhanced the response to PModS, suggesting a potential synergism between PModS and FSH in prepubertal-age animals. In 20-day-old rats (pubertal), FSH treatment of cultured Sc resulted in approximately a 2-fold elevation of Trf secretion above control cells, while treatment with PModS resulted in an approximately 4-fold elevation of Trf secretion (25). In contrast to prepubertal Sc, no synergism on Trf secretion was demonstrated in 20-day-old Sc with the combined treatment of FSH and PModS. FSH treatment of 35-day-old Sc (late puberty) demonstrated no influence on Trf secretion. In contrast, PModS treatment of 35-day-old Sc resulted in a significant elevation of Trf secretion in long-term cultures. Further investigations are needed to examine the importance of PModS in the adult testis, as well as potential interactions between PModS and FSH.

The physiological effects of FSH are mediated by elevation of cAMP levels in Sc, and agents that elevate cAMP levels or cAMP analogs have been shown to mimic FSH actions. Following activation of many functional processes in Sc, FSH induces a refractory response that leads to a reduction in the number of FSH receptors (FSH-R) (26) and decreased activity of adenylate cyclase (27). In addition, gene expression for a high-affinity cAMP phosphodiesterase is induced by FSH (28). A cAMP inhibitory pathway that is activated by such agents as adenosine, acetylcholine, and β-END is also present in Sc (13, 29). Although no regulatory agent has been shown to regulate other second-messenger systems in Sc, potential interactions between second-messenger systems exist. For example, it has been shown that phosphatidylinositol hydrolysis in Sc leads to a reduction of FSH-induced cAMP levels (30).

The mechanism of action for PModS is unknown, but PModS treatment of cultured Sc leads to an increase in cellular cGMP levels (25) with no obvious change in cellular cAMP levels, phospholipid turnover, or calcium fluxes. Treatment of Sc with agents that activate guanylate cyclase or cGMP analogs, however, do not mimic the effects seen with PModS. Sc treated with a combination of FSH and a crude PModS preparation resulted in no change in PModS-stimulated cGMP levels, but the presence of crude PModS partially inhibited the FSH-induced cAMP response. Further investigation of the mechanism of action for PModS is needed to elucidate potential interactions between PModS and FSH on a pharmacological level.

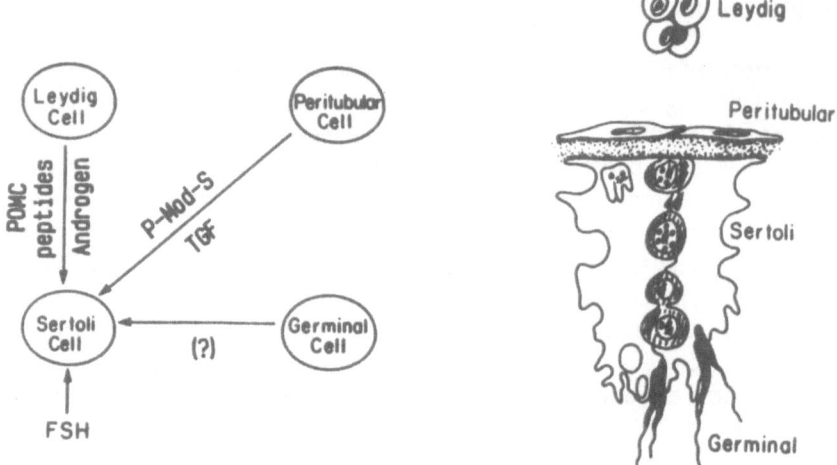

FIGURE 19.1. Current postulated cell-cell interactions of the testis that regulate FSH actions.

Summary

Interactions between the different cell types of the testis are important for normal reproductive function in the male and are speculated to be mediated by regulatory agents, such as PModS. Future identification of additional paracrine/autocrine agents will provide a better understanding of the testis cell biology. Of interest will be whether FSH stimulates the secretion of Sc products that act as paracrine agents. The paracrine factor PModS has been shown to have dramatic effects on Sc function and differentiation in culture. The speculation is made that PModS may be a differentiation factor for Sc similar to FSH. Although both FSH and PModS have been demonstrated to be important for control and maintenance of Sc function and differentiation in vitro, there is a need to examine the proposed cell-cell interactions in vivo to assess the physiological relevance of PModS and postulated interactions with FSH. The concept that FSH and androgen are the primary regulators of testis function needs to be reevaluated with a consideration of the influence of local cell-cell interactions. Data imply that these local interactions may influence the ability of FSH to regulate testis function (Figure 19.1).

References

1. Murad F, Strauch BS, Vaughn M. The effect of gonadotrophins on testicular adenylate cyclase. Biochim Biophys Acta 1969;177:591-8.

2. Kuehl F, Patanelli DJ, Humes JL, Tarnoff J. Testicular adenylate cyclase: stimulation by the pituitary gonadotrophins. Biol Reprod 1970;2:153-63.

3. Means AR, Hall PF. Effect of FSH on protein biosynthesis in testes of the immature rat. Endocrinology 1967;81:1151-60.

4. Means AR, MacDougall E, Soderling T, Corbin JD. Testicular adenosine 3',5'-monophosphate-dependent protein kinase. J Biol Chem 1974;249:1231-8.

5. Means AR. Concerning the mechanism of FSH action: rapid stimulation of testicular synthesis of nuclear RNA. Endocrinology 1971;89:981-9.

6. Janecki A, Jakubowiak A, Lukaszyk A. Stimulatory effect of Sertoli cell secretory products on testosterone secretion by purified Leydig cells in primary culture. Mol Cell Endocrinol 1985;42:235-43.

7. Wattenberg LW. Microscopic histochemical demonstration of steroid-3-ol-dehydrogenase in tissue sections. J Histochem Cytochem 1958;6:225-32.

8. Clermont Y, Harvey SG. Duration of the cycle of the seminiferous epithelium of normal, hypophysectomized and hypophysectomized-hormone treated albino rats. Endocrinology 1965;76:80-9.

9. Sanborn BM, Steinberger A, Meistrich ML, Steinberger E. Androgen binding sites in testis cell fractions as measured by a nuclear exchange assay. J Steroid Biochem 1975;6:1459-65.

10. Skinner MK, Griswold MD. Secretion of testicular transferrin by cultured Sertoli cells is regulated by hormones and retinoids. Biol Reprod 1982;27:211-21.

11. Margioris AN, Liotta A, Vaudry H, Bardin CW, Krieger DT. Characterization of immunoreactive proopiomelanocortin-related peptides in rat testis. Endocrinology 1983;113:663-71.

12. Boitani C, Mather JP, Bardin CW. Stimulation of adenosine 3',5'-monophosphate production in rat Sertoli cells by α-melanotropin-stimulating hormone (αMSH) and desacetyl αMSH. Endocrinology 1986;118:1513-8.

13. Morris D, Vola WW, Bardin CW. β-endorphin regulation of FSH-stimulated inhibin production is a component of a short loop system in rats. Biochem Biophys Res Commun 1987;148:1513-9.

14. Galdieri M, Monaco L, Stefanini M. Secretion of androgen binding protein by Sertoli cells is influenced by contact with germ cells. J Androl 1984;5:409-15.

15. Le Magueresse B, Jegou B. In vitro effects of germ cells on the secretory activity of Sertoli cells recovered from rats of different ages. Endocrinology 1988;122:1672-80.

16. Le Magueresse B, Jegou B. Possible involvement of germ cells in the regulation of oestradiol-17β and ABP secretion by immature rat Sertoli cells (in vitro studies). Biochem Biophys Res Comm 1986;141:861-9.

17. Ayer-LeLievre C, Olson L, Ebendal T, Hallbook F, Persson H. Nerve growth factor mRNA and protein in the testis and epididymis of mouse and rat. Proc Natl Acad Sci USA 1988;85:2628-32.

18. Persson H, Ayer-LeLievre C, Soder O, et al. Expression of β-nerve growth factor receptor mRNA in Sertoli cells downregulated by testosterone. Science 1990;247:704-7.

19. Skinner MK, Takacs K, Coffey RJ. Cellular localization of transforming growth factor-α gene expression and action in the seminiferous tubule: peritubular cell-Sertoli cell interactions. Endocrinology 1989;124:845-54.

20. Skinner MK, Moses HL. Transforming growth factor-β gene expression and action in the seminiferous tubule: peritubular cell-Sertoli cell interactions. Mol Cell Endocrinol 1989;3:625-34.

21. Suarez-Quian CA, Dai M, Onoda M, Kriss RM, Dym M. Epidermal growth factor receptor localization in the rat and monkey testes. Biol Reprod 1989;41: 921-32.

22. Benahmed M, Esposito G, Sordoillet C, et al. Transforming growth factor-β and its related peptides in the testis: an intragonadal polypeptide control system. Persp Androl 1989;53:191.

23. Skinner MK, Fritz IB. Testicular peritubular cells secrete a protein under androgen control that modulates Sertoli cell functions. Proc Natl Acad Sci USA 1985; 82:114-8.

24. Skinner MK, Fetterolf PM, Anthony CT. Purification of the paracrine factor, P-Mod-S, produced by testicular peritubular cells that modulates Sertoli cell function. J Biol Chem 1988;263:2884-90.

25. Norton JN, Skinner MK. Regulation of Sertoli cell function and differentiation through the actions of a testicular paracrine factor P-Mod-S. Endocrinology 1989;124:2711-9.

26. Francis GL, Brown TJ, Bercu BB. Regulation by homologous hormone exposure. Biol Reprod 1981;24:955-61.

27. Le Gac F, Attramadal H, Jahnsen T, Hansson V. Studies on the mechanism of follicle-stimulating hormone-induced desensitization of Sertoli cell adenyl cyclase in vitro. Biol Reprod 1985;32:916-24.

28. Conti M, Geremia R, Adamo S, Stefanini M. Regulation of Sertoli cell cyclic adenosine 3',5'-monophosphate phosphodiesterase activity by follicle stimulating hormone and dibutyryl cyclic AMP. Biochem Biophy Res Commun 1981; 98:1044-50.

29. Migliaccio S, Conti M. Long term treatment with adenosine analogs modifies the responsiveness of immature rat Sertoli cell in culture. Endocrinology 1990;126: 134-41.

30. Monaco L, Adamo S, Stefanini M, Conti M. Signal transduction in the Sertoli cell: serum modulation of the response to FSH. J Steroid Biochem 1989;32:129-34.

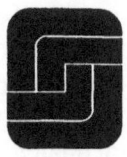

20

The Changing Functions of Follicle Stimulating Hormone in the Testes of Prenatal, Newborn, Immature, and Adult Rats

LESLIE HECKERT AND MICHAEL D. GRISWOLD

The target cells for the action of follicle stimulating hormone (FSH) in the testes of mammals are the Sertoli cells (Sc). The function of the Sc includes the physical and biochemical support for germ cell development into spermatozoa. Sc create an environment where germ cells are provided with metabolites, nutrients, and regulatory components. Thus, by exerting influence on the Sc and their functions, FSH indirectly influences spermatogenesis (1, 2). It is evident that in the rat, FSH is necessary to initiate the first wave of spermatogenesis, but its function in the adult rat testis is not well defined (3). The purpose of this manuscript is to review the probable actions of FSH during the development and maturation of the rat testes and describe recent experiments on the ontogeny and expression of the FSH receptor (FSH-R).

It has been clearly established that in the Sc, the primary action of FSH is mediated by increased concentrations of intracellular cAMP (2, 4). There is also evidence that FSH can alter intracellular calcium levels in cultured Sc, but through mechanisms that are independent of both the protein kinase C pathway and adenylate cyclase activity (5). Therefore, any influence on Sc functions by FSH appears to involve cAMP and/or possibly calcium as second messengers.

Prenatal and Newborn

FSH produced by the fetal and early postnatal rat pituitary is of critical importance in the proliferation of Sc. The proliferation of Sc is maximal in 20- and 21-day-old fetuses and declines steadily until the second week after birth, when further cell division is rare (6). Thus, the adult population of Sc is established prior to the onset of meiosis. Sc from immature rats but not from adults can be induced to divide at a low rate in culture in the presence of FSH or dibutyryl cAMP (7, 8). However, the primary evidence for the role of FSH in the proliferation of Sc comes from the laboratory of Joanne Orth. She showed that decapitation of, or addition of FSH antiserum to, day 18 rat fetuses resulted in reduced numbers of Sc in division (6). In addition, the placement of fetal testes in organ culture in the presence of FSH or dibutyryl cAMP stimulated the incorporation of radioactive thymidine into Sc nuclei when compared to controls (6). Hemicastration of immature rats resulted in an increased proliferation of Sc in the contralateral testis coincident with increased levels of serum FSH (9).

The role of FSH in the prenatal and newborn as an Sc mitogen is critical in the ultimate spermatogenic capability of the testis. Orth et al. injected cytosine arabinoside, an inhibitor of DNA synthesis, into testes of newborn rats (10). When these rats reached maturity, there was an overall 54% decrease in the size of the Sc population. However, the ratio of round spermatids to Sc in these animals was similar to controls, but the testis size was decreased proportionately. This experiment showed that the Sc population was limiting to overall sperm production and underscored the importance of FSH in the establishment of the number of Sc and, therefore, the spermatogenic capacity in the adult (10).

At 2 weeks after birth, the proliferation of Sc in vivo and in culture becomes progressively less responsive to FSH or dibutyryl cAMP. As the adult population of Sc becomes established, the primary function of FSH changes (1, 2, 4).

Immature

Most of the studies examining the actions of FSH have been done on cultured Sc from 10- to 30-day-old rats. The Sc from rats of this age are easily placed in culture and respond to FSH with increased levels of cAMP, increased protein synthesis, and increased estradiol production (11). While the cell division response is decreased and nearly finished at this age, it appears that the FSH may be required for maturation of the Sc. FSH appears to be essential for the formation of the tight junctional complexes between adjacent Sc and for the initiation of the first wave of spermatogenesis. It is generally assumed that the action of FSH on spermatogenesis results from the stimulation of Sc to produce proteins, such as androgen binding protein (ABP), plasminogen activator (PA), transferrin (Trf), sulfated glycoproteins 1 and 2, and a number of mitogens or growth factors (1, 12). FSH antisera was administered to 20-day-old rats for a period of 14 days; the testis weight was reduced by 50%, and the number of spermatids was reduced by 67%, with no effect on other parts of the reproductive system (13). A number of morphological maturation-like features of Sc, such as the pattern of chromatin condensation, the development of large nucleoli and nuclear infoldings, and the accumulation of smooth endoplasmic reticulum, also appear to require the action of FSH (14).

A large number of studies have characterized ABP as a model FSH-regulated product of Sc (1). FSH increased ABP levels in cultured cells from young animals and in vivo. A recent study showed that in culture, the initial ABP mRNA levels were maintained but not stimulated by FSH (15). In the same cell cultures, PA mRNA, inhibin α subunit mRNA, and c-*fos* mRNA were markedly increased by FSH. Since the ABP was increased in the culture medium but the mRNA levels were simply maintained by FSH, the possibility exists that the effect of FSH on ABP mRNA is at the translational or posttranslational level. Transferrin and Trf mRNA levels are increased—but only to a small extent—in Sc from 20-day-old rats cultured in the presence of FSH (16).

Adult

As the age of the rat increases to 40 days or more, the response of Sc both in culture and in vivo changes again. There is a large increase in the phosphodiesterase activity in the cells, and the accumulation of cAMP and the subsequent stimulation of specific protein synthesis is curtailed (2, 4, 16). Responses to FSH in Sc from the adult rat can usually only be measured in the presence of a phosphodiesterase inhibitor. When adult rats are hypophysectomized, spermatogenesis can be maintained by testosterone (T) in the absence of added FSH. However, if hypophysectomized rats are allowed to regress for 20 days before hormone treatment , both FSH and T are necessary to reinitiate spermatogenesis (17). Long-term passive immunization of adult rats with antiserum to FSH had little or no effect on spermatogenesis (18). These experiments have led to the concept that in the rat, FSH is not required for adult spermatogenic function. The hormonal requirements of spermatogenesis in the adult rat can be satisfied by T alone.

The experiment described in Table 20.1 is a clear example of the decreased response of adult rats to FSH and the increased response to T. Rats were hypophysectomized at 40 days of age or at 60 days of age and maintained for 20 days with no treatment or daily injections of FSH or T (19). Daily treatment with FSH increased the testis weight, total RNA per testis, and Trf mRNA in rats that were 40 days old at the time of hypophysectomy. FSH had no effect on rats that were 60 days old at the time of hypophysectomy. In turn, daily injections of T had no effect on these parameters in the younger group, but increased all three parameters in older rats.

All of the information presented so far suggests that FSH may not play a role in normal function of the adult rat testis. However, several other factors need to be considered. First, spermatogenesis can be maintained in hypophysectomized rats in the absence of FSH, but this maintenance is only qualitatively normal, and the total sperm output is greatly reduced (20). Second, FSH receptors, measured by binding studies, appear to be present in the adult testis (21, 22). Third, a recent report shows that FSH in conjunction with low levels of T is more effective in maintaining quantitatively normal spermatogenesis than T alone (23). Finally, the situation is much clearer in primates, where the action of FSH on spermatogenesis in the adult is easily demonstrated (24).

We were interested in the expression of FSH receptors (FSH-R) in the adult rat, so we have utilized a cDNA probe to quantify the mRNA for FSH-R. The probe was obtained by utilizing 2 synthetic oligonucleotides corresponding to conserved regions of the LH receptor (LH-R) in a polymerase chain reaction (PCR)-directed amplification of mRNA from Sc. PCR of the Sc mRNA yielded a single predominant species of cDNA that was cloned and sequenced (25). The sequence was identical to that reported for a region of the FSH-R. The cDNA was used to screen a genomic library, and several clones containing regions of the genomic DNA were isolated. The cloned genomic DNA was then used as a probe on Northern blots, which examined the expression of the FSH-R.

TABLE 20.1. FSH or testosterone actions on hypophysectomized rats (n = 6).

Treatments	Testis wt (g)	Total RNA (μg/testis)	Trf mRNA
40 days old			
Untreated control	1.5 ± 0.10	3.9 ± 0.6	1.00
Hypox	0.1 ± 0.02	2.7 ± 0.2	0.05
Hypox + FSH	0.4 ± 0.10	3.8 ± 0.5	0.20
Hypox + T	0.1 ± 0.10	2.8 ± 0.4	0.08
60 days old			
Untreated control	2.4 ± 0.20	3.1 ± 0.5	1.00
Hypox	0.4 ± 0.04	1.6 ± 0.4	0.03
Hypox + FSH	0.4 ± 0.02	2.1 ± 0.3	0.08
Hypox + T	1.1 ± 0.10	3.6 ± 0.5	0.40

Rats were hypophysectomized at 40 or 60 days of age and maintained for 20 days with no treatment or daily injections of FSH (0.2-U NIH S13) or testosterone (T) proprionate (2 mg). Testes were removed, the RNA was isolated, and the Trf mRNA was determined by solution hybridization. Trf mRNA values are given as the ratio of the total testicular levels in treated animals to control animals.

Source: Hugly, Roberts, and Griswold (19).

Sc were found to contain a major transcript of 2.6 kb and a minor transcript of 4.5 kb, which hybridized to the FSH-R DNA sequence. We found that both transcripts were present in mRNA from testes of rats from 10 to 60 days of age. In the adult rats, the relative amount of FSH-R mRNA was decreased, but this may have been due to the increase in testicular mRNA coming from the large number of germinal cells. Sc from 20-day-old rats were placed in culture and treated with different combinations of hormones and vitamin A. The amount of FSH-R mRNA in these cells was then assayed by Northern blots. The data were normalized to SGP2 mRNA levels, which has been shown not to change in cell culture in the presence of different hormones. It was found that after 3 days in culture, FSH, insulin, retinol, or T added individually had no affect on the FSH-R levels (relative to total poly(A) + mRNA). Addition of all 4 reagents resulted in an approximately 2-fold increase in the relative FSH-R levels. In summary, these experiments showed that FSH-R mRNA is present in adult Sc and that the relative levels can be affected in cell culture by a combination of hormones.

Spermatogenesis in the adult rat is organized into a series of 14 stages that are defined by the germinal cell composition of the tubule (26). All 14 stages are present at different regions along the length of the tubule, and the production of spermatozoa is asynchronous. It has been shown using microdissected tubules that the functions of Sc change with their association with different stages of the cycle of the seminiferous epithelium (27). Recently, we have developed a method utilizing retinol deprivation and repletion that results in the synchronization of the testis to 3 or 4 related stages of the cycle (28, 29). Spermatogenesis appears to proceed normally, but since the entire testis is in roughly the same stages, sperm are produced only every 12 to 13 days. Because of the synchronization, we can utilize testes that represent all parts of the cycle and obtain sufficient amounts of tissue to carry out biochemical analyses (30).

Utilizing the FSH-R cDNA and mRNA isolated from synchronized testes, we were able to examine the expression of the FSH-R mRNA during the different stages of the cycle of the seminiferous epithelium. The mRNA was isolated from the testes of stage-synchronized rats and analyzed by Northern blots probed with nick-translated FSH-R cDNA (Fig. 20.1). It was found that the relative levels of FSH-R mRNA varied in a cyclic manner, with low levels in the middle stages (V–IX) and 5-fold-higher levels in stages XIII, XIV, I, and II. In a recent publication, the binding of labeled FSH to dissected tubules of defined stages was determined and found to vary in a similar cyclic manner—that is, greater binding in stages XIII, XIV, I and II (31). It has also been reported that FSH maximally stimulated cAMP production in stages XIV to VI and that the tubules in stages VII–VIII were essentially refractory to FSH stimulation of cAMP levels (32).

Thus, the accumulated evidence suggests that the primary action and

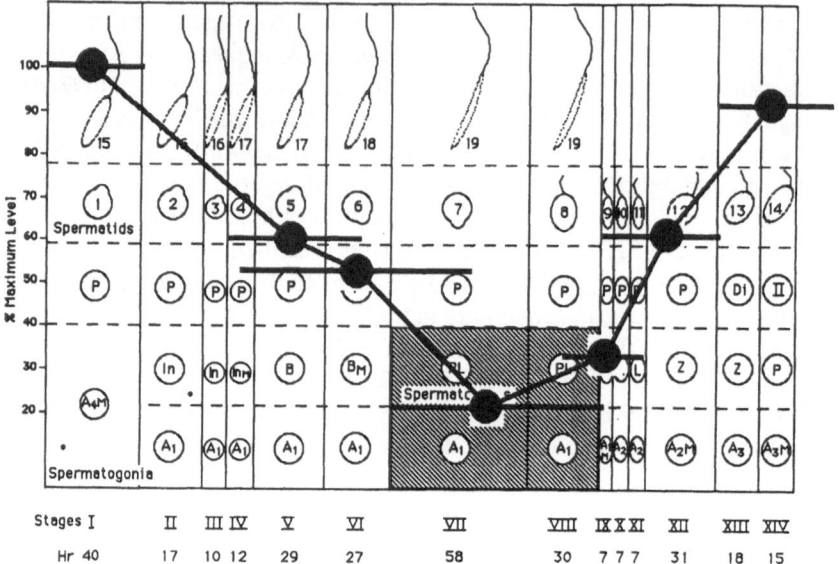

FIGURE 20.1. The relative levels of FSH-R mRNA in the stages of the cycle of the seminiferous epithelium. The mRNA was obtained from the testes of stage-synchronized rats and subjected to Northern blot analysis using FSH-R cDNA as a probe. The film from the Northern blot was scanned with a laser densitometer, and the relative densities were determined. The same amount of mRNA was loaded in each lane of the gel. All of the densities were normalized to the levels found in the sample containing stage I. The black horizontal bar indicates the stages in the sample that were present with a frequency of greater than 10%. The black circle is the approximate midpoint of the distribution of the synchronous tubules. The data are plotted over a background depicting the cycle of the seminiferous epithelium, with each stage having a width relative to its duration (26). (A and B = spermatogonia; PL, Z, P, preleptotene, zygotene, and pachytene = spermatocytes; Di = diakinesis; II = secondary spermatocyte; and numbers 1 to 19 = steps of spermatid development.)

binding of FSH in the adult rat is coincident with the maximal levels of FSH-R mRNA and is confined to stages XIII to IV. As pointed out by Sharp, these are the stages that encompass a number of the spermatogonial divisions, and an effect of FSH on these mitotic divisions would explain why there is a decrease in the efficiency of spermatogenesis in FSH- deprived animals (3). If it is assumed that the primary actions of FSH are modulated by cAMP, then the presence of a cAMP phosphodiesterase could be inhibitory to this action. The phosphodiesterase activity increases in the adult Sc and appears to be maximal during the middle (stages VII–VIII) of the cycle (27). Again, this would be consistent with a lack of FSH action during stages VI–XI.

Summary

FSH has multiple and changing roles in the regulation of spermatogenesis. The first function of FSH is to increase the number of Sc by stimulation of their mitotic activity. During the prepubertal phase of development FSH is important for the maturation of the Sc. Hormonal stimulation of tight-junction formation and specific protein secretion are essential. In the adult rat, some of the functions carried out by FSH in prepubertal animals are assumed by T. However, there is evidence that even in the rat, FSH is important for quantitatively normal spermatogenesis. Our work shows that the FSH-R mRNA is present in the testes of the adult rat and that the levels of this mRNA are changing during the cycle of the seminiferous epithelium. The presence of relatively high levels of FSH-R mRNA in stages XIV–II of the cycle and the presence of relatively low levels in stages VII–VIII suggest that the FSH-R is carefully regulated in the adult rats and, presumably, has an important function in spermatogenesis.

References

1. Fritz I. Sites of actions of androgens and follicle stimulating hormone on cells of the seminiferous tubule. In: Litwack G, ed. Biochemical actions of hormones; vol V. New York: Academic Press, 1978:249-78.
2. Means AR, Dedman JR, Tash JR, Tindall DJ, van Sickle M, Welsh MJ. Regulation of the testis Sertoli cell by follicle stimulating hormone. Annu Rev Physiol 1980;42:59-71.
3. Sharpe RM. Follicle-stimulating hormone and spermatogenesis in the adult male. J Endocrinol 1989;121:405-7.
4. Means AR, Fakunding JL, Huckins C, Tindall DJ, Vitale R. Follicle-stimulating hormone, the Sertoli cell and spermatogenesis. Recent Prog Horm Res 1976;32: 477-527.
5. Grasso P, Reichert LE. Follicle-stimulating hormone receptor-mediated uptake of $^{45}Ca^{2+}$ by cultured rat Sertoli cells does not require activation of cholera toxin- or pertussis toxin-sensitive guanine nucleotide binding proteins or adenylate cyclase. Endocrinology 1990;127:949-56.
6. Orth JM. The role of follicle-stimulating hormone in controlling Sertoli cell proliferation in testes of fetal rats. Endocrinology 1984;115:1248-55.
7. Griswold MD, Solari A, Tung PS, Fritz IB. Stimulation of the mitosis of cultured Sertoli cells by FSH. Mol Cell Endocrinol 1977;7:151-65.
8. Griswold MD, Mably E, Fritz IB. FSH stimulation of DNA synthesis in Sertoli cells in culture. Mol Cell Endocrinol 1976;4:139-49.
9. Orth JM, Higginbothem C, Salisbury R. Hemi-castration causes and testosterone prevents enhanced uptake of 3H-thymidine by Sertoli cells of immature rats. Biol Reprod 1984;30:263-70.

10. Orth JM, Gunsalus GL, Lamperti LA. Evidence from Sertoli cell-depleted rats indicates that spermatid number in adults depends on numbers of Sertoli cells produced during the prenatal period. Endocrinology 1988;122:787-94.

11. Fritz KB, Rommerts FG, Louis BG, Dorrington JH. Regulation by FSH and dibutyryl cyclic AMP of the formation of androgen-binding protein in Sertoli cell-enriched cultures. J Reprod Fert 1976;46:17-24.

12. Griswold MD, Morales C, Sylvester S. Molecular biology of the Sertoli cell. Ox Rev Reprod Biol 1988;10:124-61.

13. Raj HGM, Dym M. The effects of selective withdrawal of FSH or LH on spermatogenesis in the immature rat. Biol Reprod 1976;14:489-94.

14. Solari AJ, Fritz IB. The ultrastructure of immature Sertoli cells. Maturation-like changes during culture and the maintenance of mitotic potentiality. Biol Reprod 1978;18:329-45.

15. Hall SH, Conti M, French FS, Joseph DR. Follicle-stimulating hormone regulation of androgen-binding protein messenger RNA in Sertoli cell cultures. Mol Cell Endocrinol 1990;4:349-62.

16. Huggenvik JI, Idzerda RL, Haywood L, Lee DC, McKnight GS, Griswold MD. Transferrin messenger ribonucleic acid: molecular cloning and hormonal regulation in rat Sertoli cells. Endocrinology 1987;120:332-40.

17. Steinberger E. Hormonal control of mammalian spermatogenesis. Physiol Rev 1971;51:1-22.

18. Dym M, Raj HGM, Lin YC, et al. Is FSH required for maintenance of spermatogenesis in adult rats? J Reprod Fertil 1979;26:175-81.

19. Hugly S, Roberts K, Griswold MD. Transferrin and sulfated glycoprotein-2 mRNA levels in the testis and in the isolated Sertoli cells of hypophysectomized rats. Endocrinology 1988;122:1390-6.

20. Sharpe RM. Testosterone and spermatogenesis. J Endocrinol 1987;113:1-2.

21. Abou-Issa H, Reichert LE. Properties of follitropin-receptor interaction. Characterization of the interaction of follitropin with receptors in purified membranes isolated from mature rat testes tubules. J Biol Chem 1976;251:3326-37.

22. Yoon DJ, Reggiardio D, David R. Available FSH receptors in adult rat testis in vivo. J Endocrinol 1990;125:293-9.

23. Bartlett JMS, Weinbauer GF, Nieschlag E. Differential effects of FSH and testosterone on the maintenance of spermatogenesis in the adult hypophysectomized rat. J Endocrinol 1989;121:49-58.

24. Wickings EJ, Usadel KH, Dathe G, Nieschlag E. The role of follicle stimulating hormone in testicular function of the mature rhesus monkey. Acta Endocrinol (Copenh) 1980;95:117-28.

25. Heckert L, Griswold MD. Cloning and expression of FSH receptor mRNA in rats. 1990.

26. Leblond CP, Clermont Y. Definition of the stages of the cycle of the seminiferous epithelium in the rat. Ann NY Acad Sci 1952;55:548-73.

27. Parvinen M. Regulation of the seminiferous epithelium. Endocr Rev 1982;3:404-17.

28. Morales C, Griswold MD. Retinol-induced stage synchronization in seminiferous tubules of the rat. Endocrinology 1987;121:432-4.

29. Morales CR, Griswold MD. Retinol induces stage synchronization in semi-niferous tubules of vitamin A deficient rats. Ann NY Acad Sci 1987;513:292-3.
30. Morales CR, Alcivar AA, Hecht NB, Griswold MD. Specific mRNAs in Sertoli and germinal cells of testes from stage synchronized rats. J Mol Endocrinol 1989; 3:725-33.
31. Kangasniemi M, Kaipia A, Toppari J, Perheentupa A, Aniemi I, Parvinen M. Cellular regulation of follicle-stimulating hormone (FSH) binding in rat seminiferous tubules. J Androl 1990;11:336-43.
32. Kangasniemi M, Kaipia A, Mali P, Toppari J, Huhtaniemi I, Parvinen M. Modulation of basal and FSH-dependent cyclic AMP production in rat seminiferous tubules stages by an improved transillumination technique. Anat Rec 1990;227: 62-76.

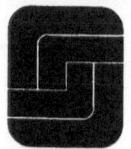

21

Novel Testicular Products of the Human SHBG/ABP Gene

GEOFFREY L. HAMMOND

The blood of most mammalian species contains a binding protein for the sex-steroid hormones; in humans, this protein is most often referred to as sex-hormone binding globulin (SHBG). Rodents are notable exceptions to this rule, and it is well known that adult rats lack a plasma equivalent of SHBG. A similar protein has, however, been found in fetal rat blood during late gestation and is probably produced by the liver (1). In humans and other primates, the protein exhibits a high affinity for both androgens and estrogens (2), and plasma concentrations of SHBG determine the distribution of these hormones between the various protein-bound and nonprotein-bound fractions in the blood (3). As a result, SHBG influences the bioavailability of sex steroids at the target cell level (4). More recently, evidence has accumulated to support the concept that SHBG may play a more direct role in the actions of sex steroids, and a plasma membrane receptor that interacts specifically with SHBG has been isolated from human prostate tissue (5). This has resulted in a reevaluation of the physiological role of SHBG in a recent comprehensive review of the subject (6).

Testicular androgen binding protein (ABP) is a Sertoli cell (Sc) product that is secreted into the seminiferous tubules where it is responsible for the transport of androgens within the male reproductive tract (7). Its physiological function is not entirely clear, but it is generally assumed that it helps maintain a highly androgenic environment for developing sperm during their passage from the testis to the epididymis (8). Once inside the caput epididymis, ABP appears to be internalized by the luminal epithelial cells (9) and may thereby promote the delivery of relatively large amounts of testosterone (T) to these cells. It is therefore possible that its ultimate function is to enhance the expression of androgen-responsive genes for secretory proteins that are important for sperm maturation.

In humans, testicular ABP is physicochemically and immunochemically almost identical to the plasma sex-steroid hormone binding globulin (SHBG)

246

produced by hepatocytes (10–12). Biochemical analyses of the purified proteins have indicated that both are homodimeric molecules of approximately 50-kD subunits, which somehow unite to form a single steroid binding site (12). When examined by polyacrylamide gel electrophoresis under denaturing conditions, both proteins exhibit subunit size heterogeneity that may be due to differences in carbohydrate composition (10), but it is not known whether this reflects catabolic modifications or differences in glycosylation during synthesis. Minor differences have also been identified in the peptide maps of both proteins (10), but these may also reflect variations in glycosylation. In this context, it is well established that SHBG in plasma binds quantitatively with concanavalin A, while ABP in human and rat testicular extracts can be separated into two forms on the basis of their ability to interact with this lectin (13, 14).

The biosynthesis of ABP and SHBG also appears to be under different hormonal control in the testis and liver, and interest has focused on the fact that the production of ABP by Sc responds specifically to FSH (15). Direct evidence that this involves an increase in ABP biosynthesis has recently been obtained using cDNA probes for rat ABP to study the accumulation of ABP mRNA in cultured Sc (16) and the testis of hypophysectomized animals (17) after stimulation with FSH in vitro and in vivo, respectively. In addition, similar studies have demonstrated that the well-established effect of T on increasing ABP levels in the rat testis (15) is probably mediated indirectly by a process that involves other androgen-responsive factors known to influence Sc function, such as the peritubular cell protein PModS (18).

Characterization of the Mammalian SHBG/ABP Gene

The gene for rat testicular ABP production has been characterized, and a potential start site for transcription has been identified by primer extension studies (16). Although the proposed promoter region in the rat ABP gene lacks the typical TATA and CAAT box sequence elements commonly found in most eukaryotic gene promoters, a potential cyclic AMP (cAMP) response element was identified 116 bp upstream from the proposed transcriptional start site (16). However, the suggestion that this may account for the induction of ABP gene expression by FSH has never been substantiated. The reason for this is unclear, but it may be that this region does not represent a functional promoter. This is supported by the fact that more than one primer extension product was actually observed when rat testis mRNA was used as a template (16). Furthermore, other rat testis (16) and fetal liver (19) ABP cDNAs have been identified with unique 5' sequences that deviate from the cDNA sequence that contains an open reading frame for the ABP precursor polypeptide, and this occurs at a potential intron-exon boundary. One way this issue might be clarified would be to define the molecular mechanisms responsible for the tissue specificity of SHBG and ABP biosynthesis. These experiments are, however, difficult to perform in the rat because the adult rat liver does not produce an SHBG-like protein, and our attention has therefore focused on defining the molecular mechanisms responsible for the biosynthesis of SHBG and ABP in human tissues.

In this regard, one of the first questions we sought to answer was whether human SHBG and ABP are the products of the same gene. This work was facilitated by the cloning of a human liver cDNA that contains the entire coding region for the SHBG subunit polypeptide (20) and that exhibits good sequence similarity with rat ABP cDNAs (17, 21). The human SHBG and rat ABP cDNAs have both been used to examine Southern blots of genomic DNA after digestion with restriction enzymes (16, 22), and the results are consistent with the presence of only a single gene in both species. This has been confirmed by the isolation and characterization of several overlapping genomic fragments that comprise part or all of the coding regions for the human SHBG and rat ABP precursors (16, 22).

In addition, we have recently examined human metaphase spreads in situ with probes prepared from two separate regions of an SHBG cDNA and have assigned the SHBG gene to the short arm of chromosome 17 (23). The mouse ABP gene has also recently been located 35 cM from the centromere of mouse chromosome 11, and this location is analogous to the region on human chromosome 17 that contains the SHBG gene (24). Taken together, these studies all support the concept that SHBG and ABP are the products of a single gene, and any differences between them may therefore be attributed to tissue-specific variations in the start of transcription and/or modifications of a common primary transcript or its translation products.

Genomic fragments of the rat and human SHBG/ABP genes that contain exons encoding the precursor polypeptides have been sequenced (16, 22), and the structural organization of both genes is remarkably similar (25). Furthermore, the coding regions for both polypeptides are distributed over 8 identically sized exons. These 8 exons are contained within approximately 3.5 kb of genomic DNA in both cases, but the sizes of the intervening sequences vary considerably between species, and there is little sequence similarity between introns that separate exons containing the protein coding sequence (25).

In contrast, there is a relatively good alignment between the first 150 bp immediately 5' to the ATG believed to represent the start of translation within the rat ABP and human SHBG mRNAs (Fig. 21.1). Therefore, even if this region does not act as a promoter, the fact that it is well conserved suggests that it may influence the expression of these genes in some way. In this context, it is interesting that the human gene contains a sequence element that binds a transcription factor known to be essential for liver-specific gene

```
                                   ___LF-A1___
TGTGACTGGGCCCCTGGGCAGGGGTCAAGGGTCAGTGCCCCTGTTTCCT--TTACCCCCTC
  :          ::  :       :       ::::::::::::: :::: : :: :        ::  ::
ATCTGCCTTCAGAGGGGCCGCATGGTCAGGGTCAGTGTCCCTATCTCTTGCCCCCCTTCTT
   cAMP


CTCCCCGGGCAACCTTTAACCCTCCACCGCCCACACGCAAGGCTGCCTGCCTCTACACATT
: :::: : :::::::::::::::::::::::: :::: :     ::::: ::: :: : ::
CCCCCGGAGCAACCTTTAACCCTCCACCACCCATGTGAGAGGCTACCTACCCCCACTGCTT
          Sp1                           SV40 promoter


                                   M    E    S ..hSHBG
CTCCCAAGAGTTGTCTGAGCCGCCGAGTGGACAGTGGCTGATTATG GAG AGC.......
: :::: :::  :  ::::::::: : : ::::::::  ::: : ::M   E   K ...rABP
CTCCTCAGATAT-TCTGAGCCACTGGGTGGACAGCTGCTAACTATG GAG AAG.......
        →
```

FIGURE 21.1. Comparison of proposed promoter sequence of rat ABP gene, as described in reference 16, with the corresponding sequence in the human SHBG gene, as described in reference 22. The location of possible regulatory sequence elements in the proposed rat ABP gene promoter (ref. 16) are underlined, and an element (LF-A1) implicated in liver-specific gene expression (ref. 22) is overlined on the human SHBG gene sequence. The arrow denotes the proposed transcription start site for rat ABP mRNA.

expression (26), and this is present at the point where these sequences diverge (Fig. 21.1). It is therefore possible that this may explain why the ABP gene is not expressed in the adult rat liver. In addition, the possible cAMP response element identified in the rat ABP gene (16) is not conserved in the human SHBG gene sequence (Fig. 21.1), and this therefore casts some doubt on its functional significance.

Identification of Novel Transcripts from the SHBG/ABP Gene

Northern blot analyses have indicated that poly(A) + RNA extracts from human testis and liver contain molecules of approximately 1.6 kb that hybridize with the human liver SHBG cDNA and that are not present in normal human ovarian RNA (22). A larger hybridizing species of approximately 2.5 kb is also present in liver RNA, but its abundance is relatively low. In order to examine in more detail the testicular mRNA that hybridized with the SHBG cDNA, it was used to screen a human testis cDNA library (22). This revealed the presence of a cDNA that is shorter but otherwise identical to the SHBG cDNA isolated from a human liver library (20) and that therefore probably corresponds to testicular ABP. Unexpectedly, it was also found that the testis is capable of producing at least two other SHBG-related mRNA species, and when their sequences were compared, it became evident that they diverge from the SHBG cDNA sequence in the same position close to its 5' end (Fig. 21.2). Furthermore, additional sequence analyses of the genomic fragment containing the SHBG gene demonstrated that these unique sequences are encoded by exons located about 1.9 kb upstream from the exon containing the coding sequence for the SHBG signal peptide (Fig. 21.2).

It is also clear that the two novel transcripts of the SHBG gene produced in human testis contain unique exons that replace the exon encoding for the start of translation for SHBG. This raises the question of whether all the mRNA species produced by the SHBG/ABP gene arise from differential exon splicing of a larger common transcript or are transcribed from separate promoters located further upstream on the SHBG gene. The fact that the exons for the 5' ends of these novel testicular transcripts are located so closely together suggests that differential exon splicing is the most likely explanation.

The tissue specificity of human SHBG gene expression has not been examined in great detail, but it is becoming increasingly apparent that the rat ABP gene may be expressed in tissues other than the adult testis and fetal liver, and an important site of ABP biosynthesis may include the brain (27). Furthermore, it appears that SHBG-related mRNAs are present in several

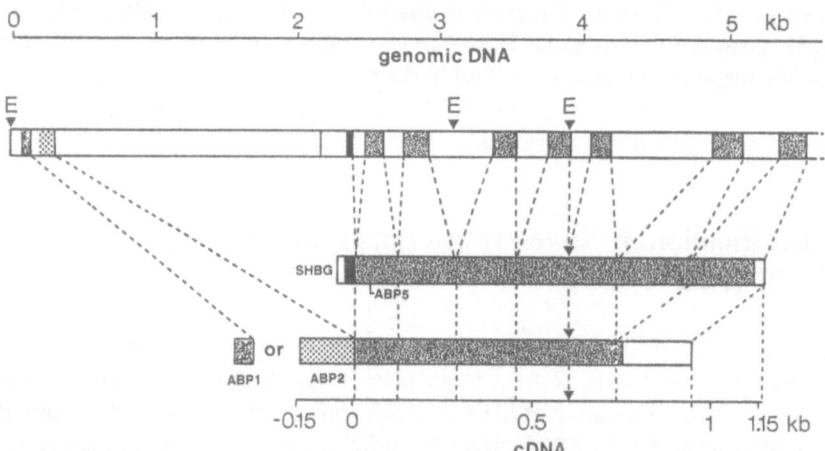

FIGURE 21.2. Organization of the human SHBG/ABP gene with reference to coding sequences in hepatic SHBG and testicular ABP cDNAs. Shaded areas represent protein sequences in both genomic DNA and cDNAs. The black area represents signal peptide sequence in SHBG promoter. Open areas represent introns in genomic DNA and noncoding regions in cDNAs. The EcoRI sites in the gene and the internal EcoRI site in the cDNAs are indicated by E.

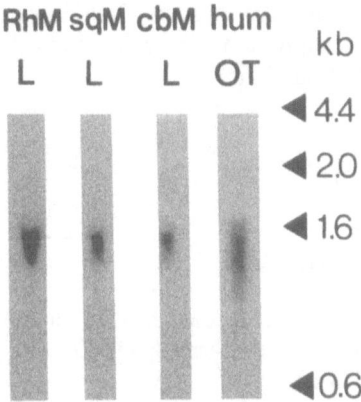

FIGURE 21.3. Northern blots of total RNA extracted from rhesus monkey (RhM), squirrel monkey (sqM), and cebus monkey (cbM) livers (L) and from a human ovarian adenocarcinoma (hum). The blot was hybridized under high-stringency conditions with a human SHBG cDNA (20). Molecular size standards are shown on the right of the blots.

human prostate tumor cell lines and that there may be variations in the size of these transcripts when compared to SHBG mRNA in human hepatoma cell lines (28). In this respect, we have also identified an SHBG mRNA in a single human ovarian tumor, the size of which was similar in size to SHBG mRNA in human and New World monkey liver samples (Fig. 21.3). Although these SHBG-related mRNA species in tumor cells remain to be characterized, it is possible that expression of the SHBG gene in hormone-dependent cells could influence the way they respond to steroid hormones.

In addition to differences at the 5' ends of the novel testicular transcripts, at least one of these SHBG-related gene products is truncated due to the deletion of the penultimate exon that makes up the SHBG cDNA sequence (Fig. 21.2). As a result, analyses of this cDNA predict a translation product that resembles SHBG with a unique aminoterminal sequence, but which lacks the carboxyterminal portion of the molecule previously implicated in steroid binding. This may explain why testicular SHBG-related peptides that lack steroid binding have not previously been detected in ABP preparations isolated from testicular tissue using steroid affinity chromatography. It will therefore be of interest to identify these SHBG-related gene products, to determine the functional significance of their expression in the testis, and to define whether their biosynthesis is regulated in the same way as ABP by hormones such as FSH. Furthermore, these novel transcripts may not be confined to the testis, and it is possible that their presence in other normal tissues or tumor cells may be physiologically or pathologically significant.

Acknowledgments. I would like to thank Gail Howard for secretarial assistance. This work was supported by grants from MRC Canada and the ArcAngelo Rea Family Foundation.

References

1. Gunsalus GL, Carreau S, Vogel DL, Musto NA, Bardin CW. Sexual differentiation: basic and clinical aspects. In: Serio M, ed. New York: Raven Press, 1984: 53-64.
2. Renoir J-M, Mercier-Bodard C, Baulieu E-E. Hormonal and immunological aspects of the phylogeny of sex steroid binding plasma protein. Proc Natl Acad Sci USA 1980;77:4578-82.
3. Anderson DC. Sex-hormone binding globulin. Clin Endocrinol (Oxf) 1974;3: 69-96.
4. Siiteri PK, Murai JT, Hammond GL, Nisker JA, Raymoure WJ, Kuhn RW. The serum transport of steroid hormones. Recent Prog Horm Res 1982;38:457-510.
5. Hryb DJ, Khan MS, Romas MA, Rosner W. Solubilization and partial characterization of sex hormone-binding globulin receptor from human prostate. J Biol Chem 1989;264:5378-83.
6. Rosner, W. The functions of corticosteroid-binding globulin and sex hormone-binding globulin: recent advances. Endocr Rev 1990;11:80-91.
7. French FS, Ritzen EM. A high-affinity androgen binding protein (ABP) in rat testis: evidence for secretion into efferent duct fluid and absorption by epididymis. Endocrinology 1973;93:88-95.
8. Bardin CW, Musto N, Gunsalus G, et al. Extracellular androgen binding proteins. Annu Rev Physiol 1981;43:189-98.
9. Pelliniemi LJ, Dym M, Gunsalus GL, Musto NA, Bardin CW, Fawcett DW. Immunocytochemical localization of androgen-binding protein in the male reproductive tract. Endocrinology 1981;108:925-31.
10. Cheng CY, Musto NA, Gunsalus GL, Frick J, Bardin CW. There are two forms of androgen binding protein in human testes. J Biol Chem 1985;260:5631-40.
11. Cheng CY, Frick J, Gunsalus GL, Musto NA, Bardin CW. Human testicular androgen-binding protein shares immunodeterminants with serum testosterone-estradiol-binding globulin. Endocrinology 1984;114:1395-401.
12. Hammond GL, Robinson PA, Sugino H, Ward DN, Finne J. Physicochemical characteristics of human sex hormone binding globulin: evidence for two identical subunits. J Steroid Biochem 1986;24:815-24.
13. Hsu AF, Troen P. An androgen binding protein in the testicular cytosol of human testis. Comparison with human plasma testosterone-estrogen binding globulin. J Clin Invest 1978;61:1611-9.
14. Cheng CY, Gunsalus GL, Musto NA, Bardin CW. The heterogeneity of rat androgen-binding protein in serum differs from that in testis and epididymis. Endocrinology 1984;114:1386-94.
15. Tindall DJ, Means AR. Properties and hormonal regulation of androgen binding proteins. In: Thomas JA, Singhal RL, eds. Advances in sex hormone research; vol 4. Baltimore: Urban and Schwarzenberg, 1980:295-327.

16. Joseph DR, Hall SH, Conti M, French FS. The gene structure of rat androgen-binding protein: identification of potential regulatory deoxyribonucleic acid elements of a follicle-stimulating hormone-regulated protein. Mol Cell Endocrinol 1988;2:3-13.

17. Reventos J, Hammond GL, Crozat A, et al. Hormonal regulation of rat androgen-binding protein (ABP) messenger ribonucleic acid and homology of human testosterone-estradiol-binding globulin and ABP complementary deoxyribonucleic acids. Mol Cell Endocrinol 1988;2:125-32.

18. Skinner MK, Fritz IB. Testicular peritubular cells secrete a protein under androgen control that modulates Sertoli cell functions. Proc Natl Acad Sci USA 1985; 82:114-8.

19. Joseph DR, Sullivan PM, Fenstermacher DA, Behrendsen ME, Zahnow CA. Alternate processed androgen-binding protein mRNAs; identification of a fusion transcript with DOPA decarboxylase-like RNA [Abstract]. Proc 71st annu meet Endocr Soc. Seattle, WA, 1989:71.

20. Hammond GL, Underhill DA, Smith CL, et al. The cDNA-deduced primary structure of human sex hormone-binding globulin and location of its steroid-binding domain. FEBS Lett 1987;215:100-4.

21. Joseph DR, Hall SH, French FS. Rat and androgen-binding protein: evidence for identical subunits and amino acid sequence homology with human sex hormone-binding globulin. Proc Natl Acad Sci USA 1987;84:339-43.

22. Hammond GL, Underhill DA, Rykse H, Smith CL. The human sex hormone binding globulin gene contains exons for androgen binding protein and two other testicular messenger RNAs. Mol Cell Endocrinol 1989;3:1869-76.

23. Bérubé D, Seralini G-E, Gagné R, Hammond GL. Localization of the human sex hormone-binding globulin gene to the short arm of chromosome 17 (17p12-p13). Cytogenet Cell Genet (in press).

24. Joseph DR, Adamson MC, Kozak CA. Cytogenet Cell Genet (in press).

25. Hammond GL. Molecular properties of corticosteroid binding globulin and the sex-steroid binding proteins. Endocr Rev 1990;11:65-79.

26. Monaci P, Nicosia A, Cortese R. Two different liver-specific factors stimulate in vitro transcription from the human α1-antitrypsin promoter. EMBO J 1988;7: 2075-87.

27. Wang Y-M, Bayliss DA, Millhorn DE, Seroogy KB, Joseph DR. The androgen-binding protein gene is expressed in rat brain. [Abstract 195]. 71st annu meet Endocr Soc. Seattle, WA, 1989.

28. Plymate SR. Effects of sex hormone binding globulin (SHBG) on human prostate carcinoma [Abstract 109]. J Steroid Biochem 1990;36:40S.

Part V

Clinical Implications of FSH and Gonadal Peptide Secretion

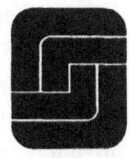

22

Follicle Stimulating Hormone and the Control of Spermatogenesis and Inhibin Secretion in Men

WILLIAM J. BREMNER AND ALVIN M. MATSUMOTO

Stimulation of the testes by the pituitary—gonadotropins, luteinizing hormone (LH) and follicle stimulating hormone (FSH)—is necessary for spermatogenesis (1). LH binds to receptors on interstitial Leydig cells of the testis and stimulates the production of testosterone (T), which in high local concentrations is thought to be important in the initiation and maintenance of sperm production. FSH binds to receptors on Sertoli cells (Sc) and stimulates the production of a number of proteins that are thought to be important in the control of spermatogenesis. The Sc also produces inhibin, and the Leydig cell has been reported to produce both inhibin (2) and activin (3).

In previous studies, men with spontaneous hypogonadotropic hypogonadism were used as models to investigate the gonadotropin regulation of spermatogenesis (1). However, because of uncertainties regarding the degree of gonadotropin deficiency and normality of testicular responsiveness in these men and the lack of pure gonadotropin preparations for replacement therapy, the specific roles of LH and FSH in the control of sperm production in men have been unclear. To clarify the relative roles of LH and FSH in the regulation of human spermatogenesis and inhibin production, we performed a series of studies involving selective gonadotropin replacement using highly purified gonadotropin preparations in normal men in whom gonadotropin deficiency was induced by administration of T-enanthate (200 mg I.M. weekly for several months).

As a result of negative feedback at the hypothalamus and pituitary, high-dosage T-administration in normal men produces results from profound suppression of gonadotropin secretion and sperm production to severe oligozoospermia or azoospermia (1). In this setting of experimentally induced hypogonadotropism, we tested the effect of selective gonadotropin replacement on spermatogenesis. This allowed us to determine the separate roles of LH and FSH in the control of sperm and inhibin production in normal men. In contrast to previous studies in men with spontaneous hypogonadotropic hypogonadism, this experimental approach offered the advantage of determining the effect of gonadotropin treatment in men known to have normal testicular responsiveness as evidenced by normal sperm counts prior to the initiation of T.

In the initial studies, we determined whether normal blood levels of FSH were necessary for spermatogenesis. Following short-term (3–5 months) T-enanthate-induced suppression of gonadotropins and sperm and inhibin production, LH-like activity was selectively replaced in normal men. While continuing T, LH replacement was accomplished with either human chorionic gonadotropin (hCG, 5000 IU I.M. 3 times weekly for 4–6 months), which resulted in supraphysiological LH-like activity, (4, 5) or physiological dosages of human LH (hLH, 1100 IU sc daily for 4–6 months), which resulted in normal serum LH levels (6). The highly purified hLH preparation used for replacement (LER-1549) was supplied by the National Pituitary Agency and contained less than 0.2% FSH-like bioactivity. Another group of normal men received prolonged T-enanthate treatment, resulting in suppression of gonadotropin secretion for 9 months and sperm production for 6 months prior to addition of LH replacement with the same dosage of hCG (7). Despite undetectable serum and prepubertal urinary FSH levels, both supraphysiological and physiological LH replacement increased sperm concentrations significantly in all men to levels averaging 20–30 million/mL, after either short- or long-term gonadotropin suppression induced by T (Fig. 22.1).

These results demonstrated that normal FSH levels were not absolutely required for stimulation of human spermatogenesis. Similarly, serum inhibin levels were significantly increased by both LH and hCG (5). Since LH has no known direct effect on Sc, there are two other potential explanations for the LH-induced increase in inhibin levels. First, there could be an indirect effect of LH through stimulation of T-production that is known to increase peritubular myoid cell release of PModS, which has recently been shown to cause Sc secretion of inhibin (8). Second, LH could be stimulating Leydig cell production of inhibin and/or an inhibin-like substance (2).

Another study was performed to determine whether FSH replacement alone, in the presence of suppressed LH levels, was sufficient to stimulate spermatogenesis. Following suppression of gonadotropin levels and sperm production by exogenous T, human FSH (hFSH, 100 IU sc daily for 4 months) was selectively replaced in normal men (9). The highly purified hFSH preparation used for replacement (LER-1577) was also supplied by the National Pituitary Agency and contained less than 1% LH-like bioactivity. Despite markedly suppressed serum LH bioactivity, hFSH replacement stimulated sperm counts significantly in all men to mean sperm concentra-

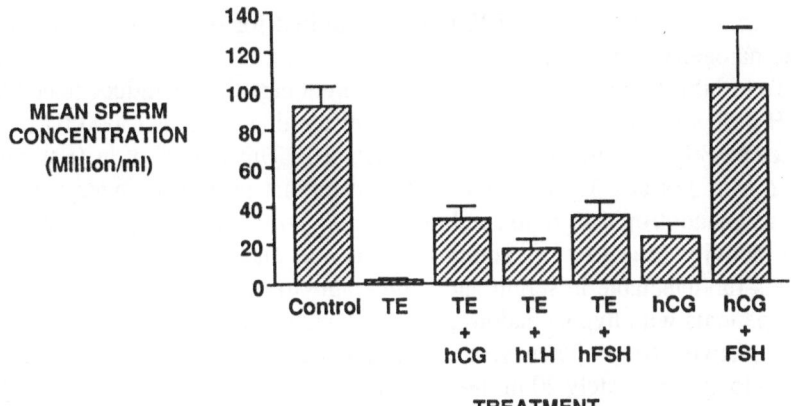

TREATMENT

FIGURE 22.1. Mean ± SEM sperm concentrations in normal men during the control period (Control) prior to hormone administration (n = 25) and with the following treatments: T-administration alone (T, 200 mg I.M. weekly for 3–9 months, n = 17); simultaneous administration of T and hCG (T + hCG, 200 mg weekly plus 5000 IU I.M. 3 times weekly, respectively, for 4–6 months, n = 17); simultaneous administration of T and hLH (T + hLH, 200 mg weekly plus 1100 IU sc daily, respectively, for 4–6 months, n = 4); simultaneous administration of T and hFSH (T + hFSH, 200 mg weekly plus 100 IU sc daily, respectively, for 4 months, n = 4); hCG administration alone (hCG, 5000 IU I.M. twice weekly for 6 months, n = 8); and simultaneous administration of hCG and FSH (hCG + FSH, hCG 5000 IU I.M. twice weekly plus hFSH, 100 IU, or hMG, 75 IU, sc daily for 4–10 months, n = 4). Experimental gonadotropin deficiency induced by T-administration alone resulted in marked suppression of sperm concentration to severely oligozoospermic or azoospermic levels. While continuing T, replacement of LH-like activity (with hCG or hLH) or FSH-like activity (with hFSH) resulted in stimulation of sperm concentrations to levels averaging 20–30 million/mL. Selective FSH deficiency induced by hCG administration alone suppressed sperm concentrations to the same level. While continuing hCG, the addition of FSH-like activity (with hFSH or hMG) restored sperm counts to control levels.

tions of approximately 30 million/mL (Fig. 22.1). These results demonstrated that FSH alone was sufficient and that normal serum LH levels were not absolutely necessary to stimulate sperm production in men. FSH also stimulated inhibin levels (5) consistent with its known effect on Sc.

In all these studies involving selective LH or FSH replacement, sperm concentrations were not consistently stimulated to control levels; instead, they averaged between 20 and 30 million/mL (Fig. 22.1). Although we demonstrated a stimulatory effect of either LH or FSH alone on spermatogenesis, neither gonadotropin was sufficient to restore completely normal numbers of sperm in all men. Therefore, we hypothesized that the stimulatory actions of both LH and FSH were required for quantitatively normal spermatogenesis in humans.

To test this hypothesis, we utilized a different paradigm to induce selective FSH deficiency in normal men. We administered hCG alone (5000 IU I.M. twice weekly for 6 months) to normal men (10). This dosage of hCG stimulated estradiol and T-production by the testis that in turn inhibited endogenous gonadotropin secretion and resulted in a hormonal setting of high LH-like activity (due to hCG administration) and markedly suppressed FSH levels (undetectable in serum and comparable to those in prepubertal boys and patients with hypogonadotropic hypogonadism in urine). In this setting of selective FSH deficiency, sperm production was partially suppressed, again to approximately 20 million/mL (Fig. 22.1).

To determine whether the suppressive effect of hCG on spermatogenesis was due to FSH deficiency induced by hCG or to a direct down-regulatory effect of hCG on the testis, FSH-like activity was replaced (with either hFSH, 100 IU, or human menopausal gonadotropin [hMG], 75 IU, sc daily for 4–10 months) in normal men receiving chronic hCG administration (10). FSH replacement restored sperm counts to control levels in all men, demonstrating that the suppression of sperm production induced by hCG was a result of FSH deficiency. These results also demonstrated the requirement of both gonadotropins for the maintenance of quantitatively normal spermatogenesis in man.

Administration of hCG alone led to a fall in inhibin levels (11) in parallel with the decrease in spermatogenesis, suggesting that the inhibin measured in blood was coming from the Sc, not the Leydig cells. When FSH administration was added to hCG, inhibin levels returned to control values (11), implying that the major source of circulating inhibin is the Sc.

Conclusion

In conclusion, our studies in normal men demonstrate that either LH or FSH when administered alone is capable of stimulating the production of normal spermatozoa; however, the total number of spermatozoa produced in the setting of stimulation by only one gonadotropin is less than normal. Similarly, either LH or FSH can stimulate inhibin secretion, but not to fully normal levels. The stimulatory effects of both FSH and LH together are required to induce quantitatively normal spermatogenesis and inhibin secretion in men. Among the practical results of these studies is the conclusion that selective suppression of FSH (e.g., by inhibin) is very unlikely to be an effective male contraceptive since the remaining LH stimulus is capable of stimulating production of spermatozoa to the level likely to cause fertility.

References

1. Matsumoto AM, Bremner WJ. Endocrinology of the hypothalamic-pituitary-testicular axis with particular reference to the hormonal control of spermatogenesis. Bailliere's Clin Endocrinol Metab 1987;1:71-87.
2. Risbridger GP, Clements J, Robertson DM, et al. Immuno- and bioactive inhibin and inhibin-subunit expression in rat Leydig cell cultures. Mol Cell Endocrinol 1989;66:119-22.
3. Lee W, Mason AJ, Schwall R, Szonyi E, Mather JP. Secretion of activin by interstitial cells in the testis. Science 1989;243:396-8.
4. Bremner WJ, Matsumoto AM, Sussman AM, Paulsen CA. Follicle-stimulating hormone and human spermatogenesis. J Clin Invest 1981;68:1044-52.
5. McLachlan RI, Matsumoto AM, Burger HG, deKretser DM, Bremner WJ. The relative roles of follicle-stimulating hormone and luteinizing hormone in the control of inhibin secretion in normal men. J Clin Invest 1988;82:880-4.
6. Matsumoto AM, Paulsen CA, Bremner WJ. Stimulation of sperm production by human luteinizing hormone in gonadotropin-suppressed normal men. J Clin Endocrinol Metab 1984;59:882-7.
7. Matsumoto AM, Bremner WJ. Stimulation of sperm production human chorionic gonadotropin after prolonged gonadotropin suppression in normal men. J Androl 1985;6:137-43.
8. Skinner MK, McLachlan RI, Bremner WJ. Stimulation of Sertoli cell inhibin secretion by the testicular paracrine factor P-Mod-S. Mol Cell Endocrinol 1989; 66:239-49.
9. Matsumoto AM, Karpas AE, Paulsen CA, Bremner WJ. Reinitiation of sperm production in gonadotropin-suppressed normal men by administration of follicle-stimulating hormone. J Clin Invest. 1983;72:1005-15.
10. Matsumoto AM, Karpas AE, Bremner WJ. Chronic human chorionic gonadotropin administration in normal men: evidence that follicle-stimulating hormone is necessary for the maintenance of quantitatively normal spermatogenesis in man. J Clin Endocrinol Metab 1986;62:1184-92.
11. McLachlan RI, Matsumoto AM, Burger HG, deKretser DM, Bremner WJ. Follicle-stimulating hormone is required for quantitatively normal inhibin secretion in men. J Clin Endocrinol Metab 1988;67:1305-8.

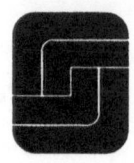

23

Gonadotropin Releasing Hormone Pulse Patterns in the Regulation of FSH Secretion

JOHN C. MARSHALL, ALAN C. DALKIN, G. TIMOTHY GOODMAN, DANIEL J. HAISENLEDER, SANDER J. PAUL, AND ROBERT P. KELCH

Reproductive function is controlled by the pituitary glycoproteins, luteinizing hormone (LH) and follicle stimulating hormone (FSH). The two hormones are composed of a common α-subunit and distinct β-subunits (1, 2). LH and FSH are secreted by the same pituitary gonadotrope cells, and their synthesis and secretion is controlled by the hypothalamic decapeptide gonadotropin releasing hormone (GnRH). GnRH is secreted into the hypophysial-portal blood in an intermittent manner (3, 4), and this pulsatile secretion is essential for maintaining gonadotropin synthesis and release (5–7). The pattern of pulsatile GnRH secretion changes in various physiologic circumstances (8, 9), and differential secretion of LH and FSH also occurs. Thus, it appears that a single gonadotropin releasing hormone can effect differential secretion of LH and FSH by the pituitary gonadotrope cell. Gonadal steroids can alter the pattern of GnRH secretion and also modify gonadotrope responses to GnRH. Inhibin, a gonadal polypeptide, acts directly on the pituitary to selectively inhibit FSH secretion. Other gonadal peptides, such as activin, may also be involved in modifying gonadotrope responses to GnRH. Thus, the differential regulation of LH and FSH synthesis and secretion appears to result from changes in the pattern of the GnRH stimulus together with the direct feedback effects of gonadal steroids and peptides on the gonadotrope.

In this chapter, we examine the potential role of altered GnRH stimulation of the gonadotrope with emphasis on the preferential synthesis and secretion of FSH. In vivo data from human and primate studies are reviewed to address the changes that occur in pulsatile LH (and by inference, hypothalamic GnRH) secretion. In the subsequent section, we review experimental data in animals, in which the effects of different GnRH pulse stimuli in regulating expression of the gonadotropin subunit genes were examined.

Normal human physiologic data were obtained in studies in the Clinical Research Center at the University of Michigan. Most studies of gonadotropin subunit gene expression examined steady state mRNA concentrations that were measured using cDNA clones originally provided by Dr. W.W. Chin (rat α and LHβ [10, 11]) and Dr. R.A. Maurer (FSHβ [12]). Measurements of α, LHβ and FSHβ gene transcription rates were made in collaborative studies with Dr. M.A. Shupnik (13).

In Vivo Studies of Pulsatile GnRH and FSH Secretion

Secretion of GnRH by the hypothalamus cannot be measured directly in humans, but data from animals have shown that pulses of LH in peripheral plasma reflect pulsatile secretion of GnRH by the hypothalamus (3, 4). Thus, in human studies, changes in pulsatile LH secretion are used to infer GnRH secretion by the hypothalamus.

Pubertal Maturation

During the first few months of life, gonadotropin secretion occurs in a pulsatile manner, and plasma gonadotropins are elevated. Data from infant monkeys suggest that GnRH is secreted at approximately 1 pulse/h in males and at a somewhat slower frequency of 1 pulse every 3–4 h in females (14, 15). By the end of the first year of life, plasma gonadotropin levels, particularly those of LH, decline (which results in a high FSH:LH ratio), and LH responsiveness to exogenous GnRH falls. Gonadotropins remain low during the first decade of life. In prepubertal children, gonadotropins, presumably responding to hypothalamic GnRH pulses, are secreted at a low level (16–18). Recent studies using frequent sampling have shown that the frequency of GnRH pulses is slow in prepubertal children, occurring approximately every 3–4 h during the day (19, 20), with a small augmentation of both frequency and amplitude during sleep (21). At this stage of development, gonadotropin responses to exogenous GnRH show predominant secretion of FSH rather than LH, and this is particularly pronounced in girls (22).

Pubertal maturation is initiated by amplification of gonadotropin secretion, which first occurs during sleep. This nocturnal increase in gonadotropins is consequent upon an increase in the frequency and amplitude of GnRH release (19–23). The frequency of LH pulses approximates 1/h during the early part of sleep. LH pulse frequency tends to fall during the early morning hours, coincident with the rise in plasma testosterone (T) consequent upon enhanced gonadotropin secretion (19). Serial studies of responses to exogenous GnRH have revealed that the initial prepubertal predominance of FSH secretion diminishes and LH responsiveness increases as puberty advances.

In humans, the mechanisms involved in changing the patterns of GnRH secretion remain uncertain, but do not appear to involve opiates (24, 25). However, a consistent association between GnRH stimulatory pattern and gonadotropin secretion appears to be present. Prepubertally, when GnRH pulses are of low amplitude and slow frequency, the predominant gonadotropin secreted is FSH. With the increase in amplitude and frequency of GnRH stimulation during puberty, FSH release diminishes, whereas that of LH increases. These data suggest a potential relationship between the pattern of the GnRH stimulus and the predominant gonadotropin released.

Ovulatory Menstrual Cycles in Women

Several studies have used multiple sampling techniques to document the changes in pulsatile LH (GnRH) secretion during ovulatory menstrual cycles (26–30). In the early follicular phase, LH pulses occur every 90–100 min, and, as plasma estradiol and inhibin levels are low, GnRH effects release of both FSH and LH. Mean plasma FSH concentrations often exceed those in LH in view of the longer half-life of FSH (approximately 3 h). By the midfollicular phase, GnRH pulses occur every 60–90 min, and the increasing estradiol (perhaps in concert with inhibin from the enlarging follicle) inhibits FSH release, and plasma FSH falls. GnRH pulses continue to occur at a rapid frequency of approximately 1 pulse/h in the presence of the rising plasma estradiol. As estradiol concentrations rise further, the positive feedback effects of estradiol become manifest, and LH responsiveness to each GnRH pulse is enhanced, leading to the midcycle preovulatory (PO) LH surge. The increase in FSH released during the surge may be consequent upon increased amplitude of GnRH stimulation (31) at a time when plasma levels of estradiol are falling and those of progesterone (P) are rising (32, 33).

The frequency of GnRH secretion slows after ovulation, and by the midluteal phase, LH pulses of irregular amplitude occur every 3–5 h. This slowing of pulsatile GnRH release appears to reflect the effects of P and estradiol acting to increase hypothalamic opioid tone, with subsequent reduction in GnRH pulse frequency (34–38).

As a corpus luteum regresses plasma estradiol, P and inhibin concentrations fall. The frequency of GnRH secretion increases, returning to a rapid-frequency consistent-amplitude stimulus. As noted below, the slow irregular GnRH stimulus in the midluteal phase may not be optimal for LHβ synthesis, and this, together with the intermittent release of LH, would deplete pituitary LH stores. Estradiol and inhibin selectively reduce FSH release, and as the slower irregular GnRH stimulus maintains FSH synthesis, pituitary FSH stores are maintained. Thus, the increase in GnRH pulse frequency acts on a gonadotrope cell primed to release FSH, resulting in the selective increase in plasma FSH that may be critical for initiating the development of ovarian follicles during the next cycle (7).

These data suggest that the slowing of GnRH stimulation of the gonadotrope in the luteal phase may be important in allowing selective FSH secretion to begin the next cycle (39, 40). This view is supported by studies that show that administration of GnRH at rapid frequencies in the luteal phase leads to subsequent deficient follicular development and corpus luteum function in later cycles (41, 42).

Anovulation

Abnormal patterns of pulsatile GnRH secretion have been found in several clinical conditions associated with the absence of cyclic ovulation. Hypothalamic amenorrhea (HA) is a disorder—often preceded by weight loss, strenuous exercise, or physiological stress—in which abnormalities of pituitary or ovarian function cannot be demonstrated (43, 44). In some women, removal of the precipitating factor(s) does not result in the return of ovulatory cycles, and studies of pulsatile LH secretion have shown that GnRH pulse frequency is markedly reduced in a majority of patients (43). The frequency of GnRH pulses (1 pulse every 3–4 h) is similar to that present in the luteal phase of ovulatory cycles. However, in contrast to the luteal phase, the slow GnRH pulses are commonly associated with circulating levels of FSH that exceed those of LH. GnRH pulse frequency can be increased to normal follicular frequencies by administration of the opioid receptor blocker, naloxone, in 60%–70% of women with HA (45, 46). These data indicate that anovulation in HA may reflect excess hypothalamic opioid activity that slows pulsatile GnRH secretion to a level that does not maintain the level of LH synthesis and secretion required for the PO surge.

Similar findings have been observed in women with hyperprolactinemia. LH pulses are of irregular amplitude and occur at slow frequency, but return to normal follicular phase patterns if prolactin is suppressed by a dopamine agonist (47, 48). Similar to findings in HA, mean plasma FSH concentrations are commonly in the normal range, while LH levels are low in hyperprolactinemic women. Thus, in both these anovulatory conditions, a slow-frequency GnRH stimulus is usually associated with reduced plasma LH but preserved FSH secretion.

A possible reversal of the relationship between slow GnRH pulses and maintained FSH secretion may be present in polycystic ovarian disease (PCO). The exact etiology of androgen excess in PCO may involve several mechanisms (49–51), but a majority of patients (approximately 75%) have elevated plasma LH, normal or low FSH, and rapid-frequency LH (GnRH) pulses of approximately 1 pulse/h. This increased GnRH stimulus appears to maintain the elevated LH and ovarian androgen secretion (52–54). Ovulation occurs infrequently in this women; thus, the normal slowing of GnRH pulses in the luteal phase does not occur. This may impair the ability to selectively increase plasma FSH and induce follicular development and, thus, could be an important factor in the irregular and infrequent ovulation in PCO (55).

In these anovulatory conditions, slow-frequency GnRH stimulation, such as that found in HA and hyperprolactinemia, is commonly associated with maintenance of normal FSH concentrations in plasma. In PCO, the persistent rapid GnRH stimulus and the apparent failure to slow GnRH secretion may be factors in reducing the selective secretion of FSH that occurs during the luteal-follicular transition in normal ovulatory cycles.

GnRH Pulses and Regulation of Gonadotropin Subunit Gene Expression

Quantification of gonadotropin subunit mRNA concentrations during the 4-day estrous cycle in rats has revealed evidence of both coordinate and differential changes in subunit mRNA concentrations (56, 57). On the morning of metestrus, FSHβ mRNA was increased (2-fold) and fell to basal values by evening. Alpha and LHβ mRNAs were unchanged on metestrus, but both increased 2-fold during diestrus when FSHβ remained stable. These changes occurred in the presence of low plasma concentrations of LH and FSH. On the afternoon of proestrus, LHβ mRNA increased 3-fold just prior to the PO LH surge. FSHβ mRNA also increased (4-fold), but values were maximal 2 h after the beginning of the FSH surge. Alpha mRNA was unchanged during the gonadotropin surges. Thus, coordinate increases in α- and LHβ mRNA occur on diestrus, and both β-subunit mRNAs increased during the gonadotropin surges. In contrast, FSHβ mRNA alone was elevated on metestrus.

The mechanisms involved in regulating subunit expression during the estrous cycle remain unknown, but may involve the effects of different GnRH stimulatory patterns. Pulsatile GnRH release changes during the cycle, as do circulating concentrations of inhibin. The selective increases in FSH mRNA on metestrus occurred at a time when GnRH pulses occur at low amplitude and slow frequency. Both the amplitude and frequency of GnRH pulses increase during the proestrus LH surge (58, 59), a time when both β-subunits were increased. These physiologic data have suggested that the pattern of GnRH stimulation may be one factor that determines differential expression of the gonadotropin subunit genes.

We have examined this question by administering GnRH pulses at various amplitudes and frequencies to GnRH-deficient rats. Castrate male rats were replaced with testosterone (T) from subcutaneous implants (serum T = 2.5

ng/mL). Testosterone replacement in this manner prevents the postcastration increase in gonadotropins and GnRH receptors, suggesting that T reduces or abolishes the increase in GnRH secretion after castration (60). Also, LH pulses occur infrequently in castrate T-replaced rats, with 75% of the animals having less than 4 LH pulses in 24 h (61). Thus, the castrate T-replaced rat is a convenient model for studying the effects of exogenous GnRH stimulatory patterns in the presence of a stable T-milieu.

Effects of GnRH Pulse Amplitude

GnRH pulses were given every 30 min—the frequency of GnRH pulse secretion in castrate rats—to castrate T-replaced animals. After 48 h of GnRH pulses, LH responses to GnRH, the number of pituitary GnRH receptors, and LHβ mRNA concentrations were all maximal after 25-ng GnRH pulses, with lower or higher amplitude pulses being less effective. In contrast, all doses of GnRH used (10–250 ng/pulse) increased α- and FSHβ mRNAs, indicating that these two subunits were expressed to a similar degree in response to a wide range of GnRH stimuli (62–64).

Similar effects were observed in female rats. When ovariectomized estradiol-replaced animals were given similar GnRH pulse regimens, both LHβ and FSHβ mRNAs were elevated by lower GnRH doses (0.5–25 ng/pulse) than were effective in males. Higher doses per pulse did not increase β-subunit mRNAs, but α-mRNA was increased (65). These data indicate that the amplitude of GnRH pulse stimulus can exert differential effects on subunit mRNA concentrations. Alpha and FSHβ mRNA expression appear to be relatively independent of GnRH pulse amplitude. However, LHβ mRNA expression is highly sensitive to changes in GnRH dose/pulse, and maximum concentrations only occur in response to a narrow range of GnRH pulse amplitude.

Responses of mRNA to different GnRH pulse amplitudes can be modified by the circulating concentration of plasma T. FSHβ mRNA responses were similar after T-replacement in the low or high physiologic range. Responses of α-mRNA tended to be lower in the presence of a high physiologic T, as were LHβ mRNA responses to the higher GnRH pulse amplitudes (75–250 ng/pulse) (64).

Effects of Changing GnRH Pulse Frequency

Gonadotropin subunit mRNA responses to GnRH pulses given at different frequencies were also examined in the castrate T-replaced male rat model. GnRH pulses (25 ng/pulse) were given at intervals between 8–480 min for a duration of 24–48 h. GnRH receptors (GnRH-R) were increased by GnRH pulses given at all intervals of less than 120 min, and acute LH release was maximal after pulses given every 15–60 min. GnRH given every 30 min produced maximum responses of GnRH-R and α- and LHβ subunit mRNAs, and values increased to levels similar to those present in castrate males (66, 67). Subsequent studies also examined the effect of GnRH pulse frequency on FSHβ mRNA expression. When given at constant amplitude (25 ng/pulse), fast-frequency GnRH pulses (every 8 min) maximally increased α-MRNA and also increased LHβ mRNA. All three subunit mRNAs were increased after pulses given every 30 min. In contrast, pulses given every 120 min or longer did not increase α- and LHβ mRNAs, but maintained the elevated level of FSHβ mRNA (68).

These effects of GnRH pulse frequency in differentially regulating the concentration of steady state mRNAs appear to be exerted at the level of gene transcription (69). Using the same experimental model, fast-frequency GnRH pulses increased α-transcription, while LHβ transcription rates were only increased after GnRH given every 30 min. Interestingly, FSHβ transcription rates were only elevated after 120-min pulses, similar to results observed for cytosolic mRNA concentrations. The pulsatile GnRH stimulus was essential for increasing subunit transcription rates, as continuous administration of GnRH by infusion did not increase transcription of any of the three subunit genes above control values.

Others have observed similar effects of GnRH pulse frequency in sheep models (70). Pulses given every 30 min increased α-mRNA, whereas pulses given every 60 min increased all three subunit mRNAs. Of interest, GnRH given at slower frequencies did not selectively increase FSHβ mRNA in this model. This may reflect the different steroid milieu, as P was used to inhibit endogenous GnRH secretion in sheep and P can inhibit FSHβ transcription in vitro (71).

The above results indicate that the pattern of GnRH stimulation, both amplitude and frequency, can exert differential effects on expression of the gonadotropin subunit genes. This action of GnRH was observed in the presence of T. In vivo, these responses to GnRH may well be modified by the prevailing steroid/gonadal peptide milieu, which could further modify subunit mRNA responses.

Summary

The data reviewed above suggest that the ability to change the pattern of GnRH secretion may be an important regulatory factor in allowing a single GnRH to differentially stimulate the synthesis and secretion of LH and FSH. The results from in vivo studies in humans and primates, showing changes in gonadotropin secretion and GnRH pulse frequency, are in good overall agreement with animal studies of GnRH regulation of gonadotropin subunit gene expression. Slow-frequency GnRH secretion is usually associated with maintained plasma concentrations of FSH and low levels of LH. The data in rats suggest that this effect may in part reflect the ability of slow-frequency GnRH signals of all amplitudes to maintain elevated concentrations of FSHβ mRNA. Rapid-frequency GnRH stimuli commonly are associated with elevated concentrations of LH in plasma. This is also in accord with the animal experiments whereby LHβ gene expression is increased by faster-frequency stimuli. Also, the amplitude of the GnRH signal is important in determining the magnitude of the LHβ mRNA response, which may have implications for increased LH synthesis prior to the midcycle LH surge. The mechanisms whereby altered GnRH signal patterns effect differential gonadotropin subunit gene expression remain uncertain. Our recent studies indicate that these actions are exerted at the level of transcription of the genes, though other actions, such as stabilization of FSHβ mRNA by T or activin (72–75), may also be important.

The factors involved in the differential synthesis and secretion of LH and FSH are complex and involve the actions of gonadal steroids and peptides directly on the gonadotrope cell (76). The extent and nature of these interactions remain to be clarified, but present data indicate that the pattern of the GnRH stimulus is also an important determinant of gonadotropin synthesis and secretion. Thus, the ability to change the pattern of GnRH stimulation may be an important mechanism for stimulating differential synthesis and secretion of LH and FSH. Results from clinical studies in anovulatory women suggest that the inability to change the amplitude and frequency of GnRH secretion may be associated with failure of ovarian follicular maturation and ovulation.

References

1. Pierce JG, Parsons TF. Glycoprotein hormones: structure and function. Annu Rev Biochem 1981;50:465.
2. Chin WW. Glycoprotein hormone genes. In: Habener JF, ed. Genes encoding hormones and regulatory peptides. Clifton, NJ: Human Press, 1987:137-72.
3. Clark IJ, Cummins JT. Temporal relationship between gonadotropin-releasing hormone (GnRH) and luteinizing hormone (LH) secretion in ovariectomized ewes. Endocrinology 1982;111:1737.
4. Urbanski HF, Pickle RL, Ramirez UD. Simultaneous measurement of GnRH, LH and FSH in the ovariectomized rat. Endocrinology 1988;123:413.
5. Belchetz PE, Plant TM, Nakai Y, Keogh EG, Knobil E. Hypophyseal responses to continuous and intermittent delivery of hypothalamic gonadotropin-releasing hormone. Science 1978;202:631.
6. Bergquist C, Nillius SJ, Wide L. Inhibition of ovulation in women by intranasal treatment with a LHRH agonist. Contraception 1979;19:497.

7. Marshall JC, Kelch RP. Gonadotropin-releasing hormone: role of pulsatile secretion in the regulation of reproduction. N Engl J Med 1986;315:1459.

8. Santen RJ, Bardin CW. Episodic luteinizing hormone secretion in man. J Clin Invest 1973;52:2617.

9. Yen SSC, Tsai CC, Naftolin F, Vanderberg G, Ajabor L. Pulsatile patterns of gonadotropin release in subjects with and without ovarian function. J Clin Endocrinol Metab 1972;34:671.

10. Godine, JE, Chin WW, Habener JF. Alpha subunit of rat pituitary glycoprotein hormone. Primary structure of the precursor determined from the nucleotide sequence of cloned cDNAs. J Biol Chem 1982;257:8368.

11. Jameson JL, Chin WW, Hollenberg AM, Chang AS, Habener JF. The gene encoding the beta subunit of rat LH. J Biol Chem 1983;259:15474.

12. Maurer RA. Molecular cloning and nucleotide sequence analysis of the cDNA for the beta subunit of rat follicle-stimulating hormone. Mol Cell Endocrinol 1987;1:717.

13. Shupnik MA, Gharib SD, Chin WW. Divergent effects of estradiol on gonadotropin gene transcription in pituitary fragments. Mol Cell Endocrinol 1989;3:474.

14. Plant TM. Pulsatile luteinizing hormone secretion in the neonatal male rhesus monkey. J Endocrinol 1982;93:71.

15. Plant TM. A striking sex difference in the gonadotropin response to gonadectomy during infantile development in the rhesus monkey. Endocrinology 1986; 119:539.

16. Jakacki RI, Kelch RP, Sauder SE, Lloyd JS, Hopwood NJ, Marshall JC. Pulsatile secretion of luteinizing hormone in children. J Clin Endocrinol Metab 1982; 55:453.

17. Penny R, Olambiwonnu NO, Frasier SD. Episodic fluctuations of plasma gonadotropins in pre and postpubertal girls and boys. J Clin Endocrinol Metab 1977;45:307.

18. Wennink JMB, Delemarre-Van deWaal HA, Van Kessel H, Mulder GH, Foster JP, Schoemaker J. LH secretion patterns in boys at the onset of puberty using a highly sensitive immunoradiometric assay. J Clin Endocrinol Metab 1988;67: 924.

19. Hale PM, Khoury S, Foster CM, et al. Increased LH pulse frequency during sleep in early to mid-pubertal boys: effects of testosterone infusion. J Clin Endocrinol Metab 1988;66:785.

20. Wu FCW, Borrow SM, Nicol K, Elton R, Hunter WM. Ontogeny of pulsatile gonadotropin secretion and pituitary responsiveness in male puberty in man: a mixed longitudinal and cross sectional study. J Endocrinol 1989;123:347.

21. Kelch RP, Khoury SA, Hale PM, Hopwood NJ, Marshall JC. Pulsatile secretion of gonadotropins in children. In: Crowley WF, Hoffer JG, eds. The episodic secretion of hormones. New York: Churchill Livingstone, 1987:187.

22. Kelch RP, Marshall JC, Sauder SE, Hopwood NJ, Reame NE. Gonadotropin regulation during human puberty. In: Reid RL, ed. Neuroendocrine aspects of reproduction. New York: Academic Press, 1983;25:229-56.

23. Wu FCW, Butler GE, Kelnar CJH, Sellar RE. Patterns of pulsatile LH secretion before and during the onset of puberty in boys: a study using an immunoradiometric assay. J Clin Endocrinol Metab 1990;70:629.

24. Sauder SE, Case GD, Hopwood NJ, Kelch RP, Marshall JC. The effects of opiate

antagonism on gonadotropin secretion in children and in women with hypothalamic amenorrhea. Pediatric Res 1984;18:322.

25. Mauras N, Veldhuis JD, Rogol L. Role of endogenous opioids in pubertal maturation: opposing actions of naltrexone in prepubertal and late pubertal boys. J Clin Endocrinol Metab 1986;62:1256.

26. Backstrom CT, McNeilly AS, Leask RM, Baird DT. Pulsatile secretion of LH, FSH, prolactin, estradiol and progesterone during the human menstrual cycle. Clin Endocrinol (Oxf) 1982;17:29.

27. Santen RJ, Bardin CW. Episodic luteinizing hormone secretion in man. J Clin Invest 1973;52:2617.

28. Reame N, Sauder SE, Kelch RP, Marshall JC. Pulsatile gonadotropin secretion during the human menstrual cycle—evidence for altered frequency of gonadotropin-releasing hormone secretion. J Clin Endocrinol Metab 1984;59:328.

29. Crowley WF, Filicori M, Spratt DI, Santoro NF. The physiology of GnRH secretion in men and women. Recent Prog Horm Res 1985;41:473.

30. Yen SSC, Tsai CC, Naftolin S, Vandenberg G, Ajabor L. Pulsatile patterns of gonadotropin-release in subjects with and without ovarian function. J Clin Endocrinol Metab 1972;34:671.

31. Sarkar DK, Chiappa SA, Fink G, Sherwood NM. Gonadotropin-releasing hormone surge in proestrus rats. Nature 1974;264:461.

32. Liu JH, Yen SSC. Induction of the mid-cycle gonadotropin surge by ovarian steroids in women—a critical evaluation. J Clin Endocrinol Metab 1983;57:797.

33. Hoff JD, Quigley ME, Yen SSC. Hormonal dynamics at mid cycle: a reevaluation. J Clin Endocrinol Metab 1983;57:792.

34. Soules MR, Steiner RA, Clifton DK, Cohen NL, Aksel S, Bremner WJ. Progesterone modulation of pulsatile luteinizing hormone secretion in normal women. J Clin Endocrinol Metab 1984;58:378.

35. Nippoldt TB, Reame NE, Kelch RP, Marshall JC. The roles of estradiol and progesterone in decreasing LH pulse frequency in the luteal phase of the menstrual cycle. J Clin Endocrinol Metab 1989;69:67.

36. Wardlaw SL, Wehrenberg WB, Ferin M, Antunes, JL, Frantz AG. Effect of sex steroids on beta endorphin in hypophyseal-portal blood. J Clin Endocrinol Metab 1982;55:877.

37. VanVugt DA, Lam NY, Ferin M. Reduced frequency of pulsatile LH secretion in the luteal phase of the rhesus monkey—involvement of endogenous opiates. Endocrinology 1984;115:1095.

38. Quigley ME, Yen SSC. The role of endogenous opiates on LH secretion during the menstrual cycle. J Clin Endocrinol Metab 1980;51:179.

39. Mais V, Cetel NS, Muse KN, Quigley ME, Reid RL, Yen SSC. Hormone dynamics during luteal-follicular transition. J Clin Endocrinol Metab 1987;64:1109.

40. Filicori M, Santoro N, Merriam G, Crowley WF. Characterization of the physiologic pattern of episodic gonadotropin secretion throughout the human menstrual cycle. J Clin Endocrinol Metab 1986;62:1136.

41. Lam NY, Ferin M. Is the decrease in the hypophysiotropic signal frequency normally observed during the luteal phase important for menstrual cyclicity in the primate? Endocrinology 1987;120:2044.

42. Soules MR, Clifton DK, Bremner WJ, Steiner RA. Corpus luteum insufficiency

induced by rapid GnRH induced gonadotropin secretion pattern in the follicular phase. J Clin Endocrinol Metab 1987;65:475.

43. Reame NE, Sauder SE, Case GD, Kelch RP, Marshall JC. Pulsatile gonadotropin secretion in women with hypothalamic amenorrhea: evidence that reduced frequency of GnRH secretion is the mechanism of persistent ovulation. J Clin Endocrinol Metab 1985;61:851.

44. Schwartz B, Cumming DC, Riordan E, Selye M, Yen SSC, Rebar RW. Exercise associated amenorrhea: a distinct entity? Am J Obstet Gynecol 1981;141:662.

45. Khoury SA, Reame NE, Kelch RP, Marshall JC. Diurnal patterns of pulsatile LH secretion in hypothalamic amenorrhea: reproducibility and responses to opiate blockade and an alpha 2-adrenergic agonist. J Clin Endocrinol Metab 1987;64: 755.

46. Wildt L, Leyendecker G. Induction of ovulation by chronic administration of naltrexone in hypothalamic amenorrhea. J Clin Endocrinol Metab 1987;64: 1334.

47. Klibanski A, Beitins IZ, Merriam GR, McArthur JW, Zervas MT, Ridgway EC. Gonadotropin and prolactin pulsations in hyperprolactinemic women before and during bromocroptine therapy. J Clin Endocrinol Metab 1984;58:1141.

48. Sauder SE, Frager M, Case GD, Kelch RP, Marshall JC. Abnormal patterns of pulsatile luteinizing hormone secretion in women with hyperprolactinemia and amenhorrhea: responses to bromocriptine. J Clin Endocrinol Metab 1984;59:941.

49. Barnes R, Rosenfield RL. The polycystic ovary syndrome: pathogenesis and treatment. Ann Intern Med 1989;110:386.

50. Dunaif A, Graf M. Insulin administration alters gonadal steroid metabolism independent of changes in gonadotropin secretion in insulin resistant women with polycystic ovary syndrome. J Clin Invest 1989;83:23.

51. Erikson GF, Magoffin DA, Cragun JR, Chang RJ. The effects of insulin and insulin-like growth factor I and II on estradiol production by granulosa cells of polycystic ovaries. J Clin Endocrinol Metab 1990;70:894.

52. Chang RJ, Laufer LR, Meldrum DR. Steroid secretion in polycystic ovarian disease after ovarian suppression by a long-acting GnRH agonist. J Clin Endocrinol Metab 1983;56:897.

53. Kazer RR, Kessel B, Yen SSC. LH pulse frequency in women with PCO. J Clin Endocrinol Metab 1987;65:223.

54. Waldstreicher J, Santoro NS, Hall JE, Filicori M, Crowley WF. Hyperfunction of the hypothalamic-pituitary axis in women with PCO. J Clin Endocrinol Metab 1988;66:165.

55. Christman GM, Randolph JF, Kelch RP, Marshall JC. Reduction of GnRH pulse frequency induces preferential FSH secretion and follicular development in women with polycystic ovarian disease [Abstract 990]. Proc 71st meet Endocr Soc. 1989:270.

56. Zmeili SM, Papavasiliou SS, Thorner MO, Evans WS, Marshall JC, Landefeld TD. Alpha and LH beta subunit mRNAs during the rat estrous cycle. Endocrinology 1986;119:1867.

57. Ortolano GA, Haisenleder DJ, Dalkin AC, et al. FSH beta subunit mRNA concentrations during the rat estrous cycle. Endocrinology 1988;123:2149.

58. Fox SE, Smith MS. Changes in the pulsatile pattern of LH secretion during the rat estrous cycle. Endocrinology 1985;116:1485.

59. Levine JE, Ramirez VD. LHRH release during the rat estrous cycle and ovariectomy as estimated with push-pull cannulae. Endocrinology 1982;111: 1439.

60. Garcia A, Schiff M, Marshall JC. Regulation of pituitary GnRH receptors by pulsatile GnRH injections in male rats—modulation by testosterone. J Clin Invest 1984;74:920.

61. Steiner RA, Bremner WJ, Clifton DK. Regulation of LH pulse frequency and amplitude by testosterone in the adult male rat. Endocrinology 1982;111:2055.

62. Haisenleder DJ, Katt JA, Ortolano GA, et al. Influence of GnRH pulse amplitude, frequency and treatment duration on the regulation of LH subunit mRNAs and LH secretion. Mol Cell Endocrinol 1988;2:338.

63. Haisenleder DJ, Ortolano GA, Dalkin AC, Paul SJ, Chin WW, Marshall JC. GnRH regulation of gonadotropin subunit gene expression: studies in T_3 suppressed rats. J Endocrinol 1989;122:117.

64. Iliff-Sizemore SA, Ortolano GA, Haisenleder DJ, Dalkin AC, Krueger KA, Marshall JC. Testosterone differentially modulates gonadotropin subunit mRNA responses to GnRH pulse amplitude. Endocrinology 1990.

65. Haisenleder DJ, Ortolano GA, Dalkin AC, Ellis TR, Paul SJ, Marshall JC. Differential regulation of gonadotropin subunit gene expression by GnRH pulse amplitude in female rats. Endocrinology 1990.

66. Haisenleder DJ, Khoury S, Zmeili SM, et al. The frequency of GnRH secretion regulates expression of alpha and LH beta subunit mRNAs in male rats. Mol Cell Endocrinol 1987;1:834.

67. Katt JA, Duncan JA, Herbon L, Barkan A, Marshall JC. The frequency of GnRH stimulation determines the number of pituitary GnRH receptors. Endocrinology 1985;116:2113.

68. Dalkin AC, Haisenleder DJ, Ortolano GA, Ellis TR, Marshall JC. The frequency of GnRH stimulation differentially regulates gonadotropin subunit mRNA expression. Endocrinology 1989;125:917.

69 Haisenleder DJ, Dalkin AC, Ortolano GA, Marshall JC, Shupnik MA. A pulsatile GnRH stimulus is required to increase transcription of the gonadotropin subunit genes: evidence for differential regulation of transcription by pulse frequency. Endocrinology 1990.

70. Leung K, Kaynard AH, Negrini BP, Kim KE, Maurer RA, Landefeld TD. Differential regulation of gonadotropin subunit mRNAs by GnRH pulse frequency in ewes. Mol Cell Endocrinol 1987;2:724.

71. Phillips CL, LeeWen L, Wu JC, Guzman K, Milsted A, Miller WL. 17-Beta estradiol and progesterone inhibit transcription of the genes encoding the subunits of ovine FSH. Mol Cell Endocrinol 1988;2:641.

72. Carroll RS, Corrigan AZ, Gharib SD, Vale W, Chin WW. Inhibin, activin and follistatin-regulation of FSH beta mRNA levels. Mol Cell Endocrinol 1989;3: 1969.

73. Carroll RS, Corrigan AZ, Chin WW. Effect of activin on FSH beta mRNA stability in cultured pituitary cells [Abstract 777]. Proc 72nd annu meet Endocr Soc. 1990:219.

74. Paul SJ, Ortolano GA, Marshall JC. Testosterone selective increases FSH beta mRNA in the absence of GnRH stimulation of the gonadotrope. Clin Res 1990; 38:297A.

75. Perheentupa A, Huhtaniemi I. Gonadotropin gene expression and secretion in GnRH antagonist treated male rats—effects of sex steroid replacement. Endocrinology 1990;126:3204.
76. Gharib SD, Wierman ME, Shupnik MA, Chin WW. Molecular biology of the pituitary gonadotropins. Endocr Rev 1990;11:177.

24

Hypergonadotropic Forms
of Amenorrhea

ROBERT W. REBAR, JANET M. CARTER, JUNG GU KIM,
CYNTHIA K. SITES, DINA Y. SONG, AND ANDREW R. LABARBERA

Circulating concentrations of follicle stimulating hormone (FSH) increase dramatically following both bilateral oophorectomy and the menopause. Thus, by definition, young women with hypergonadotropic amenorrhea should have premature ovarian failure (POF). This belief was based on the findings of Goldenberg et al. (1), who reported that without exception, individuals with FSH levels of greater than 40 mIU/mL 2nd IRP-hMG (International Reference Preparation-human menopausal gonadotropins) had no viable follicles on ovarian biopsy.

That this POF might not always be permanent was first suggested by a number of isolated case reports documenting the initiation or resumption of cyclic menses and/or pregnancy. Several larger series have confirmed these reports (2). O'Herlihy and coworkers (3) noted that as many as 1/4 of younger women with ovulatory disorders associated with circulating FSH levels in the menopausal range will spontaneously resume ovulation, and a few will even conceive. In 1982 we reported that 9 of 18 such patients had circulating levels of estradiol typical of women with functioning ovarian follicles and that 4 of the 9 women undergoing ovarian biopsy had viable oocytes (4). Furthermore, circulating concentrations of serum progesterone (P) denoting ovulation were noted in 5 patients, and spontaneous pregnancy occurred in 1.

Aiman and Smentek (5), summarizing their own experience with 35 patients including 2 who conceived, surveyed the literature and noted that 18% of 157 women who had an ovarian biopsy had specimens that showed follicles with oocytes. Moreover, in their review, 14 women conceived after the onset of ovarian failure. More recently still, Hague et al. (6) saw resumption of ovarian follicular activity in 12 (17.1%) of 93 women with hypergonadotropic amenorrhea, as documented either by resumption of menses or by serial ultrasound scans that showed follicular and uterine growth with increasing endometrial thickness, together with a fall in serum gonadotropin concentrations.

These reports and observations have prompted us to continue to examine the clinical findings in our patients with hypergonadotropic amenorrhea, seen since 1978. We have believed that important generalizations about this clinical entity and our understanding of the role of FSH in follicular development and function might result from careful evaluation of these patients. That elevated peripheral concentrations of FSH can exist in women with viable oocytes is no longer questioned, but the etiology in the majority of cases remains to be defined. This review summarizes our investigations of these women.

Clinical Features

Between July 1, 1978, and December 31, 1989, 128 sequential women with hypergonadotropic amenorrhea were evaluated by one of us (R.W.R.). Data presented here represent an update of the series recently published by us (7). Inclusion criteria were (1) amenorrhea of 3 or more months' duration, (2) age under 40 years at onset of amenorrhea, and (3) circulating FSH levels of greater than 40 mIU/mL on at least 2 occasions.

All patients had a complete history and physical examination performed, as well as a number of routine laboratory tests. The endocrine tests included measurement of LH, FSH, and estradiol on at least 2 occasions and prolactin, tetraiodothyronine, TSH, antithyroglobulin, and antimicrosomal antibodies. Adrenal function was assessed, and diabetes mellitus and hypoparathyroidism were excluded. A number of laboratory tests were performed to test for an autoimmune disorder. Radiographs of the sella turcica were obtained to exclude a pituitary lesion. Since 1986 all new patients have undergone dual photon absorptiometry of the lower lumbar spine to evaluate bone density. Karyotypes have been determined from peripheral lymphocyte cultures for all patients presenting with primary amenorrhea. Patients with secondary amenorrhea were tested on the basis of age at presentation of less than 30 years and/or physician judgment.

Of the 128 women with hypergonadotropic amenorrhea, 18, or 14.1%, presented with primary amenorrhea. The patients with primary amenorrhea had a mean age of 22.7 years with a range of 7 11/12 to 37 years at the time of onset of amenorrhea. The remaining 110 patients, or 85.9%, presented with secondary amenorrhea beginning at a mean age of 27.9 years with a range of 12 to 39 years. It is clear that differences exist between those patients presenting with primary and those presenting with secondary amenorrhea (Table 24.1).

TABLE 24.1. Comparison of women with hypergonadotropic amenorrhea presenting with primary or secondary amenorrhea.

	Primary amenorrhea		Secondary amenorrhea		Significance (chi-square)
Total number of patients (%)	18	(14.1%)	110	(85.9%)	
Symptoms of estrogen deficiency	4	(22.2%)	91	(82.7%)	P < 0.001
Incomplete sexual development	16	(88.9%)	8	(7.3%)	P < 0.001
Chromosomal abnormalities	10	(55.6%)	6/49	tested (12.2%)	P < 0.010
Immune abnormalities[†]	4	(22.2%)	21	(19.1%)	NS
Spinal bone density < 90% of controls	3/4	(75.0%)	16/33	(48.5%)	NS
Withdrawal bleeding after progestin	2/9	(22.2%)	41/75	(54.7%)	NS
Pregnancies prior to diagnosis	0		41	(37.3%)	P < 0.025
Evidence of ovulation after diagnosis	0		27	(24.5%)	P < 0.050
Pregnancies after diagnosis	0		9	(8.2%)	NS

[†]Not including any test for antiovarian antibodies.

Source: Updated data from Rebar and Connolly (7).

In just under 75% of the women studied, symptoms of intermittent estrogen (E) deficiency—typically hot flushes and/or dyspareunia—were reported. These were far more common in the women with secondary amenorrhea. On the other hand, failure to complete sexual development and chromosomal abnormalities were significantly more common in those patients with primary amenorrhea. Chromosomal abnormalities occurred in more than half those women with primary amenorrhea. Individuals with primary amenorrhea have tended to suffer from deletions of an X chromosome or a portion thereof, whereas women with secondary amenorrhea have been more apt to have additional X chromosomes.

Immune disturbances were present in approximately 20% of our patients, with 10 of the 25 women having abnormalities on laboratory testing only (Table 24.2). Such tests do not include any evaluation for the presence of antiovarian antibodies. Such a test has been developed by us, and its potential utility will be discussed subsequently. Thirteen patients had documented thyroid disturbances, making this the most commonly associated glandular disorder. Three of the 13 individuals actually developed thyroiditis after the diagnosis of hypergonadotropic amenorrhea was made.

Seven patients, all with secondary amenorrhea, had received chemotherapy with alkylating agents and, in some cases, radiation therapy as well prior to the diagnosis of hypergonadotropic amenorrhea. Six of these indi-

TABLE 24.2. Women with hypergonadotropic amenorrhea with various immune abnormalities.

Immune abnormalities[†]	Primary amenorrhea 4	Secondary amenorrhea 21
Thyroid disturbances	3	10
Addison's disease		1
Hypoparathyroidism		1
Vitiligo		1
Diabetes mellitus	1	
Polymyositis		1
+ANA	1	5
+RF		2

[†]More than 1 abnormality per individual possible.
Source: Updated data from Rebar and Connolly (7).

viduals received chemotherapy for Hodgkin's disease and 1 for breast cancer. All 7 patients became amenorrheic directly following chemotherapy.

Four patients demonstrated a temporal relationship between the development of secondary amenorrhea and infections: 1 with chicken pox, 1 with
severe shigellosis, 1 with malaria, and 1 with an undefined viral syndrome.
All reported becoming amenorrheic immediately following their illness.

Four patients with normal karyotypes had a family history of early menopause prior to age 40. All 4 developed secondary amenorrhea.

Nineteen of the 37 women—over 50%—undergoing dual photon absorptiometry had bone densities that were less than 90% of the mean value
observed in age-matched control subjects (data not shown). For the small
number of patients studied to date, no statistical difference exists in the
percentage of women with decreased bone density who have primary as
opposed to secondary amenorrhea.

Withdrawal bleeding in response to progestin occurred in just over 50% of
the women tested. Withdrawal bleeding even occurred in 2 of the 9 patients
with primary amenorrhea tested. There was, however, no correlation between response to progestin and subsequent ovulation.

Not surprisingly, none of the women with primary amenorrhea had conceived prior to diagnosis, but more than 1/3 of those with secondary
amenorrhea had prior pregnancies. Likewise, evidence of at least sporadic
ovulation was not detected after diagnosis in any of the women with primary
amenorrhea, but was noted in almost 1/4 of the patients with secondary
amenorrhea. Presumptive evidence of ovulation consisted of serum progesterone (P) concentrations of 5 ng/mL or greater followed in 2 weeks or
less by menstrual bleeding or by documented pregnancy. None of the pa-

tients resumed monthly menses after diagnosis; thus, it may be inferred that ovulation was only sporadic. One-ninth of the women with secondary amenorrhea (8.2%) later conceived.

As expected, basal LH and FSH concentrations were markedly increased over values commonly observed in the follicular phase of the menstrual cycle, with LH equal to 90 ± 5.9 (SE) and FSH equal to 107.9 ± 8.5 mIU/mL for all the patients with hypergonadotropic amenorrhea. Concentrations of estrone and estradiol were similar to those observed in the early follicular phase of the normal menstrual cycle.

Twenty-seven of the women with secondary amenorrhea were treated with clomiphene citrate in an attempt to induce ovulation, but only 4 (14.8%) ovulated based on serial ultrasound and P-concentrations. Because each of the 4 women who ovulated had evidence of spontaneous episodic ovulation before therapy, it is unclear if the clomiphene therapy actually induced ovulation or by chance was given at a time when spontaneous ovulation occurred. Nineteen of the women were suppressed for 1–3 months with either exogenous E or a gonadotropin releasing hormone agonist and then administered exogenous hMG, generally from 50 to 100 ampules. Only 2 patients (both suppressed with the agonist) had evidence of significant follicular activity and ovulation, and only 1 conceived. Thus, ovulation induction is not likely to be successful in these patients. In contrast, with the use of donor oocytes, pregnancy rates are much higher: of the 4 such patients to whom we have given donor oocytes, 2 have delivered normal children.

Fourteen of the patients with secondary amenorrhea underwent ovarian biopsy, with apparently viable follicles noted in 9 of the specimens. Yet 2 of the 9 pregnancies occurred in women with no follicles observed on biopsy. Seven of the 9 pregnancies involving the patient's own oocytes occurred while the patients were taking exogenous E, with the remaining 2 pregnancies occurring, as noted, with ovulation induction. One-third of the patients with primary amenorrhea underwent gonadal biopsy. The 2 with 46,XY karyotypes proved to have dysgerminomas. One additional patient was found to have only fibrous streaks present.

From our clinical observations, we have concluded that the women with hypergonadotropinism who present with primary and secondary amenorrhea have distinctive features. Apparently, this is a heterogeneous disorder. It is clear that the term *premature ovarian failure* to describe all young women with hypergonadotropic amenorrhea is inappropriate because significant percentages of these women will ovulate and conceive after elevated gonadotropin levels are identified. Ovarian biopsy, however, is of little benefit in predicting pregnancy and cannot be recommended. Because almost all women have conceived while taking E and because of the increased risk of osteoporosis, we now recommend exogenous E to all patients. We discourage ovulation induction, but do inform patients about the possibility of oocyte donation. Our clinical observations also indicate the need for measuring basal gonadotropin concentrations in all amenorrheic women. Progestin withdrawal, ultrasound, and other tests do not accurately identify patients with hypergonadotropic amenorrhea.

Classification

A consideration of the clinical features of affected individuals and of the literature indicates that hypergonadotropic amenorrhea has many possible explanations. A tentative classification is listed in Table 24.3.

Genetic and Cytogenetic Etiologies

Theoretically, premature loss of oocytes might result from failure of all germ cells to migrate to the genital ridges, from a reduced complement of oogonia, or accelerated loss of oocytes (atresia) arising on a genetic basis. Accelerated loss of oocytes theoretically might result from an increased rate of atresia or

TABLE 24.3. Tentative classification of hypergonadotropic amenorrhea.

I. Genetic and cytogenetic etiologies
   A. Reduced germ cell number
   B. Accelerated atresia (?)
   C. Structural alterations or absence of an X-chromosome
   D. Trisomy X with or without mosaicism
   E. In association with myotonia dystrophica
II. Enzymatic defects
   A. 17α-hydroxylase deficiency
   B. Galactosemia
III. Environmental insults
   A. Ionizing radiation
   B. Chemotherapeutic agents
   C. Viral infection
   D. Cigarette smoking
   E. Surgical extirpation
IV. Defective gonadotropin secretion or action (?)
   A. Secretion of biologically inactive gonadotropin
   B. α- or β-subunit defects
   C. Gonadotropin receptor or postreceptor defects
V. Idiopathic
VI. Immune disturbances
   A. In association with other autoimmune disorders
   B. Isolated
   C. Congenital thymic aplasia

from recruitment of an increased number of oocytes within each cohort, which then undergo atresia at the normal rate. Because each cohort is larger in this model, the oocytes are depleted more quickly.

A number of reports (8–10) have described the familial occurrence of POF with vertical transmission of the trait, suggesting autosomal dominant, sex-linked inheritance. Moreover, the ovaries of 45,X fetuses contain a normal number of follicles at 5–6 months' gestation, but these rapidly undergo atresia so that virtually all oocytes are gone by birth (11). Structural abnormalities of the X-chromosome also have been found in women with premature ovarian failure (4, 5, 12). Recent studies of a family in which 3 women had POF revealed submicroscopic deletions of the DNA in Xq26-27 (13), suggesting that other affected individuals may have similar molecular defects in chromosomal structure. Apparently, an excess of X-chromosomes also may be associated with decreased germ cell number or accelerated atresia as well (14–16). In addition, the etiology of the POF that coexists with the neurological disorder myotonia dystrophica (17) is unknown, but may well be on the basis of decreased germ cell number or accelerated atresia.

Enzymatic Defects

Sexual infantilism and primary amenorrhea occur together with increased circulating gonadotropin levels, hypertension, hypokalemic alkalosis, and increased circulating levels of deoxycorticosterone and P in girls with 17α-hydroxylase deficiency who survive until the expected age of puberty (18–20). Ovarian biopsy of affected individuals has revealed numerous large cysts and primordial follicles with an absence of orderly follicular maturation (20).

It has only recently been appreciated that individuals with galactosemia have POF with elevated gonadotropin levels, even when a galactose-restricted diet is introduced early in infancy (21, 22). The etiology of the ovarian failure in galactosemia is unknown. It is tempting to suggest that the carbohydrate moieties on gonadotropin molecules are altered, either rendering the LH and FSH biologically inactive or altering their metabolism. On the other hand, a direct effect of galactose on the oocyte is suggested by the experimental finding that pregnant rats fed a 50% galactose diet delivered offspring with markedly reduced oocyte number, apparently as a result of decreased germ cell migration to the genital ridges (23).

Environmental Insults

Destruction of oocytes by various environmental conditions is one cause of POF (24). Although unequivocal proof has been difficult to obtain, condi-

tions that have been implicated include ionizing radiation, various chemotherapeutic agents, certain viral infections, and cigarette smoking.

Antineoplastic regimens involving multiple drugs or alkylating agents
have induced amenorrhea in up to 50% of patients. The amenorrhea may be
transitory, and younger women appear to be affected less than older women.
Ionizing radiation will also cause amenorrhea, with the duration and dose of
radiation important in determining the extent and duration of amenorrhea.
On rare occasions, viral infections, particularly mumps (25), may cause
ovarian failure. Lastly, Jick et al. (26) have concluded that cigarette smokers
experience menopause at an earlier age than nonsmokers.

Defective Gonadotropin Secretion or Action

It is possible to speculate that some women with hypergonadotropic amenorrhea may have ovaries that are unable to respond to gonadotropin. The
gonadotropin or their subunits themselves might be structurally defective.
The receptors for LH (LH-R), FSH (FSH-R), or for some other gonadotropic
factor might be absent or defective. Postreceptor cellular components, including systems that generate mediators of hormone action, might be
impaired. Alternatively, extracellular molecules that block binding of gonadotropic factors such as LH or FSH to ovarian plasma membrane receptors
might account for the inability of ovarian cells to respond appropriately to
extracellular signals. Evidence to substantiate these theoretical possibilities
has not yet been obtained.

Idiopathic POF

At present, the diagnosis of idiopathic POF must be regarded as a diagnosis
of conclusion. Unfortunately, no obvious cause for hypergonadotropic
amenorrhea is found in the majority of cases. No doubt other causes not even
listed will be identified as more is learned about this entity.

Immune Disturbances

Premature ovarian failure has been observed in association with a number of
autoimmune disorders (Table 24.4) (27). Most commonly, ovarian failure
has been observed in patients with polyglandular failure, including hypoparathyroidism, hypoadrenalism, and mucocutaneous candidiasis. That the
autoimmune ovarian failure is heterogeneous is suggested by the numerous
other immune disorders with which it is associated. In addition, it seems
reasonable to surmise that autoimmune ovarian failure may occur independently of any other autoimmune disorder.

TABLE 24.4. Reported cases of autoimmune diseases associated with POF.

Thyroid	26
Adrenal	8
Polyendocrinopathy (type I)	20
Polyendocrinopathy (type II)	19
Diabetes mellitus	3
Multiple endocrinopathy	6
Myasthenia gravis	9
Pernicious anemia	2
Idiopathic thrombocytopenia	1
Glomerulonephritis	1
Rheumatoid arthritis	1
Crohn's disease	1
Vitiligo	1
Systemic lupus erythematosus	2
Asthma	1
Ovarian lymphocytic infiltrate	3
Unspecified	15
	119 of 380 cases

Source: Data tabulated from LaBarbera et al. (27).

Antireceptor antibodies have been implicated in the pathogenesis of several autoimmune disorders, such as myasthenia gravis and Graves' disease. Thus, antibodies to ovarian gonadotropin receptors might block gonadotropin action and follicular maturation in some women with early ovarian failure. The intermittent nature of autoimmune disorders and fluctuating antibody levels might well result in sporadic ovulation and occasional pregnancies.

Several investigators have utilized qualitative methods to detect circulating antibodies to human ovarian tissue in the sera of women with POF (28–31). The cytotoxic effects of serum from a few affected individuals on human granulosa cells (GC) in culture has been noted (32). In addition, Chiauzzi and colleagues (33) have demonstrated apparent FSH-R antibodies in 2 women with myasthenia gravis and hypergonadotropic amenorrhea. Clearly, additional efforts to determine the frequency of antiovarian antibodies in women with hypergonadotropic amenorrhea are warranted. Such considerations have led us to develop a quantitative test to evaluate sera for such antibodies, as discussed subsequently.

Individuals in whom the premature ovarian "failure" has an autoimmune basis might well be treated effectively. That such is the case is suggested by sequential studies in one teenage patient whose gonadotropin levels decreased when corticosteroids prescribed for adrenal insufficiency were taken regularly (34). In other reports, ovulation returned temporarily following plasmapheresis in a woman with myasthenia gravis (35) and with glucocorticoid therapy in a woman with a perifollicular lymphocytic infiltrate (36).

That a normal thymus gland and a normal immune system are required for normal follicular development is suggested by the observation that congenitally athymic girls who died before puberty had ovaries devoid of oocytes on autopsy (37). Consistent with this view is the observation that thymic extirpation in rhesus monkeys in utero is associated with a markedly reduced number of oocytes in the ovaries at birth (38).

Even if autoantibodies to ovarian tissue are present, this does not mean that the antibodies cause the ovarian failure. It would be necessary to document that a circulating immunoglobulin interferes with ovarian function. It is possible that the ovarian failure is due to cell-mediated autoimmunity and that autoantibodies appear only because of the cytotoxicity.

Antiovarian Antibodies

In autoimmune diseases such as Graves' disease, the abnormal expression of major histocompatibility (MHC) class II antigens on the surface of a target cell such as the thyrocyte is thought to allow presentation of target cell proteins to the T-helper lymphocytes (39). T-lymphocyte recognition of normal target cell proteins as foreign antigens is thought to allow presentation of these "antigens" to antibody-producing B-lymphocytes.

Expression of MHC class II antigens may be induced by cytokines such as γ-interferon (γ-IFN), which can be produced by T-helper lymphocytes. Normally, T-helper lymphocyte function is modulated by T-suppressor lymphocytes. T-suppressor lymphocyte function in patients with Graves' disease, however, is abnormally low. Hill et al. recently reported that MHC class II surface antigens were expressed intensely in ovarian GC of 4 women with POF (40). In addition, the same investigators found that γ-IFN could induce expression of MHC class II antigens in human GC from normal subjects in vitro. It is not known whether the autoantibodies resulting from the aberrant interaction between B-lymphocytes and T-lymphocytes cause the symptoms of autoimmune disease or merely are markers of autoimmunity. In Graves' disease, however, thyroid stimulating autoantibodies appear to be responsible for hyperthyroidism.

We have developed a solid-phase enzyme-linked immunosorbent assay (ELISA) to estimate titers of antibodies to ovarian tissue in sera of women with POF. The incidence of such antiovarian antibodies in women with the disorder was compared with that in normally menstruating control subjects. Blood samples were obtained with informed consent from the following groups of subjects, allowed to clot, and centrifuged at 1000 × g for 15 min; sera were stored at –20°C until use: (1) POF patients (n = 21) ≤35 years old seen in the Reproductive Endocrinology and Infertility Service of the University of Cincinnati Medical Center, with documented normal karyotypes and serum FSH levels >40 mIU/mL 2nd IRP-hMG; and (2) normal, premenopausal women (n = 11) ≤35 years old with regular menses, normal levels of serum FSH and LH and no history of autoimmune disease.

For ELISA, the wells of flat-bottomed microplates (NUNC, Denmark) were coated with 20,000 × g particulate preparations of whole porcine ovary. The concentration of coating antigen protein was 100 µg/mL in 0.1-M carbonate buffer, pH 9.6. Alternate wells were coated with bovine serum albumin (BSA) to serve as negative controls. Plates were incubated overnight at 4°C and washed 3 times in phosphate-buffered saline (PBS), pH 7.4. Antigen-coated plates were backcoated with PBS containing 1% (w/v) BSA and 0.02% sodium azide at 37°C for 60 min. All assays were performed in triplicate.

Fifty µL of patient or control serum—undiluted or diluted appropriately with PBS containing 1% BSA, 0.1% Tween-20, 0.02% sodium azide (PBSAT), and 0.3% denatured BSA—was added to each well, and the plates were incubated at 37°C for 2 h. Plates were washed 3 times with PBSAT, and 50 µL of goat antihuman IgG (F_c)-biotin conjugate (Vector Laboratories, Burlingame, CA) diluted 1:2000 with PBSAT was added to each well. The plates were incubated at 37°C for 1 h and washed, and 50 µL of streptavidin-β-galactosidase conjugate (Bethesda Research Laboratories, Gaithersburg, MD) diluted 1:2000 with PBSAT was added. Plates were incubated at 37°C for 60 min and washed 6 times with PBSAT, and 50 µL of o-nitrophenyl-β-D-galactopyranoside (4 mg/mL, freshly prepared) was added as substrate. Plates were incubated for 45 min at room temperature, and optical absorbance was determined at 405 nm using a Biotek microplate reader. Each plate included 8 blank wells with only substrate and 8 wells coated only with antigen (no antibody). Pilot experiments had indicated that coating of wells with either porcine GC membranes or porcine ovarian membranes yielded comparable results. Use of human ovarian membranes yielded unacceptably high nonspecific absorbance, presumably due to endogenous immunoglobulin G.

As demonstrated by ELISA, approximately 22% of karyotypically normal women with POF have detectable antibodies to ovarian tissue (41). These patients frequently have autoantibodies to other tissues as well. In a representative patient (Fig. 24.1), antibodies to kidney, liver, and spleen, as well as to ovary, were detected. Absorbance in the ELISA was related to serum concentration and decreased as the serum was diluted. The antibody profile varied from patient to patient, with some patients showing the greatest reactivity to ovarian tissue and others to kidney, liver, or spleen.

Some POF patients did not have detectable antibodies to ovarian tissue. Sera from normally menstruating control subjects also produced a low reac-

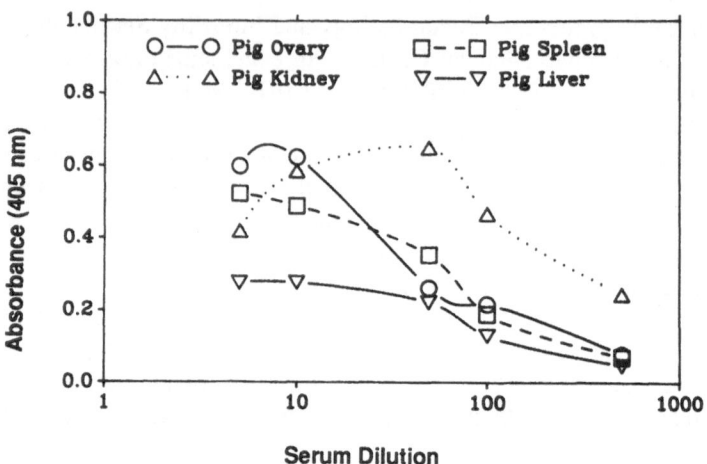

FIGURE 24.1. Detection of antibodies to kidney, liver, spleen, and ovary in a representative patient. Fifty-μL aliquots of a representative POF patient's serum diluted 1/5, 1/10, 1/50, 1/100, or 1/500 were assayed by ELISA for immunoglobulin G reactive with 20,000 × g particulate membrane preparations (5-μg protein/well) of porcine GC (circle), porcine kidney (triangle), porcine spleen (square), or porcine liver (upside-down triangle). Absorbance at 405 nm is graphed vs. serum dilution on a logarithmic scale. Each point is the mean of triplicate determinations.

tivity in the ELISA. The serum dilution curves for the POF and control groups are illustrated in Figure 24.2. The groups were significantly different (P < 0.05) by ANOVA and Neuman-Kuehl's test at serum dilutions of 1/5, 1/10, and 1/50. The reactivities of the sera (1/10 dilution) from control subjects and from POF patients with ovarian, kidney, spleen, and liver tissue are illustrated in Figure 24.3. The POF group had significantly higher titers of antibodies to ovarian and kidney tissue than did the control group (P < 0.05). The apparent reactivity of antibodies with multiple tissues does not necessarily indicate that the same antibodies react with each tissue. However, it does suggest that autoantibodies may be a marker, rather than a cause, of aberrant immune function. Ovarian failure may occur because ovarian cells are more susceptible to perturbation than other cells.

Sera from POF patients and control subjects were also analyzed using Western immunoblotting in order to begin to identify antigenic proteins. Proteins in aliquots of either 20,000 × g membrane preparations or Triton X-100 extracts of GC or 20,000 × g membrane preparations of liver, kidney, or spleen from pigs were solubilized either by boiling for 10 min in 2% sodium dodecyl sulfate (SDS) containing 10% glycerol, 62.5-mM Tris, and 10% 2-mercaptoethanol (reduced) or simply by incubation at 4°C in SDS-glycerol-Tris solution (nonreduced). Solubilized proteins or standard mo-

100 µg/mL Pig Ovary

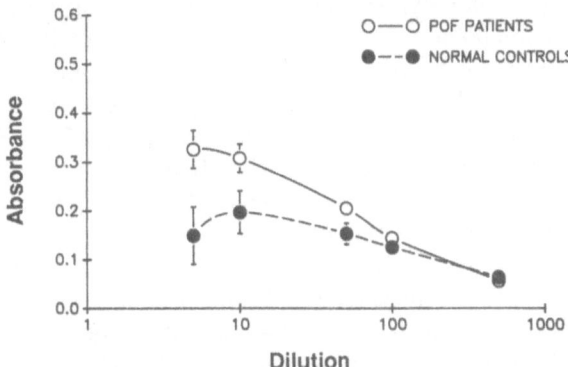

FIGURE 24.2. Serum dilution curves for POF and control groups. Fifty-µL aliquots of sera diluted 1/5, 1/10, 1/50, 1/100, or 1/500 from 11 control subjects (solid circle) and 21 POF patients (open circle) were assayed by ELISA for immunoglobulin G reactive with 20,000 × g particulate membrane preparations (5-µg protein/well) of porcine GC. Absorbance at 405 nm is graphed vs. serum dilution on a logarithmic scale. Each point is the mean of the determinations for each group, and the bars are the SEs.

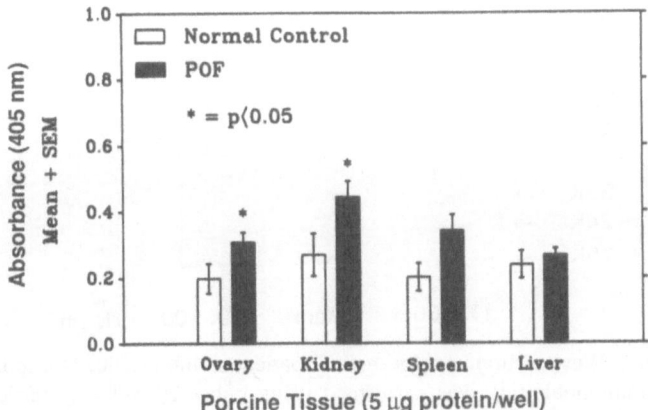

FIGURE 24.3. Comparison of sera (1/10 dilution) from POF patients and normal control subjects by enzyme immunoassay. Fifty-µL aliquots of sera diluted 1/10 from 11 control subjects (open bars) and 21 POF patients (closed bars) were assayed by ELISA for immunoglobulin G reactive with 20,000 × g particulate membrane preparations (5-µg protein/well) of porcine ovary, porcine kidney, porcine spleen, or porcine liver. Absorbance is graphed on the vertical axis. The bars represent the means for each group, and the vertical lines represent the SEs.

lecular weight markers were electrophoresed (SDS-PAGE) on 7.3 × 8.5 cm, 7.5%–12% gradient polyacrylamide slab gels according to Laemmli (42).

Western immunoblots were performed according to Towbin et al. (43). Transfer of proteins from electrophoretic gels to Immobilin PVDF membranes (Millipore, New Bedford, MA) was carried out for 1.5 h at 100 V in 6.25-mM Tris-buffered 1.375% glycine containing 0.01% SDS and 20% methanol using a Transblot chamber (Bio-Rad). Membranes with adsorbed proteins were blocked with 10-mM Tris (pH 8.0)-buffered 150-mM NaCl containing 0.05% Tween-20 (TBST) and 3% Knox gelatin at 37°C for 1 h. Membranes were incubated with serum (1:100–1:500) for 30 min at room temperature, washed 6 times for 30 min with TBST, and incubated overnight at room temperature with goat antihuman immunoglobulin G conjugated with alkaline phosphatase (Promega) diluted 1:7500. Membranes were washed 6 times for 30 min with TBST and incubated for 5 min with a substrate mixture containing 0.33-mg/mL nitro blue tetrazolium and 0.165-mg/mL 5-bromo-4-chloro-indolyl phosphate to develop a color product.

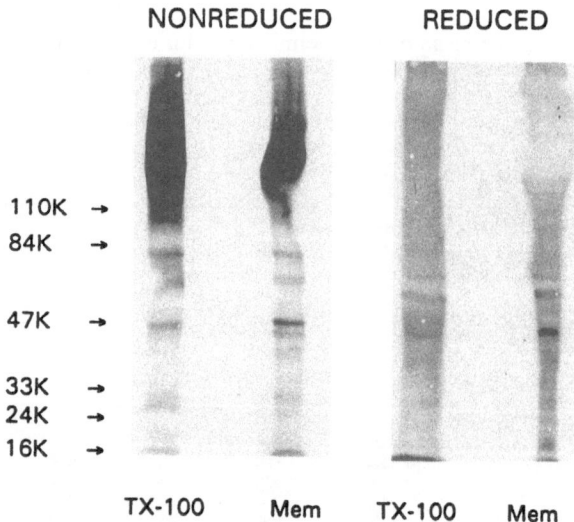

FIGURE 24.4 Western immunoblot of POF patient serum (1:500) with porcine GC. Western immunoblotting was performed using either 20,000 × g particulate GC membranes (Mem) or detergent-solubilized GC proteins (TX-100). Each preparation was incubated with SDS either at 4°C in the absence (nonreduced, 40-μg protein/ lane) or at 90°C in the presence (reduced, 80-μg protein/lane) of β-mercaptoethanol, electrophoresed by SDS-PAGE and electrolytically transferred to Immobilon PVDG membranes as antigen. Blots were incubated with serum (1:500 dilution) from a POF patient who tested positive for antiovarian antibodies by ELISA. Antigen-antibody complexes were identified by sequential incubation with a second antibody-alkaline phosphatase conjugate and color reagent. Positions of molecular weight standards are indicated at the left.

Where indicated, POF patient serum was preincubated with a particulate preparation of porcine GC membranes to preabsorb antibodies to GC membrane proteins. An aliquot (0.6 mL) of serum was incubated with 4 mL (1-mg protein/mL) of GC membranes and 7.4-mL TBST for 2 h at 37°C and centrifuged at 20,000 × g for 10 min. The supernatant was diluted 1/6.65 so that the final serum dilution used for Western blotting was 1/133.

An immunoblot using serum from a POF patient who tested positive for antiovarian antibodies by ELISA is illustrated in Figure 24.4. Using nonreduced GC proteins (40-μg protein/lane) as antigen, a very prominent band was visualized at 130 kD, and lesser bands were visualized at 81 kD and 47 kD. After reduction (80 μg/lane), which can disrupt epitopes, all bands were faint and major bands were visualized only at 52 kD and 40 kD.

Only proteins solubilized without reduction were used in subsequent experiments. Serum (1/100) from a control patient who tested negative in the ELISA reacted intensely with a 135-kD band in GC membranes, but reacted only slightly with liver, spleen, or kidney membrane proteins (Fig. 24.5). Reaction with a 57-kD band in spleen and kidney membranes was observed. The results with the control serum suggested either that asymptomatic women have detectable autoantibodies to various bodily tissues or that the goat antihuman IgG used to visualize antigen-antibody complexes bound nonspecifically to endogenous immunoglobulins in the porcine tissues or to other proteins. Therefore, we omitted the incubation with patient or control serum (first antibody) from an immunoblot. As seen in Figure 24.6, bands were visualized at 130 kD in GC and kidney membranes, at 120 kD in liver

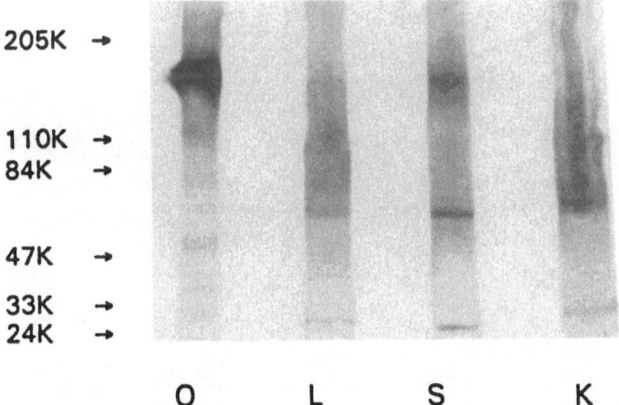

FIGURE 24.5. Western immunoblot of negative control serum (1:100 dilution). Western immunoblotting was performed using 20,000 × g particulate membrane preparations (40-μg protein/lane) of porcine GC (O), porcine liver (L), porcine spleen (S), or porcine kidney (K) as antigen without reduction. Blots were incubated with serum (1:100) from a control subject who did not have antiovarian antibodies by ELISA.

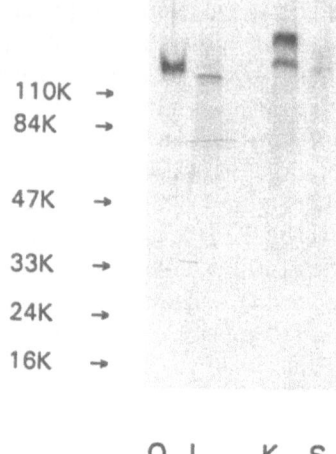

O L   K S

FIGURE 24.6. Control Western immunoblot (without first antibody). Western immunoblotting was performed as for Figure 24.5 except that serum (first antibody) was
omitted.

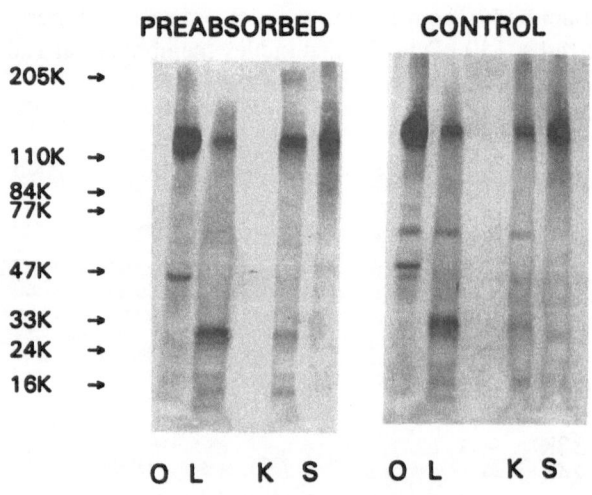

FIGURE 24.7. Western immunoblot of POF patient serum (1:133 dilution). Western
immunoblotting was performed as for Figure 24.5 except that the POF patient serum
was preincubated with either control buffer (control) or porcine GC membranes
(preabsorbed) prior to incubation with membrane blots.

membranes, and at 165 kD in kidney membranes; no bands were visualized in spleen membranes. Thus, it appears the control subject had circulating autoantibodies to ovarian tissue.

Serum from the same patient as shown in Figure 24.4 was tested by immunoblotting for reactivity to different proteins from GC, liver, kidney, or spleen membranes (Fig. 24.7, control). Although the 130-kD band was most prominent using GC membranes, it was also visualized using liver, kidney, and spleen membranes. The patient's serum also reacted strongly with GC proteins at 51 kD, 47 kD, and 44 kD. The 51-kD band was also observed using liver and kidney membranes; the 44-kD band was also observed using kidney membranes; and a prominent 33-kD band was observed using liver and, to a lesser extent, kidney. When the patient's serum was preabsorbed with porcine GC membranes (Fig. 24.7, preabsorbed), reactivity with the 61-kD band in GC, liver, and kidney was abolished. Likewise, the 44-kD band present in GC was not observed, and the 47-kD band decreased in intensity. The 33-kD band in liver and kidney was not altered by preabsorption with GC membranes.

These results indicate that the serum of a patient with POF contained GC-specific autoantibodies. The significance of these autoantibodies in the etiology of the disorder is unknown, however. In the future, we hope to establish the identity of the antigens targeted by the circulating autoantibodies. For example, we hope to determine whether the FSH-R is one of the antigenic proteins in the membrane of the GC in some, many, or all patients with autoimmune POF. Identification of the antigen would allow us to determine whether T-helper lymphocytes are sensitized specifically to the antigen and whether the ability of T-suppressor lymphocytes to hold the T-helper cells in check is compromised in these patients. Such information would facilitate identification of genetic factors responsible for the disorder.

References

1. Goldenberg RL, Grodin JM, Rodbard D, Ross GT. Gonadotropins in women with amenorrhea. Am J Obstet Gynecol 1973;116:1003-12.
2. Rebar RW, Erickson GF, Coulam CB. Premature ovarian failure. In: Gondos B, Riddick D, eds. Pathology of infertility. New York: Thieme-Stratton, 1987: 123-42.
3. O'Herlihy C, Pepperell RJ, Evans JH. The significance of FSH elevation in young women with disorders of ovulation. Br Med J 1980;281:1447-50.
4. Rebar RW, Erickson GF, Yen SSC. Idiopathic premature ovarian failure: clinical and endocrine characteristics. Fertil Steril 1982;37:35-41.
5. Aiman J, Smentek C. Premature ovarian failure. Obstet Gynecol 1985;66:9-14.
6. Hague WM, Tan SL, Adams J, Jacobs HS. Hypergonadotropic amenorrhea—etiology and outcome in 93 young women. Int J Gynaecol Obstet 1987;25:121-5.

7. Rebar RW, Connolly HV. Clinical features of young women with hypergonadotropic amenorrhea. Fertil Steril 1990;53:804-10.

8. Mattison DR, Evans MI, Schwimmer WB, White BJ, Jensen B, Schulman JD. Familial premature ovarian failure. Am J Hum Genet 1984;36:1341-8.

9. Starup J, Philip J, Sele V. Oestrogen treatment and subsequent pregnancy in two patients with severe hypergonadotrophic ovarian failure. Acta Endocrinol (Copenh) 1978;89:149-57.

10. Coulam CB, Stringfellow S, Hoefnagel D. Evidence for a genetic factor in the etiology of premature ovarian failure. Fertil Steril 1983;40:693-5.

11. Singh RP, Carr DH. The anatomy and histology of XO human embryos and fetuses. Anat Rec 1966;155:369-81.

12. Kinch RAH, Plunkett ER, Smout MS, Carr DH. Primary ovarian failure: a clinicopathological and cytogenetic study. Am J Obstet Gynecol 1965;91:630-44.

13. Krauss CM, Turksoy RN, Atkins L, McLaughlin C, Brown LG, Page DC. Familial premature ovarian failure due to an interstitial deletion of the long arm of the X chromosome. N Engl J Med 1987;317:125-31.

14. Villanueva AL, Rebar RW. The triple X syndrome and premature ovarian failure. Obstet Gynecol 1983;62:70S-4S.

15. Day RW, Larson W, Wright SW. Clinical and cytogenetic studies on a group of females with XXX sex chromosome complements. J Pediatr 1964;64:24-33.

16. Gordon DL, Paulsen CA. Premature menopause in XO/XX/XXX/XXXX mosaicism. Am J Obstet Gynecol 1967;97:85-90.

17. Harper PS, Dyken PR. Early onset dystrophia myotonica. Lancet 1972;2:53-5.

18. Biglieri EG, Herron MA, Brust N. 17-hydroxylase deficiency in man. J Clin Invest 1966;45:1946-54.

19. Goldsmith O, Solomon DH, Horton R. Hypogonadism and mineralocorticoid excess. The 17-hydroxylase deficiency syndrome. N Engl J Med 1967;277:673-7.

20. Mallin SR. Congenital adrenal hyperplasia secondary to 17-hydroxylase deficiency. Two sisters with amenorrhea, hypokalemia, hypertension, and cystic ovaries. Ann Int Med 1969;70:69-75.

21. Hoefnagel D, Wurser-Hili D, Child EL. Ovarian failure in galactosaemia. Lancet 1979;2:1197.

22. Kaufman F, Kogut MD, Donnell GN, et al. Ovarian failure in galactosaemia. Lancet 1979;11:737-8.

23. Chen Y-T, Mattison DR, Feigenbaum L, Fukui H, Schulman JD. Reduction in oocyte number following prenatal exposure to a diet high in galactose. Science 1981;214:1145-7.

24. Verp MS. Environmental causes of ovarian failure. Semin Reprod Endocrinol 1983;1:101-11.

25. Morrison JC, Givens JR, Wiser WL, Fish SA. Mumps oophoritis: a cause of premature menopause. Fertil Steril 1975;26:655-9.

26. Jick H, Porter J, Morrison AS. Relation between smoking and age of natural menopause. Lancet 1977;1:1354-5.

27. LaBarbera AR, Miller MM, Ober C, Rebar RW. Autoimmune etiology in premature ovarian failure. Am J Reprod Immunol Microbiol 1988;16:115-22.

28. Irvine WJ, Chan MMW, Scarth L, et al. Immunological aspects of premature ovarian failure associated with idiopathic Addison's disease. Lancet 1968;2:883-7.

29. Vazquez AM, Kenny FM. Ovarian failure and antiovarian antibodies in association with hypoparathyroidism, moniliasis, and Addison's and Hashimoto's diseases. Obstet Gynecol 1973;41:414-8.

30. De Moraes-Ruehsen M, Blizzard RM, Garcia-Bunuel R, Jones GS. Autoimmunity and ovarian failure. Am J Obstet Gynecol 1972;112:693-703.

31. Coulam CB, Ryan RJ. Premature menopause, I. Etiology. Am J Obstet Gynecol 1979;133:639-43.

32. McNatty KP, Short RV, Barnes EW, Irvine WJ. The cytotoxic effect of serum from patients with Addison's disease and autoimmune ovarian failure on human granulosa cells in culture. Clin Exp Immunol 1975;22:378-84.

33. Chiauzzi V, Cigorraga S, Escobar ME, Rivarola MA, Charreau EH. Inhibition of follicle-stimulating hormone receptor binding by circulating immunoglobulins. J Clin Endocrinol Metab 1982;54:1221-8.

34. Lucky AW, Rebar RW, Blizzard RM, Goren EM. Pubertal progression in the presence of elevated serum gonadotropins in girls with multiple endocrine deficiencies. J Clin Endocrinol Metab 1977;45:673-8.

35. Bateman BG, Nunley WC, Kitchin JD, III. Reversal of apparent premature ovarian failure in a patient with myasthenia gravis. Fertil Steril 1983;39:108-10.

36. Coulam CB, Kempers RD, Randall RV. Premature ovarian failure: evidence for the autoimmune mechanism. Fertil Steril 1981;36:238-40.

37. Miller ME, Chatten J. Ovarian changes in ataxia telangiectasia. Acta Paediatr Scand 1967;56:559-61.

38. Healy DL, Bacher J, Hodgen GD. Thymic regulation of primate fetal ovarian-adrenal differentiation. Biol Reprod 1985;32:1127-33.

39. Volpé R. Autoimmune thyroid disease. In: Volpé R, ed. Autoimmunity and endocrine disease. New York: Marcel Dekker, 1985:109-285.

40. Hill JA, Welch WR, Faris HM, Anderson DJ. Induction of class II major histocompatibility complex antigen expression in human granulosa cells by interferon gamma: a potential mechanism contributing to autoimmune ovarian failure. Am J Obstet Gynecol 1990;162:534-40.

41. Kim JG, Anderson BE, Rebar RW, LaBarbera AR. Determination by ELISA of antiovarian antibodies in premature ovarian failure [Abstract]. Proc 45th annu meet Am Fertil Soc, 1989.

42. Laemmli UK. Cleavage of structural proteins during the assembly of the head of bacteriophage T_4. Nature 1970;227:680-5.

43. Towbin HO, Staehnlin T, Gordon T. Electrophoretic transfer of proteins from polyacrylamide gels to nitrocellulose sheets: procedure and some applications. Proc Natl Acad Sci USA 1979;76:4350-4.

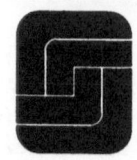

25

Use of Purified FSH for In Vitro Fertilization in Humans

Zev Rosenwaks

The goal of ovarian stimulation for in vitro fertilization (IVF) and embryo transfer (ET) procedures is the recruitment of multiple fertilizable (viable) oocytes. It has long been recognized that patients respond differently in terms of peripheral estradiol levels, number of recruited follicles, and number and quality of oocytes harvested, even when the same stimulation protocols are utilized. Estradiol response patterns have been classified as high, intermediate, or low, depending on the height of the peripheral E_2 response levels. We and others have correlated the estradiol response to the quality and number of oocytes retrieved, as well as to the pregnancy outcome. In certain circumstances, manipulation of the stimulation protocols by increasing the dosage of gonadotropin administered in the early follicular phase of the menstrual cycle can improve the stimulation response and pregnancy outcome.

Most IVF programs use a basic "standard" stimulation protocol for all first-time patients. Adjustments are made in ensuing IVF attempts based on the previous stimulation response, the number of oocytes retrieved, and oocyte or embryo quality.

Stimulation Protocols

The following two protocols are the most common stimulation protocols utilized in our unit.

Gonadotropins Only

On day 3 of the cycle, baseline ovarian ultrasound is performed and pretreatment estradiol and gonadotropin levels are determined. Stimulation is not begun if an ovarian cyst(s) is observed or if serum E_2 levels are <100 pg/mL as these findings are associated with poor stimulation response. Two ampules each of pure FSH (Metrodin) and Pergonal are administered daily, usually in split doses. When an appropriate follicular response, characterized by an adequate estradiol concentration is achieved, the dosage of gonadotropins is decreased to 2 ampules per day until the day of hCG administration.

The usual day for hCG administration (10,000 U I.M.) is day 10 + 1 day, when at least 2 lead follicles of an average diameter of approximately 16 mm are attained, which are associated with appropriate estradiol rise. Typically, hCG is administered when estradiol levels of 500–1200 pg/mL are achieved. Vaginal ultrasound-guided ovum retrieval takes place approximately 35 h after hCG administration, and for purposes of data compilation, this day is designated as day 14. If the Metrodin-hMG combination protocols yield poor results, we may in subsequent cycles utilize Metrodin alone or a combination of Lupron and gonadotropins. Progesterone (P) administration, 25–50 mg I.M. daily, is begun on day 15 (one day before embryo transfer) and is continued until menses or if a negative pregnancy test is obtained on day 28. In pregnancy, P-supplementation is continued until a fetal heartbeat is seen on ultrasound at 6 1/2-weeks gestation.

hMG + GnRHa

A GnRH analog (GnRHa) may be started on day 1 or 2 of the cycle to take advantage of the early agonistic effects of the medication (the so-called flare protocol). Most often, we begin treatment with the GnRHa (luprolide acetate) in the luteal phase, on day 21 of the cycle prior to stimulation, at a dose of 1 mg sc until E_2 and FSH levels are suppressed, usually by day 3 of the next menstrual cycle. At that time (or any chosen day thereafter to "program" a cycle), the dose is decreased to 0.5 mg, and hMG administration is begun in a protocol similar to that described above. GnRHa and Pergonal are then continued concomitantly until the day of hCG. Progesterone supplementation is begun the day following egg retrieval.

The midluteal GnRHa protocol is the treatment of choice for women with premature LH surges and single dominant follicle development. However, it increases drug costs by increasing hMG requirements, and in poor responders, it may be virtually impossible to effect ovarian stimulation successfully. These problems can be overcome by starting GnRHa on day 2 of the cycle; hMG (or hMG/hFSH) may be added anywhere from day 3 to day 5. This allows for determination of a baseline FSH level, which is not possible on the luteal GnRHa protocol. In addition, the early agonistic phase can be used to advantage to enhance early follicular recruitment while still obtaining the benefits of pituitary suppression later in the follicular phase of the cycle.

TABLE 25.1. Pregnancy outcome by day 3 FSH levels and high gonadotropin stimulation (6 ampules daily).

Day 3 FSH	<20 mIU/mL	>20 mIU/mL
Stimulation attempts	33	39
Clinical pregnancies	3 (11.0%)	2 (5.1%)
Ongoing pregnancies	2 (6.6%)	1 (2.5%)

Predictive Value of Day 3 Gonadotropins

It has been recently suggested that baseline day 3 FSH concentrations can be utilized to prognosticate stimulation response and IVF outcome. Presumably, FSH, representing a marker of ovarian reserve, is a most important prognosticator of ovarian response to stimulation and IVF outcome. Our continuing experience suggests that when high, FSH concentrations are predictive of poor stimulation response. Moreover, stimulation with high gonadotropin dosages in patients with elevated FSH (>20 mIU/mL) does not appreciably alter the outcome (Table 25.1).

Study Population

From January, 1989, to March, 1990, 784 ovarian stimulation cycles for IVF/ET were initiated at the Center for Reproductive Medicine and Infertility of The New York-Cornell Medical Center. Of these, 647 underwent oocyte harvest (82.4%), and 566 underwent embryo transfer (Table 25.2). The 143 ongoing pregnancies resulted in an ongoing rate of 25.2/transfer. In 484 stimulation attempts, gonadotropins were utilized in various combinations (in 53 attempts, clomiphene and gonadotropins were used), while in 247 cycles, stimulation was accomplished with concomitant GnRHa (Lupron) plus gonadotropins.

TABLE 25.2. IVF cycle 1–5 (January–March, 1990), Cornell University Medical College, Center for Reproductive Medicine and Infertility.

	Number of cycles	A (%)	B (%)	C (%)	D (%)
A. Attempts	786				
B. Retrievals	648	82.4			
C. Transfers	568	72.2	87.6		
D. Pregnancies	207	26.3	32.0	36.5	
E. Clinical pregnancies	181	23.0	28.0	31.9	87.4
F. Ongoing pregnancies	143	18.2	22.1	25.2	69.1

Note: Data exclude 1 case of GIFT and 1 case of embryo storage.

FSH and LH concentrations were measured on day 3 of the stimulation cycle in 531 of the 537 cycles. Table 25.3 depicts the clinical and ongoing pregnancy rates per attempt, retrieval, and transfer by day 3 FSH concentration group.

Patients with FSH concentrations of 0–10 mIU/mL on day 3 had a clinical pregnancy rate of 27.2% per stimulation attempt with an ongoing pregnancy rate of 20.2%/attempt, while the ongoing pregnancy rate per transfer for this group was 28.7%. Progressively higher day 3 FSH concentrations, reflecting diminished ovarian reserve, were associated with diminishing pregnancy rates. No viable pregnancies resulted when serum FSH was greater than 25 mIU/mL on day 3 of the cycle, whereas the viable pregnancy rate when FSH was between 21 and 25 mIU/mL on day 3 was 2.7% per stimulated cycle and 5.3% per ET.

Impact of Stimulation Protocol in High-FSH Patients

In an effort to improve stimulation response in poor responders and in patients with elevated day 3 FSH concentrations (>20 mIU/mL)—a level previously shown to be associated with a poor E_2 response—higher gonadotropin dosages were administered in the recruitment phase of the menstrual cycle. In 73 stimulation cycles, 6 ampules of gonadotropins were administered daily (either 2 hMG and 4 FSH, 3 hMG and 3 FSH, or 6 ampules of pure FSH) (Table 25.4). The high cancellation rate before retrieval (36%) and the poor pregnancy outcome suggest that increasing the dosage of gonadotropins does not alter the stimulation response appreciably, nor does it improve the pregnancy prognosis in this group of patients. Rather, the patients' diminished ovarian reserve (as reflected by the high FSH levels) dictates the outcome.

That chronological age is not as important as ovarian age (reflected by day-3 FSH) is illustrated in Table 25.5. In women >40 years of age, IVF prognosis is excellent when the serum FSH is less than 10 mIU/mL on day 3. Indeed, it is similar to pregnancy rates for the general IVF population in our unit.

Impact of GnRHa on IVF Outcome

We have observed that women with elevated or borderline FSH concentration, defined as a level >18 mIU/mL on day 3, respond poorly to GnRHa and concomitant gonadotropin regimen. Thus, only women with day-3 FSH levels of <18 mIU/mL are stimulated with the GnRHa and gonadotropins. In this highly selected group of patients, the pregnancy outcome is excellent, with a relatively low pregnancy loss during Lupron-stimulated cycles (Table 25.6). The GnRHa and gonadotropin stimulation protocol decreases the cancellation rate and improves the pregnancy rate per stimulation cycle.

TABLE 25.3. Pregnancy outcome by day 3 FSH concentration group.

Day 3 FSH (mIU/mL)	Simulation attempts (a)	Retrievals (b)	Transfers (c)	Clinical pregnancies			Ongoing pregnancies			Age (X ± SD)
				(a)	(b)	(c)	(a)	(b)	(c)	
0–10	173	142	122	47 (27.2)	(33.0)	(38.5)	35 (20.2)	(24.7)	(28.7)	34.7 ± 3.8
11–15	194	160	141	41 (21.1)	(25.6)	(29.1)	30 (15.5)	(18.8)	(21.3)	35.5 ± 5.1
16–20	91	77	67	13 (14.3)	(16.9)	(19.4)	11 (12.1)	(14.3)	(16.4)	36.3 ± 3.8
21–25	37	22	19	3 (8.1)	(13.6)	(15.8)	1 (2.7)	(4.6)	(5.3)	37.0 ± 3.2
26–30	16	6	3	0 (0.0)	(0.0)	(0.0)	0 (0.0)	(0.0)	(0.0)	37.2 ± 3.3
31–35	8	2	2	0 (0.0)	(0.0)	(0.0)	0 (0.0)	(0.0)	(0.0)	38.3 ± 2.3
>36	12	6	4	0 (0.0)	(0.0)	(0.0)	0 (0.0)	(0.0)	(0.0)	39.7 ± 2.3

Note: Pregnancy rates are expressed in parentheses per stimulation attempt (a), per retrieval (b), and per transfer (c).

TABLE 25.4. Pregnancy outcome with high gonadotropin stimulation.

Stimulation protocol	Stimulation attempts	Retrievals	Transfers	Ongoing pregnancies			
					(a)	(b)	(c)
2 hMG + 4 FSH	34	19	13	2	(5.7)	(10.5)	(15.4)
3 hMG + 3 FSH	23	16	14	1	(4.4)	(6.7)	(7.2)
6 FSH	16	12	12	1	(6.3)	(8.3)	(8.3)
Total	73	47	39				

Note: Pregnancy rates in parentheses are presented per stimulation attempt (a), per retrieval (b), and per transfer (c).

TABLE 25.5. Pregnancy outcome by day 3 FSH in women over 40 years of age.

Day 3 FSH (mIU/mL)	Simulation attempts	Retrievals	Transfers	Clinical pregnancies				Ongoing pregnancies			
					(a)	(b)	(c)		(a)	(b)	(c)
0–10	19	18	15	5	(26.3)	(27.8)	(33.3)	4	(21.0)	(22.2)	(26.7)
11–15	35	27	23	3	(8.6)	(11.1)	(13.0)	3	(8.6)	(11.1)	(13.0)
16–20	21	16	13	2	(9.5)	(12.5)	(15.4)	2	(9.5)	(12.5)	(15.4)
21–25	9	4	4	1	(11.1)	(25.0)	(25.0)	0	(0.0)	(0.0)	(0.0)
26–30	2	0	0	0	(0.0)	(0.0)	(0.0)	0	(0.0)	(0.0)	(0.0)
>30	10	4	3	0	(0.0)	(0.0)	(0.0)	0	(0.0)	(0.0)	(0.0)

Note: Pregnancy rates are expressed in parentheses per stimulation attempt (a), per retrieval (b), and per transfer (c).

TABLE 25.6. Pregnancy results in Lupron vs. non-Lupron cycles.

	Non-Lupron gonadotropin only	Lupron
Attempts	537	247
hCG injection day	8.9 ± 5.4	11.5 ± 2.7
Retrievals	420	226
Transfers	362	204
E_2 on day of hCG injection (pg/mL)	747 ± 593	1015 ± 613
Follicles aspirated	7.5 ± 6.9	12.2 ± 9.5
Oocytes harvested	5.1 ± 4.6	9.5 ± 6.9
Embryos transferred	2.0 ± 1.7	2.7 ± 1.6
Clinical pregnancies	108 (20.1) (25.7) (29.8)	72 (29.1) (31.9) (35.3)
Ongoing pregnancies	80 (14.9) (19.0) (22.1)	62 (25.1) (27.4) (30.4)

Note: Pregnancy percentage rates are expressed in parentheses and are presented per stimulation attempt, per retrieval, and per transfer, respectively.

Summary

Experience has shown that individualization of stimulation protocols is most rewarding in treating the patient undergoing IVF. While GnRHa treatment appears to offer distinct advantages (ablation of premature luteinization and decreasing cancellation rates before retrieval), not all patients do well with this regimen. It appears that more often than not, the patient's own ovarian reserve dictates the outcome. Day 3 serum FSH concentration appears to be an excellent marker for stimulation response and pregnancy prognosis.

No ideal, universal, stimulation protocol has been identified to date. Based on day 3 FSH concentrations and empirical practice, individualization of stimulation protocol is recommended. However, we must continue to search for better prognostic markers, as well as more precise stimulation response parameters, in an effort to optimize our treatment protocols and improve our clinical results.

Part VI

Poster Presentation Manuscripts

Part VI

Poster Presentation Manuscripts

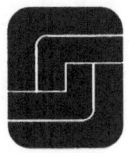

26

Regulation of Follicle Stimulating Hormone Secretion by Natural and Synthetic Corticosteroids

DARRELL W. BRANN, CARLA D. PUTNAM,
AND VIRENDRA B. MAHESH

A preeminent role has been given to the ovary as the source of steroids in the regulation of LH and FSH secretion. However, the adrenal also has great capacity to secrete steroids and may contribute significantly to the overall steroid milieu, leading to the preovulatory (PO) surges of LH and FSH, the estrous surge of FSH, and ovulation in the female rat. Adrenalectomy before day 25 in the female rat has been shown to delay puberty, an effect that is reversed by corticosterone replacement (1). This delay in puberty may be due to decreased FSH secretion since adrenalectomy has been shown to result in the acute suppression of FSH release in the immature rat (2). In the adult cycling rat, adrenalectomy has been reported to attenuate the proestrous LH and FSH surges (3), prolong the critical period (4), increase irregular cyclicity (4), reduce ovulation number (5), and disrupt follicular development (5).

Serum levels of adrenocorticotropin (ACTH) and prolactin (PRL)—the two principal regulators of adrenal steroid secretion—are also reported to be elevated on proestrus prior to the gonadotropin surge (6, 7). Furthermore, the adrenal secretion of progesterone (P), corticosterone, and deoxycorticosterone is significantly elevated throughout the afternoon of proestrus when compared to other days of the cycle (6, 8–10). Taken as a whole, these studies suggest that the adrenal exerts an important modulatory effect over LH and FSH secretion and reproduction in the female rat. The modulatory influence of the adrenal is most likely due to its ability to secrete significant quantities of adrenal steroids, and this is discussed in the following sections.

Effect of Adrenal Steroids on the Regulation of LH and FSH Secretion

ACTH Regulation of LH and FSH Secretion

In the past, the role of adrenal steroids in reproduction has been studied using regimens of chronic ACTH or corticosteroid treatment in male rats or nonestrogen-primed ovariectomized rats. Chronic treatment was chosen so as to mimic the effects of chronic stress. In virtually every study, chronic ACTH or corticosteroid treatment was found to suppress LH and FSH secretion and inhibit ovulatory function. While these studies quite clearly explain the suppressive effects seen with chronic stress, they were poorly suited to explain the significance of acute adrenal steroid secretion that is observed on proestrus. The above models utilized chronic elevations of adrenal steroids in animals with basal or nonexistent levels of estradiol; far different from events on proestrus, in which adrenal steroids rise acutely and where estrogen (E) levels are significantly elevated. Therefore, to determine the importance of adrenal steroid secretion in the regulation of gonadotropin secretion, we utilized several different approaches and animal models that more closely mimicked the acute changes and events that occur on proestrus.

In the first approach, Brann et al. (11) examined the question of whether acute stimulation of the adrenal with ACTH, in an appropriately E-primed rat, would facilitate LH or FSH secretion. The ovariectomized immature rat (26 days old) primed with 2 injections of estradiol was utilized for this study. ACTH treatment (10 IU, porcine[1-39]) on the morning of the third day (0900 h) following 2 days of E-priming, resulted in a surge of LH and FSH 6 h after administration (11). The effect of ACTH was specific, as α-MSH and ACTH[4-10] fragment did not bring about LH and FSH release. The stimulatory effect of ACTH on LH and FSH release was mediated by adrenal steroids since the effect was blocked by both adrenalectomy and treatment with the P and corticosteroid antagonist, RU486. The stimulatory effect of ACTH was found to require E-priming since ACTH had no effect in non-E-primed ovariectomized rats (Putnam, Brann, and Mahesh, unpublished data). These studies demonstrated that upon proper stimulation, in an appropriately E-primed animal, the adrenal can stimulate LH and FSH secretion.

Progesterone and Corticosteroid Regulation of LH and FSH Secretion

In subsequent studies, it was demonstrated that serum levels of both P and corticosterone were significantly elevated 15 min after ACTH injection in E-primed ovariectomized rats (11). Hence, these adrenal steroids appeared to be the most likely candidates mediating the stimulatory effects of ACTH.

Therefore, in the next series of experiments, Brann et al. (12) examined whether natural and synthetic corticosteroids, as well as P, could regulate LH and FSH secretion using the E-primed ovariectomized rat model described above.

Progesterone treatment was found to result in a stimulation of both LH and FSH secretion 6 h after administration. Of the natural corticosteroids tested, cortisol (1 mg/kg BW) was found to inhibit LH and FSH secretion, corticosterone (1 mg/kg BW) had no effect and deoxycorticosterone at doses of 0.8 mg/kg and greater stimulated LH and FSH secretion when examined 6 h after steroid administration. Of the synthetic corticosteroids tested, triamcinolone acetonide (≥0.25 mg/kg BW) markedly stimulated LH and FSH secretion. Dexamethasone preferentially released FSH at low doses (0.01–0.1 mg/kg BW) and suppressed LH levels at high doses (≥0.5 mg/kg BW). The LH and FSH releasing effects of deoxycorticosterone and triamcinolone acetonide were biologically relevant since they were found to result in ovulation in the pregnant mare serum gonadotropin-primed immature rat (13). Furthermore, the effect of triamcinolone acetonide and deoxycorticosterone appeared to be sex dependent since these steroids had no effect on LH and FSH secretion in E-primed castrate male rats (Brann and Mahesh, unpublished data).

Therefore, with respect to the possible endogenous adrenal mediator of the stimulatory effect of ACTH, it appears that P and *not* corticosterone is the active adrenal mediator responsible for ACTH stimulation of LH and FSH secretion. Deoxycorticosterone may also participate with P in mediating the effect of ACTH since it is an endogenous adrenal steroid regulated by ACTH and since it can also stimulate LH and FSH release in vivo. The secretion of deoxycorticosterone after ACTH injection was not measured in this study. In view of the absence of corticosterone effects on gonadotropin secretion observed in this study, the reported effect of corticosterone in restoring the timing of puberty in adrenalectomized female rats (1) remained unexplained. Therefore, additional studies were undertaken.

Further Studies on the Effects of Corticosteroids on FSH Secretion

Changes in GnRH and Neuropeptide Y in Response to Progesterone and Corticosteroids

The effect of P and triamcinolone acetonide in stimulating LH and FSH secretion appears to involve modulation of GnRH secretion at the hypothalamic level. Administration of the GnRH antagonist, [D-pGlu^1, D-Phe^2, D-Trp^{3,6}]-LHRH (100 µg/rat), 1 h prior to P or triamcinolone acetonide completely abolishes the stimulating effect of P and triamcinolone acetonide on LH and FSH secretion (Brann and Mahesh, unpublished data). Furthermore, Brann et al. (14) have recently demonstrated that mediobasal hypothalamic (MBH) GnRH and neuropeptide Y (NPY) content is elevated preceding the P- and triamcinolone acetonide-induced surge of gonadotropins, and this elevation is followed by a fall in content at the time of initiation of the LH and FSH surge. The effect of P and triamcinolone acetonide may also involve catecholamine and excitatory amino acid neurotransmission, as recently suggested by Brann and Mahesh (15, 16).

Interestingly, the natural corticosteroid, cortisol, was found to have no effect on MBH GnRH and NPY content, but *did* change preoptic-area GnRH and NPY concentrations at similar times (rise at 1200 h with fall at 1300 h) and in a pattern similar to P and triamcinolone acetonide effects in the MBH. The effect of cortisol was somewhat unexpected since cortisol did not cause a gonadotropin surge on the day of administration. However, cortisol regulation of preoptic-area GnRH and NPY concentrations may have relevance in explaining our recent report that FSH levels, while unchanged on the day of cortisol administration, are significantly elevated the morning after treatment as compared to vehicle-treated controls (11). Further work has now shown that corticosterone also brings about a release of FSH in the E-primed ovariectomized rat on the morning of the next day of administration. Thus, the restoration of the timing of puberty in the adrenalectomized immature rat by corticosterone may be mediated by its ability to release FSH.

Selective Enhancement of FSH Response to GnRH after Corticosteroid Administration

In a subsequent experiment, the effect of cortisol, corticosterone, and dexamethasone upon basal and GnRH-stimulated FSH and LH release in E-primed ovariectomized rats was examined. As shown in Table 26.1, cortisol had no effect on either basal or GnRH-stimulated FSH and LH secretion. In contrast, both corticosterone and dexamethasone significantly enhanced basal FSH release with a small but significant enhancement of LH secretion. Of particular interest was the additional observation of a preferential enhancement by both corticosterone and dexamethasone of the FSH response to GnRH. This finding agrees with reports by Schwartz and coworkers (17, 18) and Kamel and Krey (19) that corticosteroids can preferentially increase both basal and GnRH-stimulated FSH secretion *directly* at the pituitary level using in vitro pituitary cell cultures. Therefore, these studies suggest that in addition to the above-mentioned effects at the hypothalamic level, corticosteroids may also act *directly* at the anterior pituitary level to modulate FSH and LH secretion.

TABLE 26.1. Effect of corticosteroids upon the in vivo pituitary response to GnRH.

	T-0		T-10	
	LH	FSH	LH	FSH
E_2-E_2-Veh	22 ± 3	433 ± 62	258 ± 45[a]	1084 ± 117[a]
Cortisol	27 ± 5	346 ± 96	351 ± 84[a]	1214 ± 209[a]
Corticosterone	76 ± 24[a]	821 ± 128[a]	308 ± 43[a]	1788 ± 236[b]
Dexamethasone	50 ± 2[a]	1212 ± 87[a]	239 ± 32[a]	1803 ± 135[b]

Immature female rats were ovariectomized at 26 days of age. At 27 and 28 days of age, the rats received 2-µg estradiol (1700 h, sc). On the third day (day 29), the animals received either vehicle or steroids (1 mg/kg BW) at 0900 h. At 1200 h the response to GnRH (10 ng/rat) was assessed via cardiac puncture. Animals were anesthetized with ether, and a time-zero (T-0) blood sample was taken followed by injection of GnRH. The animals were then sacrificed 10 min after GnRH (T-10). (n = at least 6 rats per group; a = $P < 0.05$ vs. E_2-E_2-Veh (T-0); b = $P < 0.05$ vs. E_2-E_2-Veh (T-10).)

Receptors Involved in Corticosteroid Action on Gonadotropin Secretion

The effect of triamcinolone acetonide and deoxycorticosterone on releasing FSH and LH may be mediated via the P receptor (P-R) since these steroids exhibit high affinity for the P-R as well as the corticosteroid receptor and since we have previously demonstrated their effects require E-priming (12). Conclusive determination of the precise receptor system involved in mediating the effects of triamcinolone acetonide and deoxycorticosterone on gonadotropin secretion awaits development of a specific corticosteroid receptor antagonist that does not exhibit affinity for the progestin receptor. The preferential release of FSH by corticosterone and dexamethasone would appear to be exerted through the corticosteroid receptor since corticosterone and dexamethasone exhibit little affinity for the P-R.

Conclusion

The above studies provide evidence that the adrenal can stimulate the release of FSH and LH secretion upon proper stimulation and with an appropriate E-background. Furthermore, adrenal corticosteroids were found to exert both FSH and LH releasing effects depending upon the corticosteroid employed. A preferential release of FSH by several corticosteroids was demonstrated both in vivo and in vitro. This effect could be important in instances of divergent FSH secretion, such as that observed on estrus in the rat, and may explain previous reports of delays in puberty and disruption of follicle development following adrenalectomy and restoration of those events by corticosterone treatment.

Acknowledgments. This investigation was supported by Research Grant HD-16688, NICHHD, NIH, U.S. Public Health Service.

References

1. Gelato M, Meites J, Wuttke W. Adrenal involvement in the timing of puberty in female rats: interaction with serum prolactin levels. Acta Endocrinol (Copenh) 1978;89:590-7.
2. Meijs-Roelofs H, Kramer P. Effects of adrenalectomy on the release of follicle-stimulating hormone and the onset of puberty in female rats. J Endocrinol 1977; 75:419-26.
3. Lawton IE. Facilitatory feedback effects of adrenal and ovarian hormones on LH secretion. Endocrinology 1972;90:575-9.
4. Mann DR, Korowitz C, Barraclough C. Adrenal gland involvement in synchronizing the preovulatory release of LH in rats. Proc Soc Exp Biol Med 1975;150: 115-20.
5. Peppler R, Jacobs J. The effect of adrenalectomy on ovulation and follicular development in the rat. Biol Reprod 1976;15:173-8.
6. Buckingham JC, Dohler K, Wilson C. Activity of the pituitary-adrenocortical system and thyroid gland during the oestrus cycle of the rat. J. Endocrinol 1978; 78:359-66.
7. Freeman ME. The ovarian cycle of the rat. In: Knobil E, Neill J, eds. The physiology of reproduction. New York: Raven Press, 1988:1893-928.
8. Raps S. Barthe PL, Desaulles PA. Plasma and adrenal corticosterone levels during the different phases of the sexual cycle in normal female rats. Experientia 1970;21:339-40.
9. Ogle T, Kitay J. Ovarian and adrenal steroids during pregnancy and the oestrous cycle in the rat. J Endocrinol 1977;74:89-98.
10. Parker CR, Winkel C, Rush J, Porter J, Macdonald P. Plasma concentrations of 11-deoxycorticosterone in women during the menstrual cycle. Obstet Gynecol 1981;58:26-30.
11. Brann DW, Putnam CD, Mahesh VB. Validation of the mechanisms proposed for the stimulatory and inhibitory effects of progesterone on gonadotropin secretion in the estrogen-primed rat. A possible role for adrenal steroids. Steroids 1991 (in press).
12. Brann DW, Putnam CD, Mahesh VB. Corticosteroid regulation of gonadotropin and prolactin secretion in the rat. Endocrinology 1990;26:159-66.
13. Brann DW, Putnam CD, Mahesh VB. Corticosteroid regulation of gonadotropin secretion and induction of ovulation in the rat. Proc Soc Exp Biol Med 1990; 190:176-80.

14. Brann DW, McDonald JK, Putnam CD, Mahesh VB. Changes in MBH LHRH and NPY associated with progesterone and triamcinolone acetonide-induced LH and FSH release [Abstract 3770]. Soc Neurosci, 1990.

15. Brann DW, Mahesh VB. Regulation of gonadotropin secretion by steroid hormones. Frontiers Neuroendocrinol 1991 (in press).

16. Brann DW, Mahesh VB. Endogenous excitatory amino acid regulation of the progesterone-induced LH and FSH surges in estrogen-primed ovariectomized rats. Neuroendocrinology 1990.

17. Suter D, Schwartz NB. Effects of glucocorticoids on secretion of luteinizing hormone and follicle-stimulating hormone by female rat pituitary cells in vitro. Endocrinology 1985;117:849-54.

18. Suter D, Schwartz NB. Effects of glucocorticoids on responsiveness of luteinizing hormone and follicle-stimulating hormone to gonadotropin-releasing hormone by male rat pituitary cells in vitro. Endocrinology 1985;117:855-9.

19. Kamel F, Kubajak C. Modulation of gonadotropin secretion by corticosterone: interaction with gonadal steroids and mechanism of action. Endocrinology 1987;121:561-8.

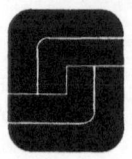

27

Modulation by Vitamin D_3 of Action of FSH on the Sertoli Cells in Immature Siberian Hamsters Raised in Long or Short Photoperiod

Subeer S. Majumdar, Andrzej Bartke, and Walter E. Stumpf

Follicle stimulating hormone (FSH) acts directly on Sertoli cells (Sc) to stimulate their secretory activity and is important for initiation of testicular growth (1, 2). A role of metabolites of vitamin D_3 (D_3) in mediating the effects of photoperiod on physiological processes has been suggested (3). Demonstration of D_3 receptors in the testes (4) and especially in the Sc (5) raised the possibility of a direct effect of D_3 on the Sc. In the present study, effects of FSH and D_3 on lactate production by the Sc were studied in vitro using cultures of Sc from juvenile Siberian hamsters (*Phodopus sungorus*). Lactate is the preferred energy substrate of the germ cells, and stimulation of Sc lactate production by FSH is believed to represent an important mechanism of FSH action on spermatogenesis (6). To further pursue the relationship between the actions of FSH and D_3, we have also examined the effects of D_3-treatment in vivo on testicular growth. The animals raised in long photoperiod (LD; 16L:8D) or short photoperiod (SD;6L:18D) were given daily injections of D_3 between 18 and 28 days of age. During this period, endogenous FSH levels in Siberian hamsters are very high in animals exposed to LD and extremely low or nondetectable in those exposed to SD (7).

Materials and Methods

Animals

Immature male Siberian hamsters (*Phodopus sungorus*) were exposed to either LD or SD from birth. The animals were weaned at the age of 18 days and thereafter maintained in all-male groups. Breeding pairs and weanlings were kept in plastic cages with constant access to pelleted food (Teklad laboratory chow, Madison, WI) and tap water in rooms with controlled photoperiod (LD or SD, lights on at 0700 h) and temperature ($22°C \pm 2°C$).

Isolation and Culture of Sc

Sertoli cells were isolated from 18- to 20-day-old hamsters and cultured following the procedure of Welsh and Wiebe (8) as modified in our laboratory (9). Cells were cultured in DMEM + HF-12 media (Sigma Chemical Company) with insulin, transferrin (Trf), and epidermal growth factor (EGF) as outlined by Mather et al. (10). The media also contained antibiotic and antimycotic compounds (9). Cells were incubated in an atmosphere of 95% air and 5% CO_2. The cells were allowed to spread for 3 days and attain confluency. Each dish contained 2-mL media that was replaced daily. The cultures were treated with 20-mM Tris (pH 7.2) for 3 min on day 3 of culture (72 h after plating) to destroy remaining germ cells. The dishes were washed once and incubated with the same media overnight. On day 4, the cells (3–5 dishes per treatment group) were incubated with media containing (1) no further additions, (2) 1-mg/mL oFSH (NIH-oFSH-16), (3) 10- to 7-M D_3 (Sigma, C-9756), and (4) oFSH 1-mg/mL and 10- to 7-M D_3. After 8-h incubation, the media were collected and assayed for lactate (9). The cells were treated with 1N.NaOH, and protein concentration was determined (11).

Treatment with D_3 In Vivo

Juvenile (18 days old) hamsters were weaned and injected (at least 6 animals in each group) with D_3 (Sigma, C-9756 and 15-mg/0.1-mL sesame oil) or with 0.1-mL of sesame oil alone. Animals were sacrificed 24 h after administration of the last injection, and body weight as well as testicular weight was determined.

Results

FSH produced the expected stimulation of lactate accumulation in the media of cultured Sc from Siberian hamsters raised in either LD or SD (Figs. 27.1 and 27.2). Vitamin D_3 failed to affect the accumulation of lactate in the media of Sc cultures when given alone, but significantly augmented the stimulatory effect of FSH.

The testicular weight of D_3-treated animals maintained in SD remained similar to control (vehicle-treated SD hamsters) values (Fig. 27.3). In contrast, testicular weight of LD-raised hamsters increased significantly upon treatment with D_3, as compared to the corresponding controls (vehicle-treated LD hamsters) (Fig. 27.4).

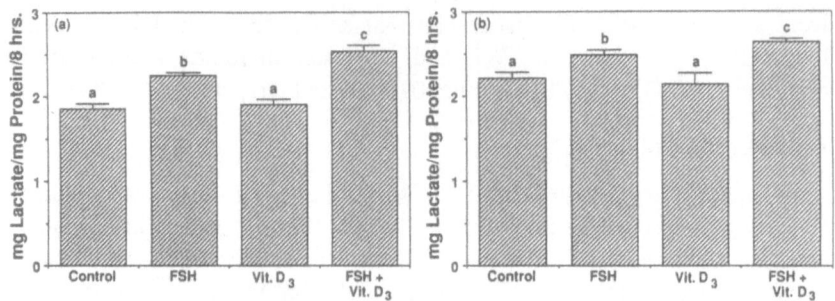

FIGURE 27.1. Secretion of lactate by cultured Sc isolated from SD-raised hamsters in control medium, upon treatment with FSH, D_3 (Vit. D_3), and a combination of FSH and D_3. Values without the same letter (a, b, and c) are significantly different ($P < 0.05$). Parts (*a*) and (*b*) are the results of replicate experiments.

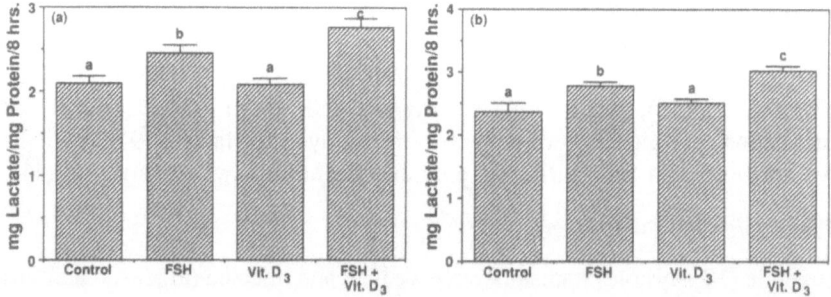

FIGURE 27.2. Secretion of lactate by cultured Sc isolated from LD-raised hamsters in control medium, upon treatment with FSH, D_3 (Vit. D_3), and a combination of FSH and D_3. Values without the same letter (a, b, and c) are significantly different ($P < 0.05$). Parts (*a*) and (*b*) are the results of replicate experiments.

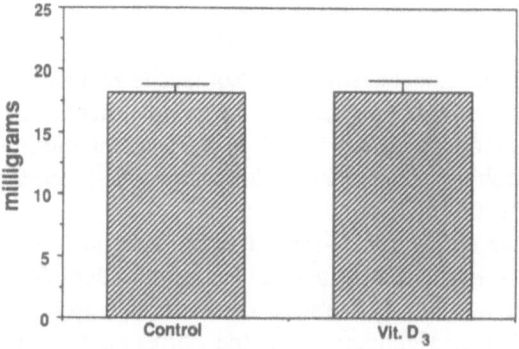

FIGURE 27.3. Effect of D_3 on the absolute testicular weight of SD-raised hamsters.

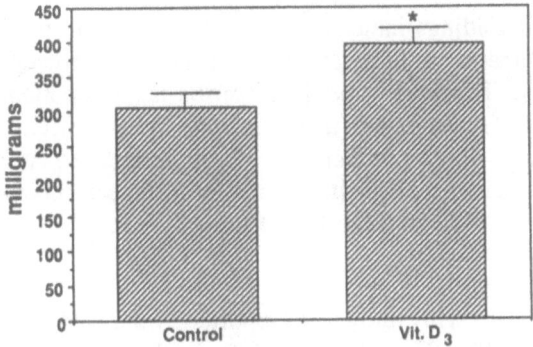

FIGURE 27.4. Effect of D$_3$ on the absolute testicular weight of LD-raised hamsters. (* represents P < 0.01.)

Discussion

There is evidence for the presence of D$_3$ receptors in the testes of rats and humans (5, 12); however, there is very little information on the possible involvement of D$_3$ in the testicular function. Since receptors for D$_3$ have been located in the seminiferous epithelium and Sc but not in the Leydig cells (5, 13), the present study was planned to examine the effects of D$_3$ on the function of the Sc.

Our observations suggest that D$_3$ does not stimulate Sc when given alone, but it amplifies the stimulatory effect of FSH on the secretion of lactate by the Sc. The presence of nuclear and cytosolic receptors for D$_3$ in Sc (5) indicates the possibility of several mechanisms of D$_3$ action, perhaps including cAMP-mediated FSH action on the synthetic activity of Sc. It is important to note that receptors for D$_3$ in human and rat testes are relatively less abundant than in other potential target tissues (12).

The results of D$_3$-treatment of LD- and SD-exposed hamsters in vivo complemented the findings in cultured Sc. Thus, hamsters raised in LD, in which endogenous FSH levels are known to be high (7), responded to D$_3$-treatment with a significant increase in the testicular weight, while hamsters raised in SD, in which the levels of FSH are very low, failed to exhibit this response. During the course of study, we found that the body weight gain in the D$_3$-treated SD animals was reduced when compared to control animals raised in SD, suggesting a possible inhibitory effect of this treatment on somatic growth of the SD-raised animals.

The present findings indicate that FSH-mediated testicular growth and Sc secretory function in Siberian hamsters can be influenced by D_3. Tsutsui et al. (14) recently reported that photoperiod is an important factor for the regulation of FSH receptors in the testis of Siberian hamsters. Therefore, we suspect that D_3, whose production is closely related to sunlight exposure, may be involved in increasing the number of FSH receptors in the testes and/ or the sensitivity of Sc to FSH stimulation.

Acknowledgments. This study was supported by the Lalor Foundation and by NIH, HD-20033. We thank Mrs. Karen Smith for typing the manuscript.

References

1. Bardin CW, Cheng CY, Musto NA, Gunsalus GA. The Sertoli cell. In: Knobil E, Neill J, eds. The physiology of reproduction. New York: Raven Press, 1988:933-74.
2. Milette JJ, Schwartz NB, Turek FW. The importance of follicle stimulating hormone in the initiation of testicular growth in photostimulated Djungarian hamsters. Endocrinology 1988;122:1060-6.
3. Stumpf WE. Vitamin D-Soltriol. The heliogenic steroid hormone: somatotrophic activator and modulator. Histochemistry 1988;89:209-19.
4. Levy FO, Eikvar L, Jutte NHPM, Froysa A, Tvermyr SM, Hansson V. Properties and compartmentalization of testicular receptors for 1,25 dihydroxy vitamin D3. J Steroid Biochem 1985;22:453-60.
5. Merke J, Hugel U, Ritz E. Nuclear testicular 1,25 dihydroxy vitamin D3 receptors in Sertoli cells and seminiferous tubules of adult rodents. Biochem Biophys Res Commun 1985;127(1):303-9.
6. Jutte NHPM, Jansen R, Grootegoed JA, Rommerts FFG, VanderMolen HJ. FSH stimulation of the production of pyruvate and lactate by rat Sertoli cells may be involved in hormonal regulation of spermatogenesis. J Reprod Fertil 1983;68: 219-26.
7. Yellon SM, Goldman BD. Photoperiod control of reproductive development in male Djungarian hamster (*Phodopus sungorus*). Endocrinology 1984;114:664-70.
8. Welsh MJ, Wiebe JP. Rat Sertoli cells: a rapid method for obtaining viable cells. Endocrinology 1975;96:618-24.
9. Newton SC, Mayerhofer A, Bartke A. Dopamine and isoproterenol stimulate lactate secretion from Sertoli cell cultures isolated from immature golden hamsters. Neuroendocrinol Lett 1989;4:207-14.
10. Mather JP, Sato GH. The use of hormone supplemented serum free media in primary cultures. Exp Cell Res 1979;124:215-21.
11. Bradford MM. A rapid and sensitive method for the quantitation of microgram quantities of protein utilizing the principal of the protein dye binding. Anal Biochem 1976;72:248-54.

12. Habib FK, Maddy SK, Gelly KJ. Characterization of receptors for 1,25 dihydroxyvitamin D3 in human testis. J Steroid Biochem 1990;35(2):195-9.
13. Stumpf WE, Sar M, Chen K, Morin J, DeLuca HF. Sertoli cells in the testis and epithelium of ductuli efferents are targets for 3H 1,25(OH)2 vitamin D3. Cell Tissue Res 1987;247:453-5.
14. Tsutsui K, Kawashima S, Masuda A, Oishi T. Effects of photoperiod and temperature on the binding of follicle stimulating hormone (FSH) to testicular preparations and plasma FSH concentrations in Djungarian hamster, *Phodopus sungorus*. Endocrinology 1988;122:1094-1102.

28

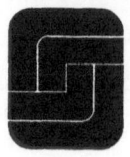

Probing Human Follicle Stimulating Hormone with Monoclonal Antibodies and Synthetic Peptides

P. BERGER, S. DIRNHOFER, R. KLIEBER, R. FRANK, AND G. WICK

The antigenic topography of the closely related molecules human follicle stimulating hormone (hFSH), human chorionic gonadotropin (hCG), and human luteinizing hormone (hLH) was previously elucidated (1–3) with extensively characterized monoclonal antibodies (MCA) against hFSH (1), hCG (4), bovine LH (bLH) (5), and the free subunits of hCG (6). The structural similarities of the glycoprotein hormones are well established (7); they all consist of 2 subunits designated α and β. In humans, the former is encoded by a single gene and is thus identical for each member of this family, whereas the latter is different from hormone to hormone and is therefore known to mediate biological specificity. Schematic epitope maps were taken as a basis for the alignment of antigenic and receptor interaction domains. The aim of the present study was to localize epitopes on hFSH at the amino acid sequence level with synthetic peptides and to describe the biological role they may play. We focused on the question of whether and, if so, in which way MCA and synthetic peptides interfere with hFSH receptor (hFSH-R) interaction.

Materials and Methods

Monoclonal Antibodies

Hybridomas producing MCA against hFSH, hCG, and hCGα were established as described previously (1, 4, 6). The MCA were directed against 9 different epitopes on the surface of hFSH: 5 on the α-subunit, 2 on the β-subunit, and 2 epitopes that were detectable only on the conformationally (c) intact holohormone (1).

One-Site Competitive Radioimmunoassay (RIA)

To localize antigenic determinants at the amino acid sequence level on the α-subunit, 3 peptides corresponding to hFSHα sequences (α11–18, α15–26, and α33–42) were synthesized according to the solid-phase 9-fluorenylmethyloxycarbonyl (Fmoc) polyamide method (8), which is characterized by reverse-phase hplc and utilized in a double-antibody competitive RIA as described previously (1).

One-Site Enzyme-Linked Immunoassay (ELISA)

The entire amino acid sequence of hFSHα was synthesized in 43 octapeptides overlapping by 2 amino acids on polypropylene pins (CRB, Cambridge, UK) essentially as described previously (8), but using Fmoc-amino acids and benzotriazole-1-yl-oxy-tris-(dimethylamino)-phosphonium hexafluorophosphate (BOP) as coupling reagent. The remaining binding sites on the peptide-coated pins were blocked by phosphate-buffered saline supplemented with 1% bovine serum albumin (PBS/BSA, pH 7.2) for 15 min at 20°C. The intra- and interspecies crossreacting MCA (INN-hFSH-132), which is directed against the epitope designated α4 (1, 6), was assayed for antipeptide response at a dilution of 10-μg IgG/mL PBS/BSA (16 h, 20°C). The peptide-bound MCA was detected by peroxidase-labeled rabbit immunoglobulins to mouse immunoglobulins (DAKO, Copenhagen) diluted 1:1000 in PBS/BSA (100 μL/well). The reaction was developed (20 min, 20°C, 150 μL/well) with 2,2'-azinobis (3-ethyl) benzthiazoline sulfonic acid (ABTS) as a substrate. The results were read at 405 nm in an automatic ELISA reader.

Competitive Radioreceptor Assay (RRA)

Decapsulated testes of Sprague-Dawley rats (200–250 g) were homogenized on ice with an Ultra Turrax tissue homogenizer (3 × 5 sec) in ice-cold 0.05-M Tris-HCl (pH 7.4). After 3 washes (20 min, 4°C), the resulting 3200 × g pellet was resuspended in Tris-HCl supplemented with BSA (1% w/v) and 30-mM $MgCl_2$ to approximately 200-mg tissue wet weight (tww)/mL.

Hormone standard hFSH-I-3 (NIADDK, AFP 4822B) in Tris-HCl/BSA or ultracentrifuged purified MCA preparations (50 μL, diluted to 10^{-8}–10^{-10}M in Tris-HCl/BSA, final assay concentration) were preincubated with 100 μL of [^{125}I]hFSH corresponding to approx 250,000 cpm for 2 h at 37°C prior to the addition of 250 μL testis receptor homogenate and 100 μL assay buffer (16 h, 20°C). After extensive washing with ice-cold Tris-HCl/BSA, pelleted radioactivity was measured in a gamma scintillation counter for 1 min. A nonrelated MCA against human prolactin and an MCA recognizing the private epitope α6 (6) served as negative controls. Nonspecific binding (NSB) was determined by competing the tracer with a 100-fold excess of unlabeled hFSH introduced in the preincubation step. The three α-peptides were tested for their ability to interfere with hormone receptor interaction in an RRA for hCG, which was performed similar to the RRA for hFSH.

Indirect Competitive RRA

The previously described inability of MCA directed against the α3 (INN-hCG-5) as well as the α5 epitope (INN-hFSH-158) to recognize radiolabeled hFSH (4, 1) might engender false-negative RRA results. Therefore, we tried to neutralize by these MCA the displacing ability of cold hFSH versus [^{125}I]hFSH in a conventional competitive RRA.

Unlabeled hFSH standard (50 μL, 10^{-8}–10^{-12}M, final assay concentration) was preincubated with 50 μL MCA (10^{-7}–10^{-10}M) for 2 h at 37°C. The subsequent incubation with 100-μL [^{125}I]hFSH, 250-μL receptor preparation, and 50-μL assay buffer, as well as the separation steps, was performed as described for the competitive RRA.

Sandwich RRA

Receptor homogenate (250 μL) was preincubated either with 100-μL hFSH-I-3 (10^{-9}M, final assay concentration) or with buffer alone for 16 h at 20°C. After extensive washing with Tris-HCl/BSA, the pellet that contained the hFSH-R complexes was resuspended in 500-μL [^{125}I]MCA (~250,000 cpm), which were directed against 9 different epitopes. The separation of bound and free radioactivity was done as described above. The functional activity of the tracers was proven by 2-site sandwich immunoassays as described previously (2).

Results

Correlation of Epitopes and FSH-R Binding Domains

Nine MCA against 9 different epitopes on hFSH were tested for their ability to interfere with hFSH-R interaction. It could be demonstrated that any of these MCA specifically inhibited binding of hFSH to its receptor in a dose-dependent manner on rat testis cell membranes, either by directly neutralizing [^{125}I]hFSH (Fig. 28.1) or by indirectly neutralizing cold hFSH standard (data not shown). The 3 peptides had no effect even in 10^6 molar excess to the tracer.

Conversely, we investigated the accessibility of epitopes on receptor-bound hFSH by [^{125}I]MCA in a sandwich-type receptor assay. None of the 9 epitopes could be detected on receptor-bound hFSH.

The peptide-spanning hFSHα residues 15–26 inhibited the binding of MCA INN-hFSH-132, which recognizes the α4 epitope (6) with an IC 50 of

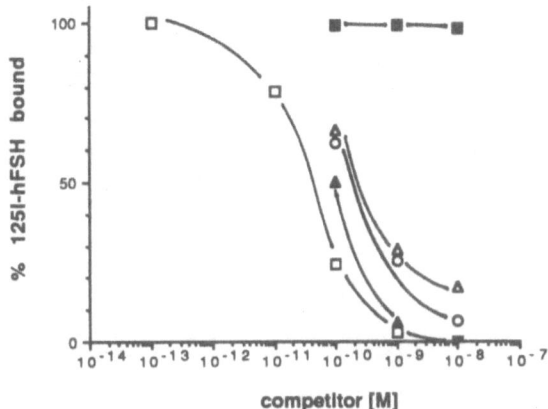

FIGURE 28.1. Competitive RRA. The binding of [^{125}I]hFSH to rat testis FSH-R was competed by MCA of different epitope specificity. One representative MCA for each main specificity group is shown (INN-hFSH-132, α-MCA, closed triangle; INN-hFSH-60, β-MCA, open triangle; and INN-hFSH-117, c-MCA, open circle). All MCA except for the control MCA, which is directed against an epitope only accessible on the free α-subunit (INN-hCG-80, closed square), were able to neutralize [^{125}I]hFSH. MCA against the epitopes α3 and α5 did not have any effect, as their epitopes are destroyed upon radioiodination as described in references (1) and (4). They were tested in the indirect RRA, where they neutralized cold hFSH (data not shown).

30 mM compared to an IC 50 of hFSH of 20 nM (Fig. 28.2a). Using the peptide-scanning method with solid-phase synthesized peptides, the epitope was narrowed down to the sequence α17–22 (FFSQPG) (Fig.28.2b).

Discussion

During the past few years, we have produced MCA against glycoprotein hormones of various species. Our original intentions were to map these hormones antigenically and to look for structure-function relationships. The first steps were to (a) investigate intra- and interspecies epitope sharing and the involvement of the carbohydrate portion in epitope recognition using 1- and 2-site RIA and ELISA, indirect immunofluorescence, and isoelectric focusing in combination with Western blotting (1–6); (b) to establish the highly specific and sensitive immunoenzymometric assay (IEMA) for holo-hFSH and free α-subunit, respectively (1, 6); and (c) to design schematic epitope maps of holo-hFSH and the free α-subunit (1, 6).

Our objective now was to specifically probe structure-function relation-

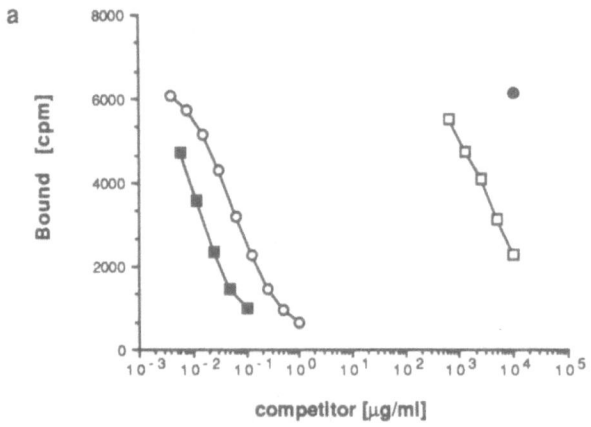

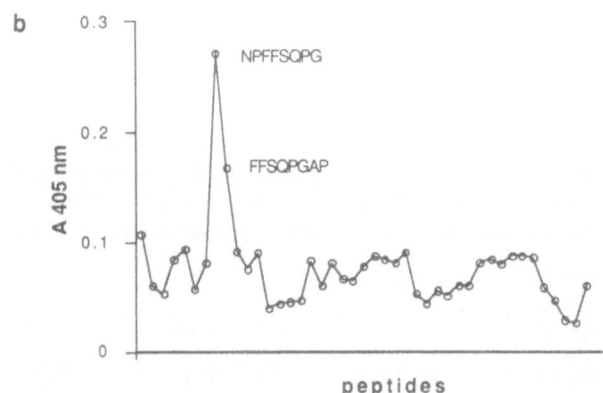

FIGURE 28.2. *a*: Identification of the epitope α4, as described in references (1) and (6), by competitive RIA. Note the specific inhibition by the free α-subunit (closed square), the holohormone (open circle), and the peptide α15–26 (open square). The peptide α33–42 had no effect (closed circle). *b*: Scan with overlapping octapeptides of the entire amino acid sequence of hFSHα for reactivity with the MCA INN-hFSH-132 (α4 epitope). Only 2 peptides (single-letter code) reacted with this MCA. Their overlapping sequence corresponds to FFSQPG.

ships of holo-hFSH by epitope-defined MCA and synthetic peptides. One epitope (α4) could be defined at the primary amino acid sequence level (FFSQPG). MCA against 9 defined epitopes on hFSH and 3 synthetic peptides of the α-subunit were used in two types of RRA: (1) in a competitive RRA, MCA and the peptides were investigated for their ability to inhibit hFSH from binding to the rat FSH receptor; and (2) in a sandwich-type RRA, the antigenic accessibility of receptor-bound hFSH was probed by

[^{125}I]MCA. Strikingly, all MCA directed against hFSH were able to specifically block hormone receptor interaction in a dose-dependent manner, whereas none of the 3 α-peptides were able to do so.

Identity between antigenic and receptor recognizing structures is based on the fulfillment of a number of prerequisites: Epitopes should be shared by FSH of other species, they should be expressed by the holohormone, and MCA directed against such determinants should inhibit the binding of the hormone to its receptor. On the other hand, epitopes should neither be accessible after hormone receptor interaction nor shared by holo-hFSH and its free subunits. Considering the intra- and interspecies presence of epitopes, most of them will not meet all of the above-mentioned criteria: Some of our MCA do not recognize FSH of other species (β2, α1, α2, α3, and all c-epitopes), do bind well to holo-hFSH and its free subunits (epitopes β2 and β3, and α1–5), and are not hormone specific, crossreacting with all human glycoprotein hormones (epitopes α1–5). Two epitopes (α3 and α5) are destroyed upon iodination, but this has no effect on hormone receptor interaction.

MCA against 9 determinants on holo-hFSH seemed to be powerful reagents to detect receptor interaction sites, but we were not able to assign them unequivocally to certain epitopes. It appeared as if our MCA provided too high a resolution, due to which, the information for receptor recognition is lost. Another explanation would be that receptor binding domains are not detectable by the immune system, either by not being sterically accessible or on the basis of "holes" in the immunological repertoire.

The fact that no antigenic determinant is detectable on the hormone receptor complex and the observation that all MCA are able to neutralize hormonal receptor binding ability speaks in favor of an involvement of the entire molecule in hormone receptor interaction. This is in agreement with previous findings for the closely related molecule hCG (3, 9).

References

1. Berger P, Panmoung W, Khaschabi D, Mayregger B, Wick G. Antigenic features of human follicle stimulating hormone delineated by monoclonal antibodies and construction of an immunoradiometric assay (IRMA). Endocrinology 1988;123: 2351.
2. Schwarz S, Berger P, Wick G. The antigenic surface of human chorionic gonadotropin as mapped by murine monoclonal antibodies. Endocrinology 1986;118: 189.
3. Schwarz S, Berger P, Nelboeck E, et al. Probing the receptor interaction of glycoprotein hormones with monoclonal antibodies. J Recept Res 1988;8:437.
4. Kofler R, Berger P, Wick G. Monoclonal antibodies against human chorionic gonadotropin (hCG): I. production, specificity, and intramolecular binding sites. Am J Reprod Immunol 1982;2:212.

5. Kofler R, Kalchschmid E, Berger P, Wick G. Production and characterization of monoclonal antibodies against bovine luteinizing hormone. Immunobiology 1981; 160:196.
6. Berger P, Klieber R, Panmoung W, Madersbacher S, Wolf H, Wick G. Monoclonal antibodies against the free subunits of human chorionic gonadotropin. J Endocrinol 1990;125:301.
7. Ryan RJ, Keutmann HT, Charlesworth MC, et al. Structure-function relationships of gonadotropins. Recent Prog Horm Res 1987;43:383.
8. Geysen HM, Rodda SJ, Mason TJ, Tribbick G, Schoofs PG. Strategies for epitope analysis using peptide synthesis. J Immunol Methods 1987;102:259.
9. Moyle WR, Ehrlich PH, Canfield RE. Use of monoclonal antibodies to subunits of human chorionic gonadotropin to examine the orientation of the hormone in its complex with receptor. Proc Natl Acad Sci USA 1982;79:2245.

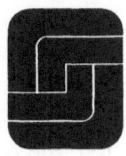

29

Prostate—An Extrapituitary Source of Follicle Stimulating Hormone

SEEMA V. GARDE AND ANIL R. SHETH

The prostate is known to synthesize and secrete various protein hormones, growth factors and neuropeptides, that without any doubt, establish the entity of the prostate as an endocrine organ (1, 2). Our earlier studies had demonstrated the presence of a protein exhibiting inhibin-like activity—prostatic inhibin peptide (PIP)—in prostates of human (3) and animal species (4) that preferentially suppressed synthesis and release of pituitary follicle stimulating hormone (FSH). Since the synthesis and secretion of FSH and inhibin are interdependent (5) and earlier studies also indicated their coexistence in various tissues (6–8), we were prompted to look for FSH in prostates of human and animal species.

The present study concerns the immunocytochemical localization of FSH, de novo biosynthesis, and its hormonal modulation in vitro in the prostates of human and animal species. In addition, the similarity between human pituitary FSH and prostatic FSH is established by immunochemical and physico-chemical criteria.

Materials and Methods

Immunohistochemistry

The paraffin sections of (1) normal, benign prostatic hyperplasia (BPH) and malignant human prostates and metastatic lymph nodes from patients having prostatic carcinoma, (2) intact and castrated langur monkey (*Presbytes entellus*) prostates (1 month after castration), and (3) rat, mouse, and guinea pig prostates were stained for FSH using the avidin-biotin system (7). The antisera of both intact and β-subunit hFSH (NIADDK, USA) and antirat FSH serum (for the rodent species) were used to localize FSH. Anti-hFSH serum absorbed with FSH and normal rabbit serum was used in place of primary antiserum and served as a control to check the nonspecific binding.

The method for in vitro biosynthesis of FSH by human prostate was essentially the same as described earlier (9). To study the hormonal modulation, the prostate tissues were incubated in the presence of either PIP or its synthetic fragments, the nonapeptide and decapeptide (10, 11).

The comparison of physicochemical characteristics of human prostatic FSH with those of human pituitary FSH was carried out using high-performance liquid chromatography (HPLC): Both prostatic tissue homogenate and pituitary extract were loaded on a preparative gel filtration column under identical conditions, and the fractions collected were assayed for FSH immunoreactivity using a radioimmunoassay. SDS-PAGE electrophoresis and Western blot analysis were also carried out for prostatic tissue extract and purified human pituitary FSH.

Results

FSH was localized in the cytoplasm of epithelial cells of the prostate gland whether they were normal, BPH (Fig. 29.1), or malignant (Fig. 29.2). The intense staining observed in BPH specimens was coarse and granular. At times, an alternating pattern of staining was observed, indicating cells in different stages of secretory activity. In some areas, blobs of FSH emerging from the apical portion of the cell were seen, indicative of FSH being secreted. The intensity of staining varied in moderately differentiated carcinoma. Some glands exhibited intense staining, whereas adjoining glands were faintly stained (Fig. 29.2). Immunostaining for FSH in poorly differentiated carcinoma was diffuse and much less intense compared to BPH. In

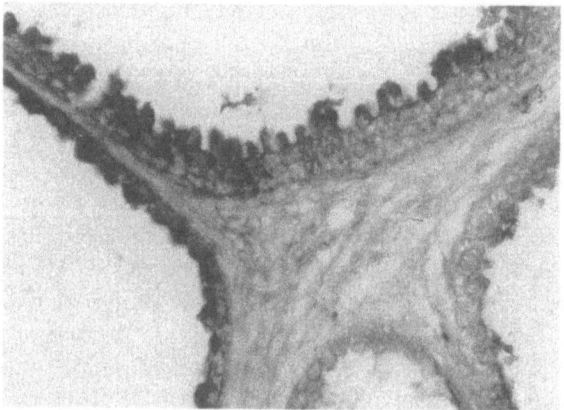

FIGURE 29.1. Benign prostatic hyperplasia. Note the strong positive staining for FSH in the cytoplasm of epithelial cells (400×).

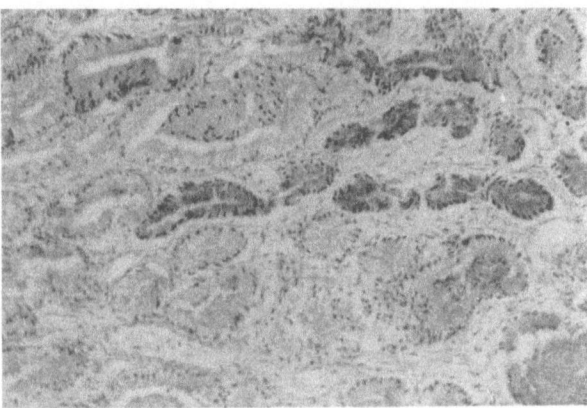

FIGURE 29.2. Moderately differentiated carcinoma. Some glands exhibit intense staining, while the adjoining glands are faintly stained for FSH (100×).

some prostate specimens besides cytoplasm, the staining was observed in the nucleus.

The epithelial cells that had been invaded in the lymph nodes of metastatic prostate tumors were positive for FSH, while the adjoining lymphatic tissue was negative. Immunoreactive FSH was not unique to human prostate, but was also present in nonhuman primates and rodents, such as rats, mice, and guinea pigs (Fig. 29.3). In langur monkey prostate, positive staining for FSH was observed even after 1 month of castration.

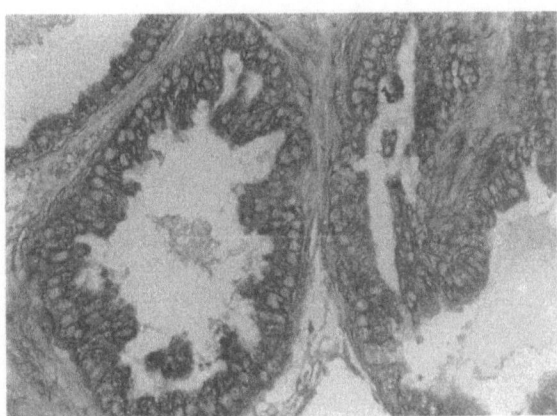

FIGURE 29.3. Mouse ventral prostate. Note the immunoreactive FSH in the cytoplasm of the epithelial cells (250×).

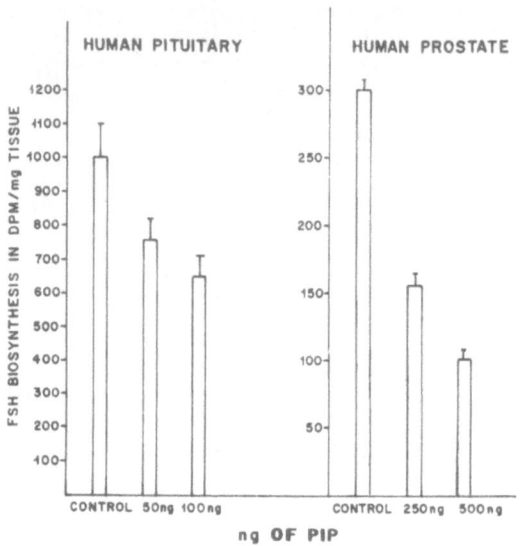

FIGURE 29.4. Effect of PIP on the biosynthesis of FSH.

The synthesis of FSH in vitro by both human pituitary and prostate tissues was modulated in a similar fashion. PIP and its decapeptide synthetic fragment suppressed the biosynthesis of FSH, while the nonapeptide increased its synthesis (Figs. 29.4–29.6).

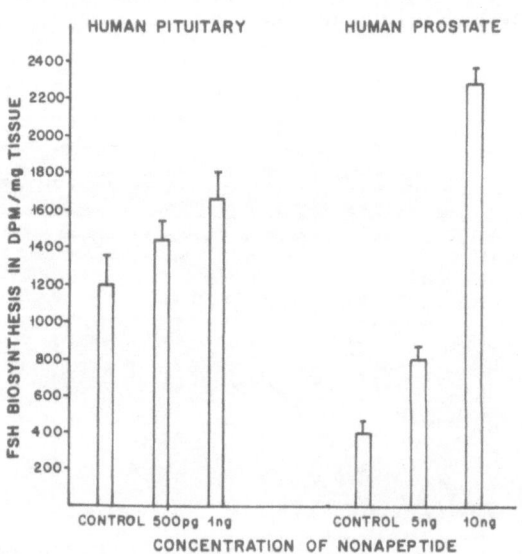

FIGURE 29.5. Effect of nonapeptide on biosynthesis of FSH.

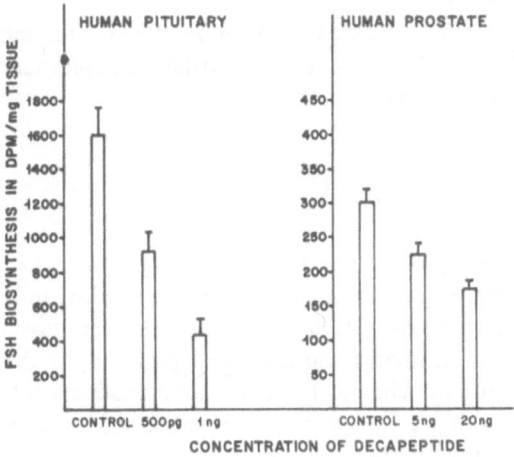

FIGURE 29.6. Effect of decapeptide on biosynthesis of FSH.

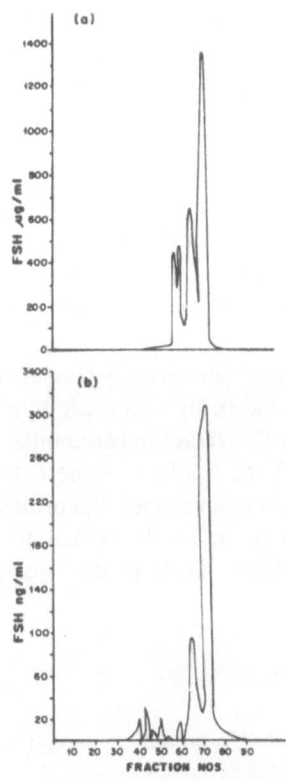

FIGURE 29.7. Elution pattern on a column of HPLC for human pituitary and prostatic FSH.

The HPLC analysis indicated the coelution of FSH of human pituitary and prostate (Fig. 29.7). The immunoblot of prostatic and pituitary extract exhibited identical protein bands.

Discussion

In the present investigation, we have presented evidence for the occurrence, de novo biosynthesis, and hormonal modulation of FSH in human prostate. Further, the occurrence of FSH is not unique to human prostates, but is also found in nonhuman primates and rodent species. The studies also demonstrated that the physicochemical and immunoreactive profile of prostatic FSH is similar to that of pituitary. Further, based on granulosa cell (GC) aromatase assay, it is biologically active.

As recently reviewed by Hsueh et al. (12), FSH was thought to be highly tissue specific. No other gland was implicated in FSH biosynthesis and action. Contrary to this concept, we demonstrated for the first time that the prostate is an extrapituitary source of FSH. It now appears that regulatory peptides are widely distributed and are involved in various functions that are beyond those classically recognized for these peptides.

In all the species studied, the localization of FSH was primarily confined to the cytoplasm of epithelial cells. However, FSH was occasionally found to be localized inside the nucleus. The physiological significance of FSH in the nucleus is rather intriguing. However, it may be mentioned that recently, inhibin and other regulatory peptides were also reported to occur in the nucleus (13). An intracrine mechanism of action for growth factors has also been reported recently (14). Whether FSH can also act in similar way needs to be elucidated.

Circulating hormones have been widely studied and compared in patients with prostatic carcinoma and benign prostatic hypertrophy. Androgens, estrogens, and FSH have similar values in carcinoma, benign hypertrophy, and the control population. These findings suggest that it is not so much the plasma concentrations of these hormones that influence the onset of prostatic cancer, but probably their tissue levels. Hence, the role of FSH directly or through modulation of inhibin levels in the etiopathology of the prostatic diseases is warranted.

References

1. Farnsworth WE, Ablin RJ. The prostate as an endocrine gland. FL: CRC Press, 1990.
2. Ablin RJ, Whyard TC. Immunological implications of select bioactive molecules in the prostate with a known and unknown target. In : Farnsworth WE, Ablin RJ, eds. The prostate as an endocrine gland. FL: CRC Press, 1990:149-72.

3. Sathe VS, Sheth NA, Sheth AR, et al. Biosynthesis and localization of inhibin in human prostate. Prostate 1987;10:33-43.

4. Garde SV, Sheth AR. Immunoperoxidase localization of prostatic inhibin peptide in human, monkey, dog and rat prostates. Anat Rec 1989;223:181-4.

5. Hurkadli KS, Sheth AR, Garde SV. Follicle stimulating hormone (FSH) modulating peptides : inhibin related peptides. Ind J Exp Biol 1989;27:303-9.

6. Garde SV, Sheth AR, Kulkarni SA. Cellular distribution of inhibin in marmoset testes during development. Anat Rec 1990.

7. Garde SV, Sheth AR, Kulkarni SA. FSH in testis of marmosets during development: immunocytochemical localization and de novo biosynthesis. Anat Rec 1990.

8. Sheth AR, Garde SV, Hurkadli KS, et al. Prostate—a nonclassical source of FSH and inhibin: are these hormones involved in the etiopathology of prostatic tumours? Proc Int Conf Perspectives Primate Reprod Biol. Bangalore, Feb 3-7, 1990.

9. Hurkadli KS, Shah MG, Pardanani DS, et al. De novo biosynthesis of FSH-like peptide by the human prostate. Life Sci 1990;47:391-400.

10. Hurkadli KS, Mahale SD, Iyer KNS, et al. Enhancement of in vitro release of FSH from rat pituitaries by a synthetic nonapeptide fragment of human seminal plasma inhibin. Life Sci 1989;45:1357-63.

11. Iyer KSN, Mahale SD, Hurkadli KS, et al. A synthetic decapeptide analogue of human seminal plasma inhibin exhibiting specific suppression of follicle stimulating hormone release in rats. Ind J Exp Biol 1989;27:10-3.

12. Hsueh AJW, Bicsak TA, Jia X, et al. Granulosa cells as hormone targets: the role of biologically active follicle stimulating hormone in reproduction. In: Clark JH, ed. Recent progress in hormone research. New York: Academic Press, 1989; 45:209-77.

13. Shaha C, Morris PL, Chen CLC, et al. Immunostainable inhibin subunits are in multiple types of testicular cells. Endocrinology 1989;125:1941-50.

14. Logan A. Intracrine regulation at the nucleus—a further mechanism of growth factor activity? J Endocrinol 1990;125:339-43.

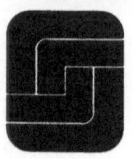

30

Biological Activities of Recombinant Human Follicle Stimulating Hormone

PETER R. SCHOFIELD, ANNE CERPA-POLJAK, MARK F. ALBRECHT, MARGARET C. STUART, AND YVONNE J. HORT

Follicle stimulating hormone (FSH), a member of the glycoprotein hormone family produced in the anterior pituitary, plays a major role in the maturation of ovarian follicles. FSH is a 32-kD heterodimer consisting of 2 non-covalently linked subunits, α and β. Each subunit contains 2 asparagine-linked carbohydrate complexes that are required for full biological activity of the hormone (e.g., circulatory half-life, signal transduction, etc.). Variation in glycosylation patterns at these sites results in multiple hormone isoforms that possess differing biological activities.

We have produced recombinant human FSH (rhFSH) by expressing the human FSH (hFSH) α- and β-subunit cDNAs in the Chinese hamster ovary (CHO) cell line. Using secreted rhFSH, we have sought to characterize the biological properties of the recombinant hormone and compare these properties to those of human pituitary and urinary FSH. In particular, we wished to identify the most potent isoforms of rhFSH by studying the involvement of carbohydrate variation on biological activity.

In Vitro Analysis of rhFSH Isoforms

Specific isoelectric (pI) isoforms of recombinant, pituitary, or urinary FSH have been obtained from preparative chromatofocusing columns (1). Quantitation is by means of an IRMA (Bioclone, Australia), which utilizes monoclonal antibodies that only recognize dimeric hormone.

Isoform fractions of rhFSH were assayed for bioactivity using the rat granulosa cell (GC) aromatase bioassay (2). Estrogen (E) production was monitored by RIA. In vitro bioassay of isoforms of rhFSH (Fig. 30.1A) demonstrates that the acidic fractions (pH 3.43) have significantly less bioactivity ($P < 0.05$) than the more basic fractions (pH 4.89).

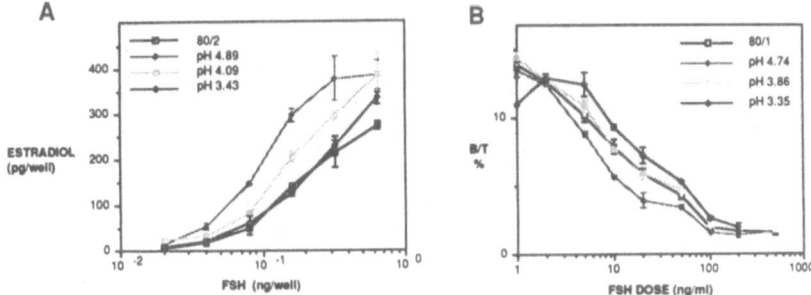

FIGURE 30.1. In vitro activity of rhFSH isoforms. *A*: In vitro bioactivity of rhFSH isoforms in the rat GC aromatase bioassay. Equivalent doses (ng protein) of 3 rhFSH isoforms (pH 3.43, pH 4.09, and pH 4.89) and a pituitary hormone standard (80/2) were incubated with primary cell cultures of rat GC, as described in reference 2. Estradiol production was determined by RIA. *B*: Displacement of iodinated pituitary FSH from rat testicular membranes by various isoforms of rhFSH. The displacement of maximal tracer binding by differing doses (ng protein) of rhFSH is displayed. Three different isoforms of pH 3.35, pH 3.86, and pH 4.74 and a pituitary hormone standard (80/1) were used. For both experiments, data are means of triplicate determinations, and the SE is indicated.

A radioreceptor assay (RRA) was established using rat testicular membranes. Radiolabeled pituitary FSH standard was used as the tracer, and rhFSH samples of differing pI were used to competitively displace the binding of the tracer. As seen in Figure 30.1B, acidic isoforms (pH 3.35) have reduced affinity for FSH receptors (FSH-R), whereas more basic isoforms (pH 4.74) have increased receptor affinities.

Combined, these two experiments support the hypothesis that basic isoforms have higher affinity for FSH-R and, accordingly, are capable of increased signal transduction when compared to acidic isoforms, which show reduced receptor affinity and decreased signal transduction.

In Vivo Analysis of FSH

The augmented ovarian weight gain assay (3) was used to monitor the potency of rhFSH. The increase in ovarian weight after administration of rhFSH clearly demonstrates that the recombinant material is biologically active in vivo (Fig. 30.2), with an apparent increase in potency over the urinary FSH tested [Metrodin (R)]. This may reflect the slight predominance of acidic isoforms in the recombinant FSH when compared to the urinary FSH, as seen by chromatofocusing (1).

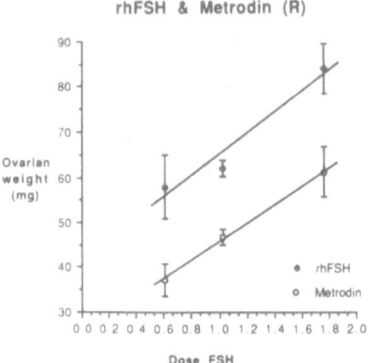

FIGURE 30.2. Ovarian weight gain bioassay of rhFSH vs. urinary FSH. FSH doses of equivalent microgram amounts were supplemented with hCG and injected daily into 21-day-old female rats, as described in reference 3. Ovaries were dissected and weighed on day 4. Data are quintuplicate determinations, and the SE is indicated.

Sections of ovaries from control and treated rats were examined by light microscopy. Marked proliferation of ovarian follicles resulting from treatment with both urinary and rhFSH was observed. Preovulatory (PO) Graafian follicles were clearly visible in the treated ovaries.

The metabolic clearance of rhFSH was determined. Two days after insertion of an indwelling cannula into the right external jugular vein of 200-g female rats, a bolus injection of 1-µg rhFSH was given. Plasma samples were obtained at varying times after injection, and FSH levels were determined. Figure 30.3 shows the percentage of the original dose of rhFSH present at various times after injection. Analysis of the data shows that the half-life of the clearance phase is between about 95 and 115 min. The clearance-phase half-lives observed lie in the middle of reported values (4, 5) that vary from 13 to 565 min. The clearance of a tracer of iodinated rhFSH closely parallels that of the unlabeled bolus, indicating that radiolabeled FSH may be used to follow the biodistribution of rhFSH.

Pituitary or recombinant FSH was iodinated and affinity purified. Radiolabeled FSH was injected via either the tail vein or an indwelling jugular vein cannula into conscious 200-g female rats. Animals were sacrificed at various time points, and organs were dissected and the total radioactivity present was determined in a gamma counter. The kidney and urine were major sites of radiolabel accumulation with about 50% of recovered radioactivity, as has been previously reported (6). On a whole-organ basis, about 25% of recovered radioactivity was found in the liver. However, when the percentage of radioactivity recovered per gram tissue is calculated (Fig. 30.4), there was a significant accumulation of radiolabel in the target tissue, the ovary. Thus, in

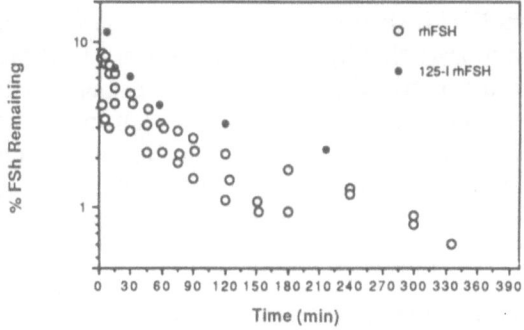

FIGURE 30.3. Plasma clearance of rhFSH from conscious adult female rats. A 1-µg bolus of rhFSH (0.5 mL in phosphate-buffered saline) was injected into the jugular vein cannula. Samples of 100 µL (open circles) were withdrawn at the time intervals shown, and FSH levels were determined. Plasma volume was replaced with PBS. Data shown are individual samplings from 3 different animals. In a separate study, affinity-purified iodinated rhFSH was injected (solid circles). Levels of injected radiolabeled rhFSH were determined using a gamma counter.

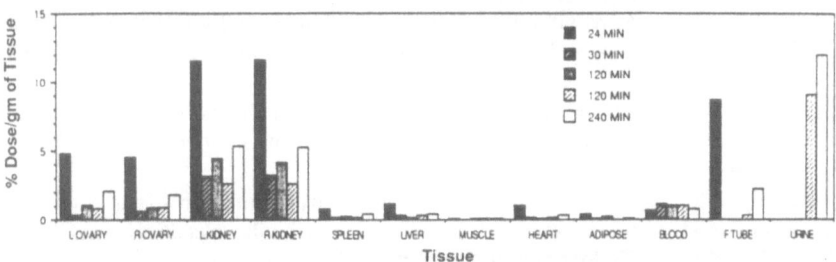

FIGURE 30.4. Biodistribution of iodinated FSH in adult female rats. Affinity-purified rhFSH (1) (24- and 240-min time points) or pituitary FSH (80/1) (30- and 120-min time points) was injected, and organs were dissected and the residual radioactivity was determined after the times indicated. Time points are from individual animals.

determining the effect of the metabolic clearance of FSH, the partitioning to the target organ needs to be considered.

Conclusions

In vitro bioassay of rhFSH and its isoforms has shown that the recombinant material is biologically active. Using both the radioreceptor and GC aromatase bioassay, it is seen that basic isoforms have higher receptor affinity and increased signal transduction (as measured by estradiol production) when compared to more acidic isoforms.

Recombinant FSH is shown to be highly potent in vivo, with activities on a gram-for-gram basis slightly higher than urinary FSH preparations. The examination of the in vivo activity and other metabolic parameters, such as biodistribution, bioavailability, and plasma half-lives of the various pI isoforms, will provide further insights into the role of the carbohydrate residues on the biological activity of FSH. Based on the results presented, recombinant human FSH should be of clinical utility.

Acknowledgments. Support was provided under the Generic Technology Component of the Industrial Research and Development Act, 1986.

References

1. Smith GM, Bishop LA, DeKroon R, Wright G, Cerpa-Poljak A, Schofield PR. Purification and characterization of recombinant human follicle stimulating hormone, Serono Symposia, USA. (See Chapter 31, this volume.)
2. Jia X-C, Hsueh AJW. Granulosa cell aromatase bioassay for follicle-stimulating hormone: validation and application of the method. Endocrinology 1986;119: 1570-7.
3. Steelman SL, Pohley FM. Assay of the follicle stimulating hormone based on the augmentation with human chorionic gonadotrophin. Endocrinology 1953;53: 604-16.
4. Blum WFP, Gupta D. Heterogeneity of rat FSH by chromatofocusing: studies on serum FSH, hormone released in vitro and metabolic clearance rates of its various forms. J Endocrinol 1985;105:29-37.
5. Sebok K, Meloche S, Sairam MR. Pharmacokinetic analysis of the plasma disappearance of ovine follitropin and analogues in the male rat. Life Sci 1990; 46:927-34.
6. Sebok K, Sairam MR, Cantin M, Mohapatra SK. Distribution of follitropin and deglycosylated follitropin in the rat: a quantitative and autoradiographic study. Mol Cell Endocrinol 1987;52:185-97.

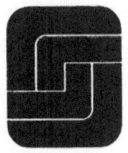

31

Purification and Characterization of Recombinant Human Follicle Stimulating Hormone

GLENN M. SMITH, LEONORA A. BISHOP, ROBERT DeKROON,
GREG WRIGHT, ANNE CERPA-POLJAK, AND PETER R. SCHOFIELD

Follicle stimulating hormone (FSH) plays a major role in the maturation of ovarian follicles. FSH, a member of the glycoprotein hormone family produced in the anterior pituitary, is a 32-kD heterodimer consisting of 2 noncovalently linked subunits, α and β. Each subunit contains 2 asparagine-linked carbohydrate complexes that are required for full biological activity of the hormone (e.g., metabolic clearance rate, signal transduction, etc.). Variation in glycosylation patterns at these sites results in multiple hormone isoforms that possess differing biological activities.

Recombinant human FSH (rhFSH) has been produced by expressing the hFSH α- and β-subunit cDNAs in a Chinese hamster ovary (CHO) cell line. Using this secreted rhFSH, we have sought to characterize the biochemical properties of the recombinant hormone and compare these properties to those of human urinary FSH.

Chromatofocusing of FSH Isoforms

Recombinant or urinary FSH isoforms were resolved using chromatofocusing. The isoelectric (pI) profiles of recombinant and urinary FSH were obtained using a Mono-P (Pharmacia) chromatofocusing column, Polybuffer 74, and 0.25-M histidine (pH 6.2) start buffer. A linear separation range of 5.5 to 3.0 was effected. FSH was quantitated by a dimer-specific immunoradiometric assay (Bioclone, Australia). As shown in Figure 31.1, the isoform profile of rhFSH was comparable to that of the urinary preparation, with the majority of the rhFSH isoforms occurring between pI 3.0 and pI 5.0. The maximal isoform concentration was at pI 4.2. This is indicative of varying numbers of sialic acid residues present on the carbohydrate struc-

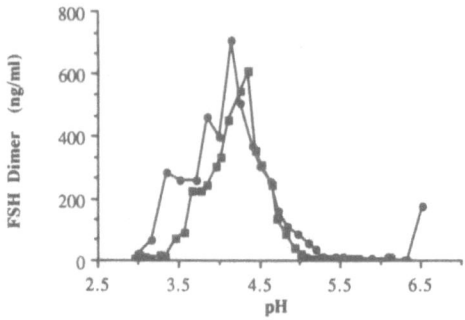

FIGURE 31.1. Comparison of the isoform profiles obtained from chromatofocusing of urinary (square) and recombinant (circle) FSH.

tures. The fractionated isoforms have been used for biological characterization of rhFSH (1).

pH and Temperature Stability of rhFSH Dimer

Subunit dissociation of gonadotropins occurs in the presence of denaturing molecules, such as urea and guanidine chloride, and also by lowering or increasing the pH or raising the temperature. Using a dimer-specific immunoradiometric assay, the hormone dissociation of rhFSH (30µg/mL) was followed as a function of pH and temperature. After incubation at the experimental pH and temperature, the sample was cooled rapidly on ice, neutralized with 0.5-M Tris-HCl (pH 8.0) and assayed for the presence of FSH dimer. Figure 31.2 shows that the dissociation of rhFSH is both pH and

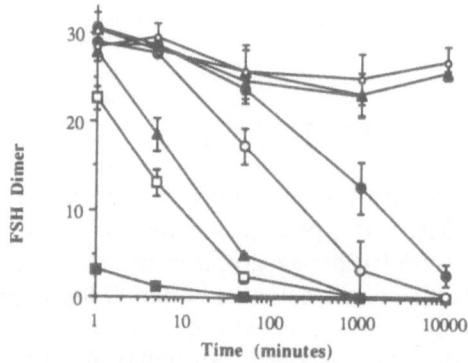

FIGURE 31.2. pH dependence of the dissociation of recombinant FSH. FSH (30µg/mL) was incubated at pH 1.0 (filled square), 2.0 (open square), 2.5 (filled triangle), 2.8 (large open circle), 3.0 (filled circle), 3.2 (open triangle), 4.2 (cross), and 7.6 (small open circle) at 25°C for various times before neutralization and assaying in a dimer-specific immunoradiometric assay.

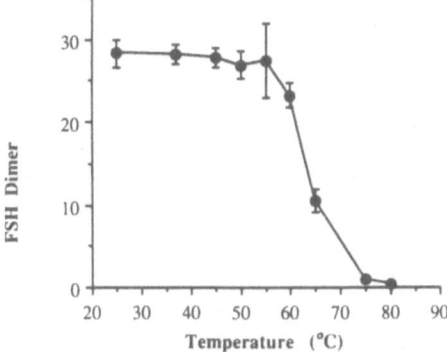

FIGURE 31.3. Temperature dependence of the dissociation of recombinant FSH. FSH (30µg/mL) was incubated at various temperatures at pH 7.6 for 1 h before cooling on ice and assaying.

time dependent. At a pH of 3.2 and above, the dimer was stable for up to 7 days, while at pHs of 3.0 and below, the dimer shows a time-dependent dissociation. The dimer was stable at pHs up to 11.5 at 25°C for 24 h. The pH dependence of dimer dissociation suggests that the association depends on ionization of aspartate and/or glutamate residues.

Figure 31.3 shows the effect of temperature on the dissociation of the FSH dimer at pH 7.6 for 1 h. The dimer was stable up to 55°C, above which, dissociation occurs.

Immunopurification of FSH

A dimer-specific monoclonal antibody (affinity = 3.0×10^{-8}M) that does not crossreact with either free α- or free β-subunits was coupled to an NHS-Sepharose column (Bio Rad). Concentrated serum-free conditioned media was loaded onto the column, and the FSH was eluted using 0.1-M glycine (pH 3.0). Using this procedure, it was possible to purify crude rhFSH to essential homogeneity (95% purity) as judged by SDS-PAGE and Western blot analysis (Fig. 31.4). The recovery of glycine-eluted FSH was 75%, and 25-µg FSH could be purified per milligram of immobilized antibody.

FSH run on SDS-PAGE under nonreducing conditions runs as a single band at ~40 kD. This band is intact dimeric hormone, as shown by Western blot analysis in which only this band interacts with the dimer-specific monoclonal antibody. Under reducing conditions, the subunits are dissociated, and a single diffuse band containing both α- and β-subunits is seen between 25 and 28 kD.

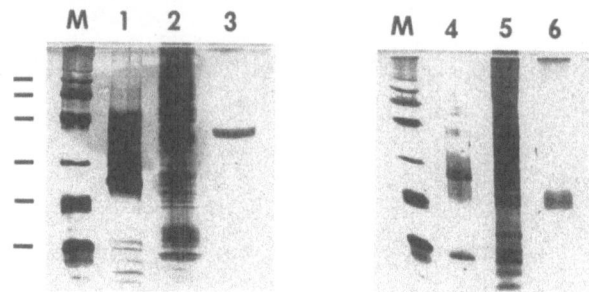

FIGURE 31.4. SDS-PAGE of affinity-purified rFSH. Column M is molecular weight standards at 94, 65, 43, 30, 20 and 14 kD; samples 1 and 4 are Metrodin; samples 2 and 5 are crude CHO-conditioned media; and samples 3 and 6 are affinity-purified rhFSH. Samples 1, 2, and 3 are nonreduced; samples 4, 5, and 6 are reduced. After running, the gels were silver stained.

Acknowledgments. Support was provided under the Generic Technology Component of the Industrial Research and Development Act, 1986.

References

1. Schofield PR, Cerpa-Poljak A, Albrecht MF, Stuart MC, Hort YJ. Biological activities of recombinant human follicle stimulating hormone, Serono Symposia, USA. (See Chapter 30, this volume.)

32

Purification and Biological Activities of Isoforms of Human FSH

P.G. Stanton, D.M. Robertson, P.G. Burgon, B. White, and M.T.W. Hearn

It is known that pituitary FSH, LH, and TSH are heterogeneous, existing as families of isoforms with respect to isoelectric point (pI), circulating half-life, in vitro and in vivo activities (for recent review, see [1]). To date, however, no systematic study has been undertaken to purify and characterize these isoforms with a view to establishing the biochemical basis for these differences. To this end, we have utilized a novel method exploiting the differences in charge-based protein separation between isoelectrofocusing and ion exchange chromatography for the purification to homogeneity of the isoforms of human pituitary FSH.

Materials and Methods

The purification procedure was based on a previously described method (2). Frozen human pituitaries supplied by the Human Pituitary Advisory Committee (HPAC, Canberra, Australia) were minced and homogenized in 50-mM phosphate buffer (pH 7.0), and a high-speed supernatant was prepared (100,000 g × 1 h at 4°C). The supernatant was applied to a gel filtration column (Sephacryl S200, Pharmacia, Uppsala, Sweden, 100 × 5 cm) in 50-mM ammonium acetate (pH 7.0), and the FSH radioreceptor active fractions were pooled and lyophilized.

Preparative Isoelectrofocusing (IEF)

The sample (400 mg dissolved in water containing 300-µM EDTA, 1.1-µM pepstatin, 1.3-µM leupeptin, and 0.2-µM phenylmethylsulphonylfluoride) was electrofocused in a 440-mL sucrose density gradient column (LKB, Bromma, Sweden) using carrier ampholytes (1% Ampholines, LKB) in the pH range from 3.5 to 10 for 17–18 h at 2000 V or 30 W at 4°C. The gradient was eluted at 100 mL/h and 1-mL fractions were collected. The pH was determined in every 5th tube. Phosphate buffer (pH 7.0) (0.5 mL, 0.3 M) was added to neutralize the pH.

High-Performance Liquid Chromatography

An FPLC (Pharmacia) system was used with a Mono Q anion exchange (HPIEX) column (HR5/5, 5×0.5 cm). The sample (50–60 mL) was sequentially fractionated with (a) a 57-min 0- to 342-mM NaCl gradient in 20-mM piperazine (pH 9.60) and 0.015% Brij-35 and (b) a 34-min 0- to 300-mM NaCl gradient in piperazine buffer (pH 6.0) at 1 mL/min at 20°C–22°C.

A TSK G3000SW column (60×0.75 cm, Toya Soda Co.) in 20-mM Tris buffer, 150-mM NaCl (pH 7.5), and 0.015% Brij-35 was employed at a flow rate of 0.4 mL/min. For SDS-PAGE, samples were reduced in dithiothreitol, electrophoresed in 16% gels using the method of Laemmli (3), and silver stained. Samples for amino acid analysis were hydrolyzed in vacuo in 6-M HCl, 0.2% phenol (22 h, 110°C) and analyzed by the Picotag method (Millipore/Waters, MA, USA).

FSH Radioreceptor Assay (RRA) and FSH In Vitro Bioassays

The FSH-RRA method of Cheng (4) was employed using calf testis membranes as the receptor source, the first IS for FSH (83/575) as standard, and iodinated human FSH isoform (pI 4.25) as tracer. The binding of tracer to an excess of membrane was 65%. A membrane dilution giving 25% binding with nonspecific binding of 1.5%–2% was used. Parallelism of logit log-dose-transformed dose-response lines was observed between preparations and standard. The between-assay variation was 7.8% (n = 6). The within-assay variation, based on the mean index of precision, was 0.048.

The FSH in vitro bioassay method of Van Damme (5) was used based on the FSH-induced aromatization of 19-hydroxyandrostenedione by immature rat Sertoli cells (Sc) in culture. All samples were assayed in the one assay. The within-assay variation, based on the mean index of precision, was 0.090.

Results

Human pituitary high-speed supernatant preparations were sequentially purified by gel filtration on Sephacryl S200, preparative isoelectrofocusing, 2 anion exchange chromatographic steps, and a final gel filtration HPLC chromatographic step (Figs. 32.1a–32.1d). Two of the FSH radioreceptor active regions (region A, pH 3.76–3.97; and region B, pH 4.07–4.34) from the preparative IEF were chosen for further processing. Following HPIEX at pH 9.6 and pH 6.0, regions A and B were further resolved into 3 isoforms

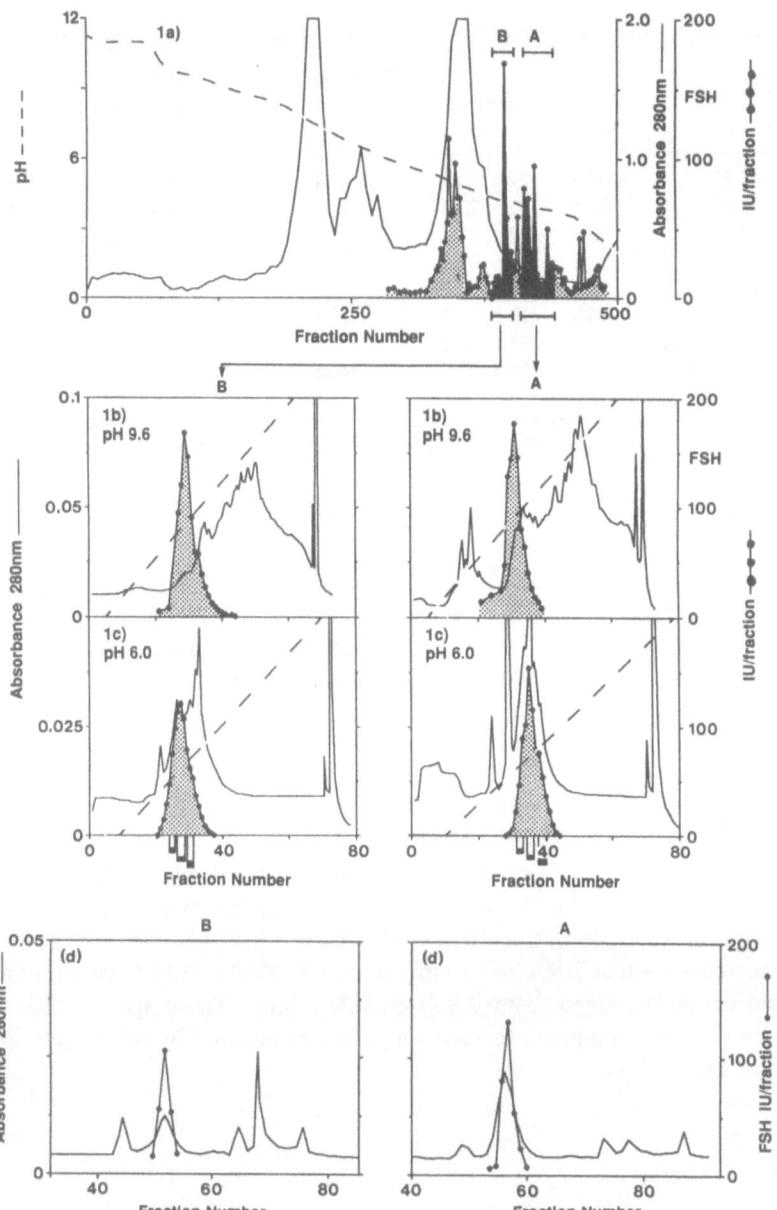

FIGURE 32.1. *a*: Isoelectrofocusing pattern of FSH radioreceptor activity from the human pituitary extract. *b*: Ion exchange chromatography (pH 9.6). Fractions containing FSH radioreceptor activity from *a* were fractionated on a Mono Q HPLC column equilibrated at pH 9.60. *c*: Ion exchange chromatography (pH 6.0). Fractions containing FSH radioreceptor activity from *b* were fractionated on the Mono Q column at pH 6.0. *d*: HPLC gel filtration FSH radioreceptor active fractions from *c* were then fractionated by HPLC gel filtration.

TABLE 32.1. Physiochemical and biological characterization of hFSH isoforms.

Isoform (pI)[a]	K_{AV}[b]	Mol wt (k)	Radioreceptor assay (IU/mg protein)	In vitro bioassay (IU/mg protein)	In vitro bioassay: RRA ratio
A1 (3.87)	0.89	22.4, 23.4	16800	21100	1.26
A2 (3.87)	0.84	22.4, 23.4	16000	17800	1.11
A3 (3.87)	0.83	22.4, 23.4	21300	24000	1.13
B1 (4.21)	0.71	19.6, 21.9	28300	44500	1.57
B2 (4.21)	0.70	19.6, 21.9	9800	21800	2.22
B3 (4.21)	0.70	19.6, 21.9	35200	64900	1.84
hFSH-I-3 (NIH)		21.5–25.5	7024		
hFSH (HPAC)		20.1–23.7	3400	3360	0.99
Pituitary extract			3.88		

[a]pI values from preparative IEF. Number of replicate assays = 2–3.

[b]K_{AV} coefficient derived from retention data on HPLC GF column.

Note: Bioactivity of NIH-FSH-I-3 by hCG-augmentation assay = 3,100 IU/mg.

each, which, when rechromatographed under identical conditions at pH 6.0, gave single peaks with retention times analagous to the previous run (data not shown), confirming isoform separation. Isoforms from regions A and B differed in apparent molecular weight, as shown by differing K_{AV}'s following gel filtration chromatography (Table 32.1) and SDS-PAGE (Table 32.1 and Fig. 32.2).

Silver stain patterns of the 3 purified isoforms from Region A (Fig. 32.2) indicated 2 diffuse staining bands in each case of 23.4 k and 22.4 k (Table 32.1). Isoforms from region B yielded 2 diffuse bands of 21.9 K and 19.6 K. A single broad band of M_r 21.6 k–25.5 k with higher molecular weight contaminants was seen in the NIH-I-3 hFSH sample. FSH-specific activities as assessed by either RRA or in vitro bioassay (Table 32.1) (based on amino acid content) ranged from 9,800–64,900 IU/mg. These specific activities were elevated compared to FSH preparations purified by other methodologies (Table 32.1).

Discussion

The isolation procedure described here gives considerably increased resolving power over other published methods for the purification of the human glycoprotein hormones. This increase in resolution is due to the sequential separation of isoforms based on (a) the pH at which they have zero mobility (i.e., zero net charge, pI) in an electric field and (b) the differences in the charged groups on the surfaces of the isoforms. Hence, we may expect

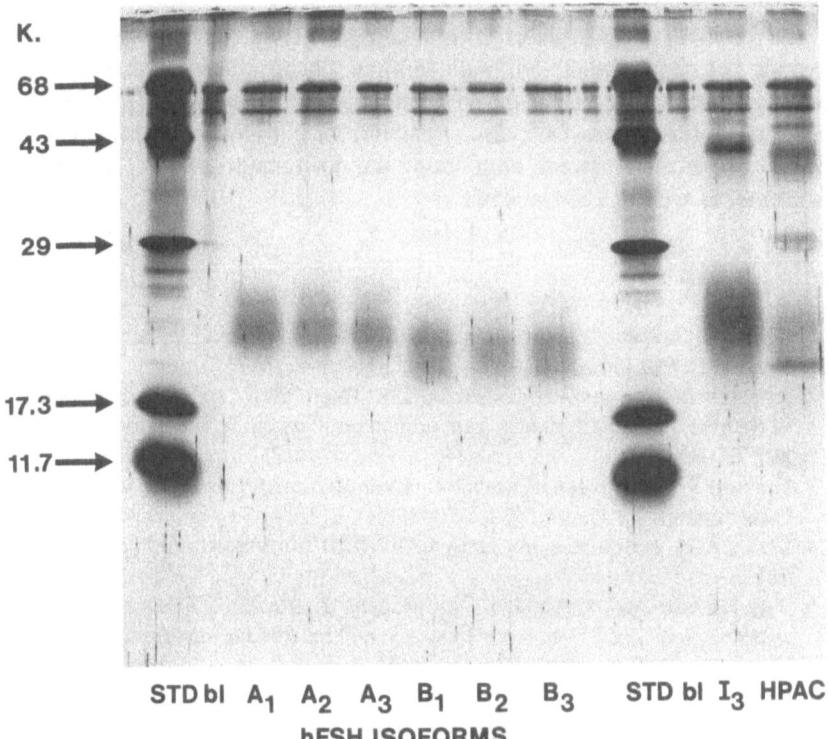

STD bl A₁ A₂ A₃ B₁ B₂ B₃   STD bl I₃ HPAC
hFSH ISOFORMS

FIGURE 32.2. Molecular weights of FSH Isoforms. Purified FSH isoforms were fractionated by SDS-PAGE under reducing conditions and visualized by silver staining. (STD = molecular weight standards; Bl = blank; I_3 = NIH FSH-I-3; and HPAC = HPAC FSH.) (The double staining lines at 50–60 k are artifacts, as seen in the blank lanes.)

HPIEX to separate proteins of similar pI where the charged groups are in different locations on the protein surface. For example, IEF region B, which is a single FSH RRA peak, was further separated into a minimum of 3 FSH isoforms by HPIEX. The selectivity of HPIEX has been extended by the use of mobile phases of 2 different pHs to further separate the hFSH isoforms (Figs. 32.1c–32.1d).

Biological specific activities of the 6 FSH isoforms by RRA and in vitro bioassay are greater than previously reported (6) and higher than the NIH-I-3 hFSH and HPAC hFSH preparations assayed concurrently. These high values are most probably due to the deliberate choice of mild purification conditions and the use of protease inhibitors throughout the procedure. The protein content of all FSH preparations was estimated by amino acid analysis without correction for the presence of cysteines or carbohydrate content, which based on literature values is likely to be approximately 20% (7).

Current data suggest that isoform heterogeneity is primarily due to carbohydrate heterogeneity (1), with concomitant changes in immunological and biological activities. Using the methodology presented here it is now possible to establish the carbohydrate structure of individual isoforms. Current studies are directed toward completing the purification of other major FSH isoforms, as well as LH and TSH.

References

1. Keel BA, Grotjan HE, eds. Microheterogeneity of glycoprotein hormones. Boca Raton, FL: CRC Press, 1989.
2. Johnston RC, Stanton PG, Robertson DM, Hearn MTW. Separation of isoforms of the glycoprotein hormones from human pituitary extracts. J Chromatog 1987; 397:389-98.
3. Laemmli UK. Cleavage of structural proteins during the assembly of the head of bacteriophage T_4. Nature 1970;227:680-5.
4. Cheng KW. A radioreceptor assay for FSH. J Clin Endocrinol Metab 1975;41: 581-9.
5. Van Damme MP, Robertson DM, Marana R, Ritzen EM, Diczfalusy E. A sensitive and specific in vitro bioassay method for the measurement of FSH activity. Acta Endocrinol 1979;91:224-37.
6. Grotjan HE. Oligosaccharide structures of the anterior pituitary and placental glycoprotein hormones. In Keel BA, Grotjan HE, eds. Microheterogeneity of glycoprotein hormones. Boca Raton, FL: CRC Press, 1989:23-52.

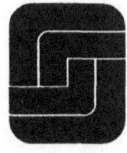

33

Expression of FSH and LH Receptor mRNAs in the Rat Ovary

TAMARA A. CAMP AND KELLY E. MAYO

The pituitary gonadotropins, follicle stimulating hormone (FSH) and luteinizing hormone (LH), play important roles in regulating the steroidogenic and gametogenic functions of the gonads. The actions of these hormones are mediated by specific cell-surface receptors, the LH/hCG receptor (LH/hCG-R), and the FSH receptor (FSH-R). Cloned cDNAs for these receptors were recently isolated in several laboratories (1–4). The deduced amino acid sequences of these two receptors predicts 7 potential transmembrane domains, indicating that they are related to the G-protein-coupled receptor family.

One particularly powerful approach to identifying new members of the G-protein-coupled receptor family has been the use of the polymerase chain reaction (PCR). Degenerate oligonucleotide primers corresponding to conserved regions of known receptors have been used to amplify cDNA from specific tissues (5). We have been utilizing this approach to isolate both known and novel members of the G-protein-coupled receptor family from ovarian tissue. In the initial pool of clones that we characterized, we identified both FSH-R and LH-R partial cDNAs. Here, we report on the identification of these cDNAs and on the localization of the FSH-R and LH-R mRNAs in the adult rat ovary.

Materials and Methods

Degenerate oligonucleotide primers to transmembrane domains 2 (GRTM-2) and 6 (GTRM-6) were designed using the known sequences of 6 members of the G-protein-coupled receptor family: rhodopsin and the β-adrenergic, muscarinic, serotonin, substance K, and LH receptors. The oligonucleotides are shown in Figure 33.1. In addition to the sequences indicated, the primers included either an *Eco*RI site (5' primer) or a *Hind*III site (3' primer) to fa-

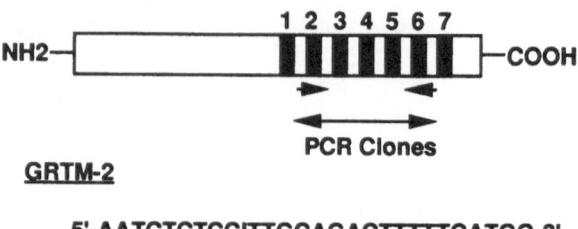

GRTM-2

5'-AATCTCTCCITTGCAGACTTTTTCATGG-3'
    C GG   G C   C C G
256-28mers (1 inosine)

GRTM-6

3'-ACGTACGGCGGGTTGITG-5'
    AC CA   AA GA
256-18mers (1 inosine)

FIGURE 33.1. Strategy for isolating G-protein-coupled receptor cDNA clones. The two oligonucleotide primers shown were made to transmembrane domains 2 and 6 of known G-protein-coupled receptors. The schematic at the top shows the location of the primers within the coding region of the rat LH-R cDNA.

cilitate cloning of the amplified fragments. Poly(A)+ rat ovarian RNA was reverse-transcribed using either oligo(dT) or random hexamer primers, and the resulting single-stranded cDNA was amplified through 35 PCR cycles at an annealing temperature of 50°. PCR products were gel purified, ligated into pGEM vectors, and sequenced.

For RNA analysis, polyadenylated RNA was isolated from rat liver, brain, pituitary, thyroid, and ovary. RNA (10 μg) from each tissue was separated by electrophoresis on a 1% agarose-formaldehyde gel, and the RNA was transferred to a nylon membrane. The receptor cDNA inserts were labeled with [^{32}P]dCTP using random hexamer primers and Klenow DNA polymerase and were used to probe identical RNA blots. Following hybridization, the filters were washed in 0.2x SSC/0.1% SDS at 65°C and were exposed to Kodak XAR-5 film for 15 h.

For in situ hybridization experiments, cycling female Sprague-Dawley rats (Charles River) were sacrificed at 1100 h on each day of the cycle, and ovaries were removed and frozen. Serum gonadotropin measurements and ovarian morphology were used to verify cycle stages. Sections (20 μm) were cut on a cryostat and were processed for in situ hybridization on microscope slides with ^{35}S-labeled FSH-R and LH-R antisense RNA probes, as described previously (6, 7). After washing the slides, they were coated with Kodak NTB-2 emulsion and exposed for 2–3 weeks. Following development, tissues were stained with hematoxylin/eosin.

Results

Numerous cDNAs of approximately 500 base pairs (bp) were isolated using the PCR procedure outlined above. DNA sequence analysis indicated that 2 of the most abundant cDNAs isolated encoded the LH-R and FSH-R. To determine whether the partial cDNA clones originally isolated were specific for the LH-R and FSH-R mRNAs, we probed RNAs isolated from a variety of rat tissues using RNA blot analysis. These results are shown in Figure 33.2. The left panel shows a blot probed with the LH-R cDNA; the right panel shows an identical blot probed with the FSH-R cDNA. In both cases, hybridization is observed only to ovarian RNA. Consistent with previous results, numerous LH-R transcripts are detected (approximately 7.0, 4.4, 2.7, and 1.5 kb). In contrast, a single predominant FSH-R transcript of about 2.7 kb is observed; in addition, the hybridization intensities indicate that the LH-R mRNA is much more abundant than the FSH-R mRNA in ovarian tissue. As an additional control for specificity of these cDNAs, a rat thyroid stimulating hormone receptor (TSH-R) cDNA, which is related to FSH-R and LH-R cDNAs and was isolated in our laboratory, was used to reprobe the RNA

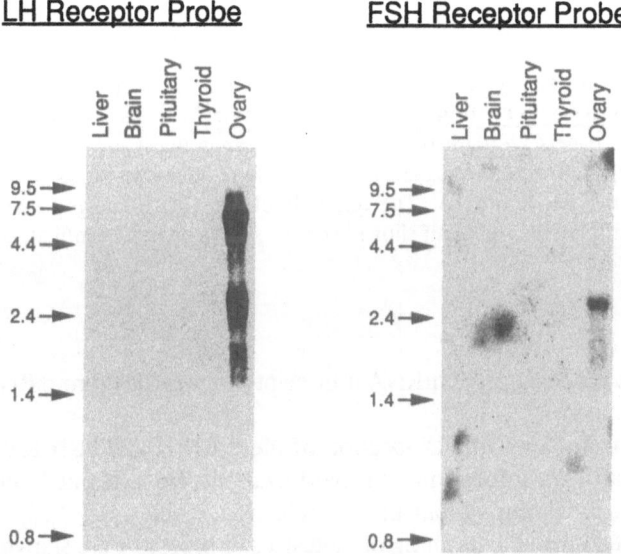

FIGURE 33.2. RNA blot analysis of rat tissues with LH-R and FSH-R cDNAs. Each lane contains 10-µg ovarian poly(A)+ RNA. Size markers are indicated next to the autoradiograms. LH-R expression is shown on the left, FSH-R expression is shown on the right. The material in the brain lane of the FSH-R blot is a film artifact and is not FSH-R mRNA.

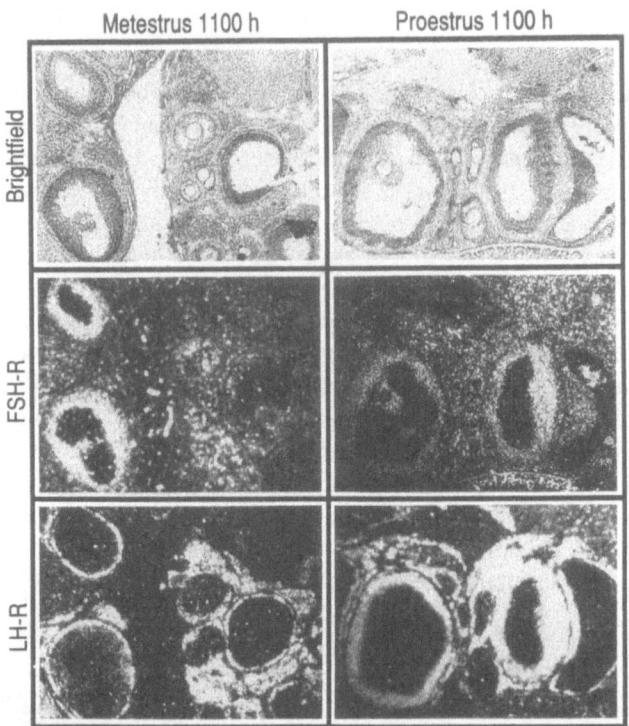

FIGURE 33.3. In situ hybridization to detect FSH-R and LH-R mRNAs in the rat ovary. The top panels are bright-field photomicrographs that show ovarian histology. The middle panels are dark-field photomicrographs that show localization of the FSH-R mRNA. The bottom panels are dark-field photomicrographs that show localization of the LH-R mRNA. The left half of the figure shows sections from a metestrus animal; the right half shows sections from a proestrus animal, as indicated.

blots. This probe detected mRNA transcripts only in the thyroid RNA sample (data not shown).

To determine the cellular location of these LH-R and FSH-R mRNAs in the rat ovary, we utilized in situ hybridization. We examined animals at a number of times throughout the 4-day estrous cycle, and 2 representative examples taken on the morning of metestrus or proestrus are shown in Figure 33.3. In the metestrous ovary, FSH-R mRNA is found localized to the granulosa cells (GC) of maturing antral follicles. In contrast, LH-R mRNA is found predominantly in the thecal cells of these same follicles, as well as in some interstitial tissues (Fig. 33.3, left panels). In the proestrous ovary, FSH-R mRNA continues to be expressed in the GC of apparently healthy follicles;

these same follicles also express the α- and β-inhibin genes (data not shown). There appears to be a slight reduction in expression of the FSH-R mRNA in the proestrous ovary. The LH-R mRNA is highly expressed in the proestrous ovary and is found in GC, thecal cells, and some interstial tissue (Fig. 33.3, right panels).

Discussion

Partial cDNA clones encoding the rat FSH-R and LH-R were isolated from ovarian mRNA by a reverse-transcription-PCR approach. These cDNA clones specifically detect the LH-R and FSH-R mRNAs as determined by RNA blot analysis. As a first step toward understanding where these receptor mRNAs are expressed and how they are regulated, we have used in situ hybridization to examine the distribution of the FSH-R and LH-R mRNA in the ovary of adult cycling rats. The results presented here indicate that the FSH-R gene is expressed in the GC of healthy follicles throughout the estrous cycle. In contrast, the LH-R gene is expressed predominantly in the thecal cells of small follicles, then gradually increases in expression in GC as follicles mature to preovulatory status.

These results agree with previous findings that have localized [^{125}I]FSH binding to the GC, [^{125}I]hCG binding to thecal cells and interstitial tissues of immature rats, and [^{125}I]hCG binding to the GC of FSH-treated rats (8). Thus, changes previously observed in binding studies appear to be due to direct changes in the expression of the genes for these two receptors. It will clearly be important to try to understand the molecular mechanisms by which these two genes are differentially expressed in ovarian cell types and are regulated during the reproductive cycle. The availability of cloned FSH-R and LH-R cDNAs will certainly facilitate these types of studies.

Acknowledgments. This work was supported by grants from the NIH, NSF, and the Searle Scholars Program to K.E.M. We thank Jason Rahal for sequencing of cDNA clones.

References

1. McFarland KC, Sprengel R, Phillips HS, et al. Lutropin-choriogonadotropin receptor: an unusual member of the G protein-coupled receptor family. Science 1989;245:494-9.
2. Sprengel R, Braun T, Nikolics K, Segaloff DL, Seeburg PH. The testicular receptor for follicle stimulating hormone: structure and functional expression of cloned cDNA. Mol Cell Endocrinol 1990;4:525-30.

3. LaPolt PS, Oikawa M, Jia X, Dargan C, Hsueh AJW. Gonadotropin-induced up- and down-regulation of rat ovarian LH receptor message levels during follicular growth, ovulation, and luteinization. Endocrinology 1990;6:3277-9.
4. Loosfelt H, Misrahi M, Atger M, et al. Cloning and sequencing of porcine LH-hCG receptor cDNA: variants lacking transmembrane domain. Science 1989; 245:525-7.
5. Libert F, Parmentier M, Lefort A, et al. Selective amplification and cloning of four members of the G protein-coupled receptor family. Science 1989;244:569-72.
6. Woodruff TK, Meunier H, Jones PB, Hsueh JW, Mayo KE. Rat inhibin: molecular cloning of α- and β-subunit complementary deoxyribonucleic acids and expression in the ovary. Mol Cell Endocrinol 1987;1:561-8.
7. Suhr ST, Rahal JO, Mayo KE. Mouse growth hormone-releasing hormone: precursor structure and expression in brain and placenta. Mol Cell Endocrinol 1989;3:1693-700.
8. Zeleznik AJ, Midgley AR, Reichert AR, Jr. Granulosa cell maturation in the rat: increased binding of human chorionic gonadotropin following treatment with follicle-stimulating hormone in vivo. Endocrinology 1974;95:818-25.

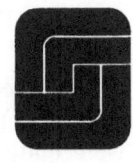

34

Regulation of Epidermal Growth Factor (EGF) Binding Sites in Rat Granulosa Cells by Follicle Stimulating Hormone (FSH)

H. Fujinaga, M. Yamoto, T. Shikone, K. Nishimori, and R. Nakano

In the present study, we examined the effect of FSH on [^{125}I]mEGF binding to rat granulosa cells (GC). The GC, isolated from diethylstilbestrol-treated immature female rats, were cultured with ovine FSH (NIADDK-oFSH-17) (1–300 ng/mL) in serum-free McCoy's 5a medium for 48 h at 37°C and then were incubated with [^{125}I]mEGF (0.05 µCi) for 18 h at 20°C to quantify EGF binding sites. After culture with oFSH for 48 h, the GC were cultured with or without mEGF (30 ng/mL) for 48 h at 37°C, then tissue plasminogen activator (tPA) activities in the conditioned media were examined by the fibrin overlay method. FSH significantly increased [^{125}I]mEGF binding to rat GC in a dose-dependent manner, and EGF produced a dose-dependent increase in tPA activity compared to the control. Our findings suggest that functional EGF binding sites in rat GC are regulated by FSH and that FSH might influence folliculogenesis by regulating EGF receptors (EGF-R).

Follicular development, steroidogenesis, and ovulation are dependent upon the actions of follicle stimulating hormone (FSH) and luteinizing hormone (LH). Growth factors, such as epidermal growth factor (EGF), also regulate ovarian follicular growth and differentiation. The binding sites for EGF have been demonstrated in rat ovary and GC (1). In addition, EGF has been thought to stimulate tPA activity (2). We examined [^{125}I]mEGF binding to rat GC cultured with oFSH and tPA activities in the conditioned media to establish the effect of FSH on EGF-R in rat GC.

Materials and Methods

GC were isolated from 25-day-old immature female rats treated with diethylstilbestrol 1 mg/day for 4 days. Iodination of mEGF was carried out by chloramine-T method, as described by Carpenter and Cohen (3). The specific activity of the labeled mEGF was 150–190 µCi/µg. GC (5×10^5 viable cells) were cultured in 1-mL serum-free McCoy's 5a medium with or without oFSH (NIADDK-oFSH-17) (1–300 ng/mL) for 48 h in a humidified atmosphere of 5% CO_2 in air at 37°C and then were incubated with [^{125}I]mEGF (0.05 µCi) for 18 h at 20°C to quantify EGF-R. Nonspecific binding was assessed in the presence of 300-ng mEGF. The incubation was stopped by the addition of 1.5-mL ice-cold 0.1% BSA-PBS (pH 7.4) and centrifugation for 10 min at 2000 × g. The pellets were washed twice with 1.5-mL 0.1% BSA-PBS and then counted in an automatic γ-counter (Aloka Co., Tokyo).

After culture with oFSH (100 ng/mL) or in medium alone for 48 h, GC were cultured with or without mEGF (30 ng/mL) for an additional 48 h. The media were collected at the end of culture and adjusted 0.01% Tween-20 before analysis of tPA activity by the fibrin overlay method (2). Statistical analyses were performed by Student's t-test.

Results

Unlabeled mEGF inhibited the binding of [^{125}I]mEGF to cultured rat GC in a dose-dependent manner. Displacement studies demonstrated that [^{125}I]mEGF was specifically bound to the GC (data not shown).

FSH treatment significantly increased [^{125}I]mEGF binding to rat GC at 48 h of culture (Fig. 34.1). The increases in [^{125}I]mEGF binding at the concentration of 3-ng/mL and 100-ng/mL oFSH were 124% (P < 0.05) and

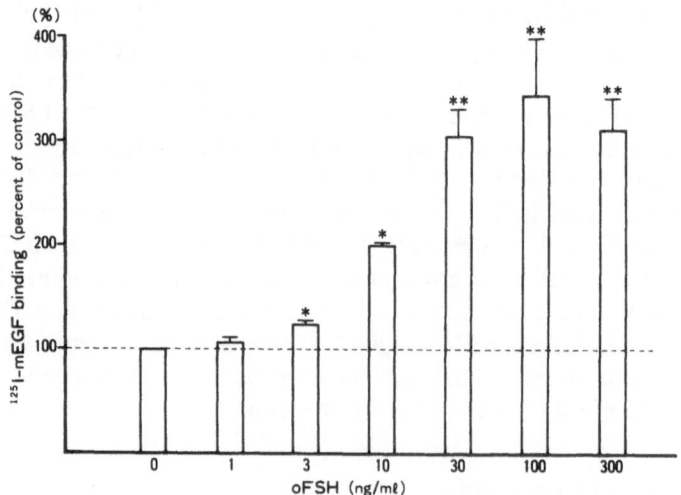

FIGURE 34.1.   Effect of oFSH (1–300 ng/mL) on [^{125}I]mEGF binding to rat GC. Mean ± SEM. (*P < 0.05; **P < 0.01.)

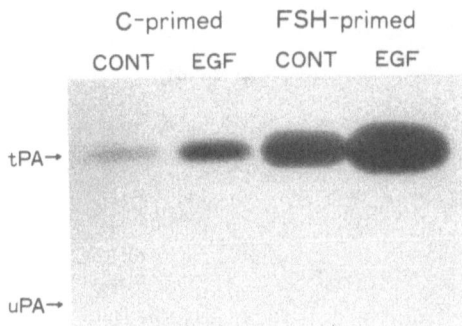

FIGURE 34.2. Effects of EGF on tPA and uPA activities in the cultured rat GC. FSH pretreatment and EGF stimulated tPA activities. EGF produced more remarkable increase in tPA activity compared to the control.

344% (P < 0.01), respectively. Maximal stimulation was produced by 50–300 ng/mL of oFSH. Thus, FSH appears to have a stimulative effect on EGF-R.

GC were cultured for 48 h in medium alone (Fig. 34.2, C-primed) or with oFSH (Fig. 34.2, FSH-primed). The media were then removed, and the GC were cultured for an additional 48 h in medium alone (Fig. 34.2, CONT) or with mEGF (Fig. 34.2, EGF) or increasing doses of mEGF (Fig. 34.3). tPA activities in the conditioned media were measured by the fibrin overlay method (Figs. 34.2–34.3). FSH pretreatment (100 ng/mL) and EGF (30 ng/mL) stimulated tPA activities (2). Additionally, EGF produced a more remarkable increase in tPA activity compared to the control, and this stimulative effect of EGF was dose dependent. FSH and EGF had no effect on urokinase plasminogen activator (uPA) activity.

Discussion

The functions of reproductive organs are regulated by several polypeptide hormones, including FSH and LH. Furthermore, it has been reported that EGF influences some FSH-mediated actions—such as suppression of FSH-induced LH receptor (LH-R) expression (4) and regulation of ovarian progestin production (5)—and that EGF-R exist in GC and are modulated by FSH (1, 6, 7). These reports suggest that the effects of EGF might be controlled by gonadotropins.

We have demonstrated that FSH increased [^{125}I]mEGF binding to the cultured rat GC in a dose-dependent manner and that EGF produced a dose-

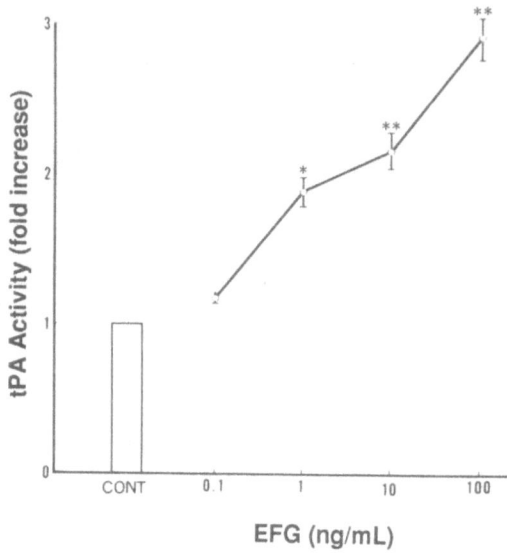

FIGURE 34.3. Effect of EGF on tPA activity in the cultured rat GC. EGF produced a dose-dependent increase in tPA activity compared to the control. Vertical bars represent SEM. (*P < 0.02; **P < 0.01.)

dependent increase in tPA activity compared to the control. EGF binding sites in the GC were up-regulated by FSH. Since FSH-induced EGF binding sites stimulated tPA activities, these FSH-induced EGF binding sites could be functional receptors. Our findings suggest that FSH might influence the growth and differentiation of GC by regulating functional EGF-R. Ovarian folliculogenesis might be regulated by the interactions of FSH and EGF or other factors. Further studies are needed to elucidate these interactions.

References

1. St Arnaud R, Walker P, Kelly PA, Labrie F. Rat ovarian epidermal growth factor receptors: characterization and hormonal regulation. Mol Cell Endocrinol 1983; 31:43-52.
2. Galway AB, Oikawa M, Ny T, Hsueh AJW. Epidermal growth factor stimulates tissue plasminogen activator and messenger ribonucleic acid levels in cultured rat granulosa cells: mediation by pathways independent of protein kinase-A and -C. Endocrinology 1989;125:126-35.
3. Carpenter G, Cohen S. ^{125}I-Labeled human epidermal growth factor binding, internalization, and degradation in human fibroblast. J Cell Biol 1976;71:159-71.
4. Mondschein JS, Schomberg DW. Growth factors modulate gonadotropin receptor induction in granulosa cell cultures. Science 1980;211:1179-80.

5. Jones PBC, Welsh TH, Jr, Hsueh AJW. Regulation of ovarian progestin production by epidermal growth factor in cultured rat granulosa cells. J Biol Chem 1982;257:11268-73.
6. Buck PA, Schomberg DW. [^{125}I]Iodo-epidermal growth factor binding and mitotic responsiveness of porcine granulosa cells are modulated by differentiation and follicle-stimulating hormone. Endocrinology 1988;122:28-33.
7. Feng P, Knecht M, Catt K. Hormonal control of epidermal growth factor receptors by gonadotropins during granulosa cell differentiation. Endocrinology 1987;120:1121-6.

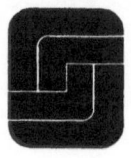

35

FSH and LH Stimulation of Granulosa Cell Prodynorphin Gene Expression Abolished by Overexpression of a Nonfunctional Mutant of the RI Subunit of Protein Kinase A

ALAN H. KAYNARD, CYNTHIA T. MCMURRAY, JAMES DOUGLASS, AND MICHAEL H. MELNER

At least three second-messenger systems are potentially involved in follicle stimulating hormone (FSH) activation of follicular development. They are cAMP/protein kinase A (cAMP-dependent protein kinase; PKA) (1), phosphoinositide turnover (2), and calcium/calmodulin(3); the latter two both act to increase the activity of protein kinase C. FSH has many actions on the ovary, and these three systems may be of different importance in contributing to each action of FSH. One mechanism by which FSH drives follicular development is its ability to stimulate the expression of mRNAs that encode important ovarian anabolic enzymes (4) and secretory products (5), including the endogenous opioid peptide genes prodynorphin (6) and proopiomelanocortin (7). To delineate the relative importance of different second-messenger systems in transducing the stimulatory effects of FSH on granulosa cells (GC) we tested the hypothesis that suppression of the cAMP/PKA system in these cells would alter FSH and luteinizing hormone (LH) stimulation of prodynorphin gene expression.

We focused on the cAMP/PKA system because cAMP is considered the major second-messenger transducing FSH stimulation of GC (for review, see [8]). FSH stimulates cAMP production and increases PKA activity in GC (1). Many actions of FSH can be mimicked in vitro by treatment with cAMP analogs (9) and adenylate cyclase stimulators (10). Expression of prodynorphin was examined because we have shown that gonadotropin treatment in vivo will affect the level of ovarian prodynorphin mRNA (6). Furthermore, others have shown that prodynorphin-derived peptides, which are

356

produced in numerous mammalian tissues, have many different sites of action, including the hypothalamic-pituitary-gonadal axis (for reviews, see [11, 12]).

Materials and Methods

Plasmids

The prodynorphin promoter/chloramphenicol acetyltransferase fusion plasmid (DYN-CAT) used in these studies contains 1994 bp of the rat dynorphin gene (including 1863 bp of the upstream promoter region and 131 bp of exon 1) inserted into the promoterless pOCAT vector (13). The MtREV expression plasmid was kindly provided by Dr. G. Stanley McKnight (University of Washington, Seattle, WA). It contains the coding region (1191 bp) of a mutated mouse gene for the RI subunit of PKA inserted between an ~700-bp segment of the mouse metallothionein-1 promoter and a 630-bp segment of the human growth hormone 3'-untranslated flanking sequence (14). The MtREV expression plasmid overexpresses a mutated form of the RI regulatory subunit of PKA that is incapable of binding cAMP, yet retains the capability of complexing with the catalytic subunit. In the absence of cAMP binding, the RI subunit irreversibly binds to and thereby inhibits the activity of the catalytic subunit (14). The control plasmid used for cotransfection controls in experiment 2 was pUC13, the core plasmid into which MtREV was inserted. All plasmids were amplified in *Eschericia coli* (DH5α) as previously described (15) and purified using pZ523 columns according to the manufacturer's protocol (5'-3', West Chester, PA) or by equilibrium gradient centrifugation in CsCl gradients. The identity of the plasmids was confirmed by restriction enzyme digestion.

GC Preparation and Culture

GC were isolated and cultured as previously described (16). Briefly, follicular development was hyperstimulated in 26-day-old rats by subcutaneous injection of 20IU PMSG. Forty-eight hours later, GC were isolated by the method of Campbell (17), and 4×10^6 viable cells were plated into 35-mm wells precoated with 35 μg of Cell-Tak (Biopolymers, Inc., Farmington, CT). Cells were cultured (37°C in 5% CO_2) in serum-free Medium 199 (Gibco, Grand Island, NY), which was minimally supplemented to maintain cell viability with corticosterone (18 ng/mL), bovine serum albumin (0.1%), insulin (1 μg/mL), transferrin (Trf) (1 μg/mL), and selenous acid (1 ng/mL) (16).

GC Transfection and Hormone Treatment

Transfection of GC with a calcium-phosphate/DNA coprecipitate was carried out as described previously (16). To summarize, freshly isolated GC were cultured for 4 h and then exposed to a DNA precipitate (45-µg DNA/ well) for 4 h followed by a 3.5-min glycerol shock. In the first series of experiments, cells were transfected with the DYN-CAT plasmid only. In the second series of experiments, cells were transfected with DYN-CAT and cotransfected with either the MtREV expression plasmid or a control plasmid (pUC13). Cells were then rinsed with phosphate-buffered saline and cultured in Medium 199 for 12 h in the absence or the presence of either FSH (human, 20 ng/mL), hCG (10 ng/mL), or cpt-cAMP (0.5 mM).

Quantification of CAT Activity and Progesterone Accumulation

After 12 h of culture, 1-mL medium was removed for progesterone (P) measurement and cells were scraped. Cells were collected by low-speed centrifugation, resuspended in 100 µL of 0.25-M Tris HCl (pH 7.4), and lysed by 3 freeze/thaw cycles. Insoluble cellular components were removed by centrifugation at $15,000 \times g$ for 5 min. Eighty-five µL of each cell extract was incubated with 10-µL FluoReporter substrate (Molecular Probes, Eugene, OR) and 30 µL of 1-M Tris HCl (pH 7.4) containing 16.67-mg/mL acetyl CoA (Sigma Chem. Co., St. Louis, MO) at 37°C for 4 h. FluoReporter substrate is a fluorescent-labeled derivative of chloramphenicol (18). Buffer controls (to determine background activity) and tubes with CAT enzyme added (0.08 U; Sigma Chem. Co., St. Louis, MO) (to assure reaction conditions were adequate) were run in triplicate in each assay. The reaction was stopped by adding 850-µL ice-cold ethyl acetate (Mallinckrodt, Paris, KT). The substrate and its acetylated reaction products (1-acetyl, 3-acetyl, and 1,3-di-acetyl chloramphenicol) were extracted into the organic phase, dried down, redissolved in 15-µL ethyl acetate, and separated by thin-layer chromotography (TLC) (LK6 plates, Whatman, Clifton, NJ). Enzyme activity was quantified by scraping and extracting each band from the TLC plate and measuring its fluorescence. Enzyme activity was calculated as the percent conversion of substrate to its acetylated derivatives. Total CAT activity was calculated as the sum of the percent conversions of substrate into each of its 3 acetylated derivatives. Nonenzymatic conversion observed in buffer control lanes (due mainly to impurities in the substrate) was subtracted from all values. Progesterone in medium samples from each experiment was measured in a single RIA (19) with an average intra-assay coefficient of variation of 7.5% ± 2.0%.

Data Analysis

Means are presented as mean ± 1 SEM. One-way analysis of variance (ANOVA) was used to test the effects of hormone and cAMP treatments in the first series of experiments (DNY-CAT transfection). In cotransfection experiments, 2-way ANOVA was used to test the effects of hormone and

TABLE 35.1. CAT activity and P-accumulation in GC cultures transfected with DYN-CAT.

Group	CAT activity	P
Control	0.80 ± 0.13	2.84 ± 0.19
FSH	$14.33 \pm 2.24^{a,b}$	11.32 ± 0.41^a
hCG	$15.37 \pm 2.93^{a,b}$	11.89 ± 0.60^a
cAMP	5.50 ± 0.74^a	11.74 ± 0.16^a

All values are means $\pm$ 1 SEM of n = 3. Treatments are: FSH (20 ng/mL), hCG (10 ng/mL), and cAMP (cpt analog, 0.5 mM). CAT activity is the sum of the percent conversions of FluoReporter CAT substrate into each of its 3 acetylated derivatives. Progesterone accumulation is presented as ng/ml of medium. ([a] $P < 0.01$ vs. control; [b] $P < 0.05$ vs. cAMP.)

cAMP treatments and their interaction with the effect of MtREV cotransfection. Specific differences between groups were made using post hoc Duncan's Multiple Range tests.

Results

FSH, hCG, and cAMP Stimulation of GC Prodynorphin Promoter Activity

CAT activity in GC transfected with DYN-CAT was stimulated by FSH, hCG, and cAMP (Table 35.1). FSH produced an 18-fold increase in total CAT activity, hCG a 19-fold increase, and cAMP a 7-fold increase ($P < 0.01$). Stimulation by FSH and hCG were significantly greater than that produced by cAMP ($P < 0.025$). In the absence of androgen precursors, cultured GC produce P de novo. Table 35.1 shows that equivalent increases in P production were produced by FSH, hCG, and cAMP treatments. This indicates that cell viability and function were not grossly impaired by transfection and that the trophic stimulation produced by the three treatments was equal.

Abolition of FSH and LH Stimulation of Prodynorphin Promoter Activity by Overexpression of a PKA Inhibitor in GC

Table 35.2 shows that overexpression of the PKA inhibiting mutant RI subunit by cotransfection with MtREV abolished FSH, hCG, and cAMP stimulation of CAT activity ($P < 0.01$ vs. same treatment without MtREV).

TABLE 35.2. CAT activity and P-accumulation in GC cultures cotransfected with DYN-CAT and either pUC13 or MtREV.

Cotransfect	Group	CAT activity	P
pUC13	Control	0.10 ± 0.09	2.50 ± 0.16
pUC13	FSH	0.99 ± 0.16[a,b,c]	8.85 ± 0.17[a]
pUC13	hCG	1.05 ± 0.13[a,b,c]	6.24 ± 0.43[a]
pUC13	cAMP	0.58 ± 0.05[a,c]	10.03 ± 0.25[a]
MtREV	Control	0.12 ± 0.04	2.29 ± 0.12
MtREV	FSH	0.20 ± 0.11	8.08 ± 0.41[a]
MtREV	hCG	0.21 ± 0.12	5.63 ± 0.04[a]
MtREV	cAMP	0.05 ± 0.04	10.82 ± 0.04[a]

All values are means ± 1 SEM of n = 3. Treatments are FSH (20 ng/mL), hCG, (10 ng/mL), and cAMP (cpt analog, 0.5 mM). CAT activity is the sum of the percent conversions of FluoReporter CAT substrate into each of its 3 acetylated derivatives. Progesterone accumulation is presented as ng/mL of medium. ([a]$P < 0.005$ vs. appropriate control; [b]$P < 0.05$ vs. cAMP; [c]$P < 0.01$ vs. MtREV treated.)

CAT activity in MtREV cotransfected cultures was not different from unstimulated controls ($P > 0.4$). When cotransfected with DYN-CAT and a control plasmid, FSH, hCG, and cAMP significantly stimulated CAT activity (10-, 11-, and 6-fold, respectively; $P < 0.005$). As in experiment 1, the effects of FSH and hCG stimulation were significantly greater than that induced by cAMP ($P < 0.05$).

Discussion

We have shown that FSH, hCG, and cAMP treatments yield a robust stimulation of prodynorphin promoter activity in transfected rat GC in primary, serum-free culture. Although cAMP produced a lower level of stimulation than gonadotropins, no conclusion can be drawn concerning their relative stimulatory properties since the time course and dose dependency of the responses may differ. Additional experiments employing several doses of cAMP and various durations of exposure are necessary to answer this question. Previous studies have demonstrated high levels of prodynorphin mRNA in the ovary, as well as in other tissues of the female and male reproductive tracts (20). We have shown that ovarian levels of prodynorphin mRNA are altered by gonadotropin treatments that cause follicular development, ovulation, development of corpora lutea, and pseudopregnancy (6). The results reported here suggest that some of ovarian prodynorphin expression may be attributed to GC/luteal cell expression.

The >10-fold increase in expression produced by FSH treatment in the present study implicates the prodynorphin gene as an important target of FSH action. The presence of specific trans-acting factors in GC may enhance transgene prodynorphin expression, as they would presumably do for the endogenous prodynorphin promoter. The magnitude of induction achieved in these studies points out the advantage of using cells that normally express the gene under study. In regards to this point, this model system is, to our knowledge, the only one that involves study of the prodynorphin promoter in a homologous transfection system in cells that normally express this neuropeptide. As such, it represents a powerful tool for the study of the physiological regulation of prodynorphin expression.

Overexpression of MtREV, which encodes a PKA inhibitor (14), eliminated FSH, LH, and cAMP stimulation of prodynorphin promoter activity. This supports our hypothesis that FSH and LH stimulation of prodynorphin promoter activity is dependent on a functional cAMP/PKA second-messenger system. Many studies using different experimental approaches have implicated PKA as an important mediator of FSH stimulation of the ovary. FSH increases cAMP levels (8, 21) and PKA activity (8, 22) in GC. Adenylate cyclase stimulators, such as forskolin, increase PKA activity and mimic the effects of FSH in vitro (10). However, for the transmission of FSH stimulation to be attributed solely to cAMP/PKA, it is necessary to selectively disrupt this system in a model in which FSH action can be accurately monitored. DYN-CAT/MtREV cotransfection provides just such a model. Since MtREV cotransfection reduced prodynorphin promoter activity to the level of unstimulated controls, it can be concluded that the cAMP/PKA second-messenger system is of primary importance for transmitting the stimulatory effect of gonadotropins to the prodynorphin promoter. Recently, Adashi et al. (23) reported that treatment with a competitive inhibitor of cAMP produced an ~70% reduction of FSH-stimulated P accumulation by GC in vitro. Incomplete inhibition observed in that study may be the result of insufficient intracellular availability of the antagonist, homeostatic responses of the cell resulting in increased endogenous cAMP production, or nonspecific effects of the cAMP antagonist used (23). However, alternate intracellular signaling systems that are not active in induction of prodynorphin expression may be involved in the stimulation of steroid hormone secretion.

It may be that the cAMP/PKA system is responsible for many more of the alterations in gene expression produced by FSH and LH stimulation; most notable of these gonadotropin effects is the regulation of genes encoding the steroid hormone anabolic enzymes (4, 25). Although this study examined only the stimulation of prodynorphin promoter activity, the results may be indicative of a generalized mechanism by which gonadotropins regulate gene transcription in the ovary.

Acknowledgments. The authors would like to thank Christian P. Neilsen for his technical assistance in preparing plasmids for these experiments. This study would not have been possible without the efforts of Steven L. Young in developing the GC transfection system. We thank Dr. David L. Hess and the RIA core facility at the Oregon Regional Primate Research Center for performance of P assays. These studies were supported, in part, by NIH DK-41035, NIH RR-00163, and ONR N-00014-90-J-1122.

References

1. Richards JS, Sehgal N, Tash JS. Changes in content and cAMP-dependent phosphorylation of specific proteins in granulosa cells of preantral and pre-ovulatory ovarian follicles and in corpora lutea. J Biol Chem 1983;258:5227-32.
2. Davis JS, Weakland LL, Farese RV, West LA. Luteinizing hormone increases inositol triphosphate and cytosolic free Ca2+ in isolated bovine luteal cells. J Biol Chem 1987;262:8515-21.
3. Carnegie JA and Tsang BK. Follicle-stimulating hormone-regulated granulosa cell steroidogenesis: involvement of the calcium-calmodulin system. Am J Obstet Gynecol 1983;145:223-8.
4. Hickey GJ, Chen S, Besman MJ, et al. Hormonal regulation, tissue distribution, and content of aromatase cytochrome P450 messenger ribonucleic acid and enzyme in rat ovarian follicles and corpora lutea: relationship to estradiol biosynthesis. Endocrinology 1988;122:1426-36.
5. LaPolt PS, Piquette GN, Soto D, Sincich C, Hsueh AJW. Regulation of inhibin subunit messenger ribonucleic acid levels by gonadotropins, growth factors, and gonadotropin-releasing hormone in cultured rat granulosa cells. Endocrinology 1990;127:823-31.
6. Kaynard AH, Melner MH. Elevation of prodynorphin mRNA levels in the rat ovary by gonadotropin stimulation [Abstract]. Soc Neurosci 1990;16(1):952.
7. Melner MH, Young SL, Czerwiec FS, et al. The regulation of granulosa cell proopiomelanocortin messenger ribonucleic acid by androgens and gonadotropins. Endocrinology 1986;119:2082-8.
8. Hsueh AJW, Adashi EY, Jones PBC, Welsh TH, Jr. Hormonal regulation of the differentiation of cultured ovarian granulosa cells. Endocr Rev 1984;5:76-127.
9. Young SL, Nielsen CP, Melner MH. Specific inhibition of protein kinase A in granulosa cells abolishes gonadotropin regulation of the proopiomelanocortin gene promoter [Abstract]. In: Prog Endocr Soc 72nd annu meet. Atlanta: 1990:291.
10. Kurten RC, Richards JS. An adenosine 3',5'-monophosphate-responsive deoxyribonucleic acid element confers forskolin sensitivity on gene expression by primary rat granulosa cells. Endocrinology 1989;125:1345-57.
11. Howlett TA, Rees LH. Endogenous opioid peptides and hypothalamo-pituitary function. Annu Rev Physiol 1986;48:527-36.
12. Howlett TA, Rees LH. Endogenous opioid peptides and human reproduction. Oxf Rev Reprod Biol 1987;9:260-93.

13. Prost E, Moore DD. CAT vectors for analysis of eukaryotic promoters and enhancers. Gene 1986;45:107-11.

14. McKnight GS, Clegg CH, Uhler MD, et al. Analysis of the cAMP-dependent protein kinase system using molecular genetic approaches. Recent Prog Horm Res 1988;44:307-35.

15. Hardy KG. Purification of bacterial plasmids. In: Hardy KG, ed. Plasmids: a practical approach. Oxford: IRL Press 1987:1-6.

16. Young SL, Neilsen CP, Lundblad JR, Roberts JL, Melner MH. Gonadotropin regulation of the rat proopiomelanocortin promoter: characterization by transfection of primary ovarian granulosa cells. Mol Cell Endocrinol 1989;3:15-21.

17. Campbell K. Ovarian granulosa cells isolated with EGTA and hypertonic sucrose: cellular integrity and function. Biol Reprod 1979;21:773-86.

18. Hruby DE, Brinkley JM, Kang HC, Haugland RP, Young SL, Melner MH. Use of a fluorescent chloramphenicol derivative as a substrate for CAT assays. BioTechniques 1990;8:170-1.

19. Resko JA, Ellinwood WE, Paztor LM, Buhl AE. Sex steroids in the umbilical circulation of fetal rhesus monkeys from the time of gonadal differentiation. J Clin Endocrinol Metab 1980;50:900-5.

20. Douglass J, Cox B, Quinn B, Civelli O, Herbert E. Expression of prodynorphin gene in male and female mammalian reproductive tissues. Endocrinology 1987; 120:707-13.

21. Kolena J, Channing CP. Stimulatory effects of LH, FSH and prostaglandins upon cyclic 3',5'-AMP levels in porcine granulosa cells. Endocrinology 1972;90: 1543-50.

22. Knecht M, Ranta T, Katz MS, Catt KJ. Regulation of adenylate cyclase activity by follicle-stimulating hormone and gonadotropin-releasing hormone agonist in cultured rat granulosa cells. Endocrinology 1983;112:1247-55.

23. Adashi EY, Resnick CE, Jastorff B. Blockade of granulosa cell differentiation by an antagonistic analog of adenosine 3',5'-cyclic monophosphate (cAMP): central but non-exclusive intermediary role of cAMP in follicle-stimulating hormone action. Mol Cell Endocrinol 1990;72:1-11.

25. Chedrese PJ, The VL, Labrie F, Juorio AV, Murphy BD. Evidence for the regulation of 3-β-hydroxysteroid dehydrogenase messenger RNA by human chorionic gonadotropin in luteinized porcine granulosa cells. Endocrinology 1990;126:2228-30.

36

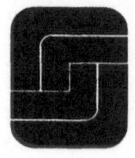

Effects of Specific FSH Deprivation on Testicular Germ Cell Transformations and on LDH-X and Hyaluronidase Activity of Immature and Adult Rats

MAHIMA Y. VAISHNAV AND N.R. MOUDGAL

Although the requirement for FSH to initiate spermatogenesis in the immature rat is well accepted (1–3), its continuous need to support quantitative sperm production in the adulthood is questioned (4, 5). It is suggested that testosterone (T) alone is adequate to maintain sperm production and testicular function in the adult state (6). Since the Sertoli cell (Sc), the primary regulator of germ cell transformation and maturation through the various factors it puts out, continues to be sensitive to both FSH and T even in the adult rat (7), we felt by corollary that FSH should have an effect on spermatogenesis even in the adult rat.

Hitherto, spermatogenesis was quantitated by morphometric analysis of testicular tissue. Compared to this semiquantitative and time-consuming procedure, the flow cytometric analysis (FCM) of germ cells, based on the ability of cells to bind fluorochromes such as diaminidophenyl indole (DAPI) as a function of their DNA content, provides an opportunity to analyze germ cell transformations quantitatively. Besides being rapid, the FCM analysis analyzes a large number of cells—more than 10,000 cells/sample—to arrive at a more meaningful quantitation of cell transformations.

In the current study, in addition to FCM analysis, we have investigated the effect of FSH deprivation on two key marker enzymes of testicular function—LDH-X and hyaluronidase. Specific FSH deprivation in both immature (35-day-old) and adult (100-day-old) rats has been achieved by injecting a minimal dose of characterized FSH antiserum (a/s) daily for a 10-day period. As a positive control to the FSH-deprived state, a separate set of rats were treated with either characterized LH a/s alone or LH a/s plus T. All animals were autopsied 24 h after the last injection of control serum or specific a/s. Methods used for the preparation and characterization of both FSH and LH a/s have been described elsewhere (8, 9). The dose of T-propionate administered where indicated was 3.0 mg or 15.0 mg per rat/day for the prepubertal and adult rats, respectively.

Effect of Gonadotropin Deprivation on Key Marker Enzymes of Testicular Function

For measuring LDH-X activity, the testicular tissue samples obtained from control as well as from FSH- or LH-deprived rats for 10 days were homogenized in 5 vol of 0.1-M phosphate buffer (pH 8.3), and the supernatants (enzyme samples) obtained on centrifugation at $10,000 \times g$ for 30 min were electrophoresed (4-μg protein/lane for each tissue sample) on 8%-25% gradient polyacrylamide minigels on a Pharmacia Phast system at $10°C$ for 600 AV h. The LDH isoenzymes were visualized by staining for LDH-X activity at $37°C$ for 10 min in the dark in a staining solution containing D-L-lactate, β-NAD+, phenazine methosulfate, and nitroblue tetrazolium in 0.1-M Tris-HCl buffer (pH 8.3). The gel was scanned in an integrated densitometer, and the relative integrated area representing the LDH-X band in each group was plotted (10). The mean $\pm$ SD of values obtained in three identical experiments is plotted.

In the case of prepubertal rats, gonadotropin deprivation (either FSH or LH) resulted in a drastic reduction (>90%) in enzyme activity. With adult rat tissues, it was observed that FSH and LH deprivation brought about 50% and 43% reduction, respectively, in activity. Interestingly, exogenous T-propionate supplementation reversed in toto the LH a/s-induced reduction in the case of adult but not prepubertal rats. All changes in enzyme activity observed were statistically significant ($P < 0.05$).

For measuring hyaluronidase activity, the testis was homogenized in 1:19 w/v acetate-buffered saline (pH 4.5) containing 0.15-M NaCl and 0.2% Triton-X-100. The specific activity was measured by estimating the amount of N-acetyl glucosamine released by the action of hyaluronidase on hyaluronic acid per mg protein/h. In the case of the adult rat, though the reduction in enzyme activity following a/s treatment was statistically significant ($P < 0.05$), it amounted to only 30% over the controls. In the case of pubertal rats, FSH deprivation led to a more marked reduction (70%) in enzyme activity. Testosterone supplementation once again was able to partially relieve the inhibition of enzyme activity caused by the lack of LH.

The results of the current study show that LDH-X, an exclusive testis-specific isozyme associated with the development of germ cells from pachytene spermatocyte stage onwards, is regulated by both FSH and LH.

The effects observed for each of these hormones is specific, as deprivation of either of the hormones did not lead to deficiency of the other. As far as we are aware, this is the first report describing gonadotropin involvement in the regulation of LDH-X activity. The effect on hyaluronidase, an acrosomal enzyme, was clearly related to the age of the test animal, the maximal effect being seen in 25-day-old rats. Since acrosome development is largely associated with spermiogenesis, could the observed effect indicate a defect in the process? Perhaps deprivation of FSH support for longer periods (>10 days) is required before a regulatory role for FSH/LH in this enzyme activity can be envisioned.

Effect of Gonadotropin Deprivation on Germ Cell Transformations

The testis of a 40- to 50-day-old rat shows the presence of spermatogonial cells (2C), preleptotene spermatocytes (S-phase), primary spermatocytes (4C), and the round spermatids (1C). The mid (0.7C) spermatids and the elongates (0.3C) are present only during adulthood (100 days and beyond). The FCM analysis permits one to quantitate the 2C, 4C, and 1C population, as they have distinctly different amounts of DNA. During spermiogenesis, because of differences in the degrees of compaction and/or condensation of nuclear chromatin, the haploid DNA picks up relatively lesser dye, permitting us to differentiate between mid and elongate spermatids.

An analysis of cell ratios gives a clearer idea of cellular transformations than the quantitations of only the different cell numbers. In the pubertal rat, FSH deprivation (Exptl) leads to over 90% reduction over controls (Ctrl) in conversion of spermatogonia (2C) to round spermatids (1C) (1C:2C of Ctrl:4.0 ± 1.2 vs. Exptl:0.1 ± 0.0; $P < 0.025$). This primarily appears to be due to a block in meiosis—that is, conversion of 4C to 1C (1C:4C of Ctrl:5.4 ± 0.3 vs. Exptl:0.4 ± 0.1; $P < 0.001$). Such a block leads to accumulation of 4C (by 90%) and 2C (by 259%) populations of cells, leading to a significant ($P < 0.025$) reduction in 4C:2C ratio (Ctrl:0.7 ± 0.1 vs. Exptl:0.3 ± 0.1). These results essentially confirm the observation made by Raj and Dym (2) and Shivashankar et al. (3) using morphometry to analyze germ cell populations.

The testis of the adult rat deprived specifically of FSH provides an entirely different picture. Within the 10-day experimental period, the overall transformation of 2C to 1C is reduced by only 26% (1C:2C of Ctrl:5.4 ± 0.5 vs. Exptl:4.0 ± 0.3; $P < 0.05$). Though the round spermatid population did not show any change, there appeared to be a deficiency in spermiogenesis, leading to a significant reduction ($P < 0.001$) in the hypofluorescent mid (0.7C) and elongate (0.3C) spermatid populations. The ratios reflecting the conversion of 1C to 0.7C and 0.3C were significantly (P < 0.001) reduced (0.7C:1C of Ctrl:0.3 ± 0.05 vs. Exptl:0.11 ± 0.02 and 0.3C:1C of Ctrl:0.7 ± 0.10 vs. Exptl:0.16 ± 0.02).

FSH deprivation did not seem to affect either spermatogonial proliferation or its conversion to primary spermatocytes (2C and 4C populations increased by 47% and 97%, respectively). This increase in 4C population (4C:2C of Ctrl:0.36 ± 0.06 vs. Exptl:0.53 ± 0.06) would suggest either a block or slowing down of meiosis (1C:4C of Ctrl:19.5 ± 1.7 vs. Exptl:8.9 ± 0.9). Perhaps this effect is marked (no change in 1C population is seen) because of further blockage in the conversion of round to elongate spermatids. FSH deficiency in the adult rat thus seems to primarily affect spermiogenesis and possibly meiosis also. This block in the latter stages of germ cell transformation could be the cause for the accumulation of spermatogonial cells as well as of primary spermatocytes.

Conclusion

The current study thus successfully demonstrates that FSH has a crucial role in regulating spermatogenesis in both the adult and prepubertal rat. The FSH need, analyzed using both biochemical markers as well as FCM analysis, appears definitely greater in the case of the pubertal state. Perhaps more severe effects could have been observed in the case of the adult rat if FSH deprivation had been continued beyond 10 days. However, the use of heterologous FSH a/s (as employed in the current study) precludes such long-term experimentation.

References

1. Lostroh AJ. Regulation of FSH and ICSH (LH) of reproductive function in the immature male rat. Endocrinology 1969;85:438-45.
2. Raj HGM, Dym M. The effects of selective withdrawal of FSH and LH on spermatogenesis in immature rat. Biol Reprod 1976;14:489-94.
3. Shivashanker S, Prasad MRN, Thampson TNRV, Sheela Rani CS, Moudgal NR. Effect of a highly purified antiserum to FSH on testicular function in immature rat. Indian J Exp Biol 1977;15:845-51.
4. Dym M, Raj HGM, Lin YC, et al. Is FSH required for maintenance of spermatogenesis in adult rats? J Reprod Fertil 1979;26(suppl):175-81.
5. Russell LD, Clermount Y. Degeneration of germ cells in normal, hypophysectomised and hormone treated hypophysectomised rats. Anat Rec 1977;187:347-53.
6. Buhl AE, Cornette JC, Kirton KT, Yuan D. Hypophysectomised male rats treated with polydimethylsiloxane capsules containing testosterone; effects on spermatogenesis, fertility and reproductive tract concentrations of androgens. Biol Reprod 1982;27:183-8.

7. Ritzen EM, Biotani C, Parvinen M, French FS, Feldman M. Stage dependent secretion of ABP by rat seminiferous tubules. Mol Cell Endocrinol 1982;25:25-33.
8. Sheela Rani CS, Moudgal NR. Advances in immunology of gonadotropins. In: Li CH, ed. Hormonal proteins and peptides. New York: Academic Press, 1983:183-4.
9. Prahalada S, Mukku VR, Rao AJ, Moudgal NR. Termination of pregnancy in macacaques (*Macaca radiata*) using monkey antiserum to ovine luteinizing hormone. Contraception 1975;12:137-47.
10. Wheat TE, Goldberg E. LDH-X: the sperm-specific C4 isozyme of lactate dehydrogenase. In: Markert CL, ed. Isozymes; II. Developmental biology. New York: Academic Press, 1974:325-45.

37

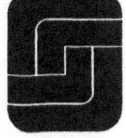

Modulation of Gonadotropin and Sex Steroid Levels by Adrenal Androgens with Osmotic Pumps

WLODZIMIERZ KOWALSKI AND ROBERT T. CHATTERTON, JR.

Chronic exposure to an excess of adrenal androgens has been linked to the pathophysiology and the clinical picture of such endocrinological disorders as polycystic ovary syndrome (1), congenital adrenal hyperplasia (2), and hirsutism (3), conditions often associated with impaired fertility. The purpose of our study was to investigate *subacute* effects of elevated adrenal androgen levels on gonadotropin secretion and sex steroid concentrations in female monkeys. Of all adrenal androgens, dehydroepiandrosterone sulfate (DS) is the most abundant in the circulation, has the lowest metabolic clearance rate, and can be converted in vivo to other adrenal androgens (4). For these reasons, this steroid was chosen as a model for studying the influence of adrenal hyperandrogenaemia on the hormones of the pituitary-ovarian axis.

Materials and Methods

Osmotic pumps (Alzet model 2ML2, Alza Corp., Palo Alto, CA) with a release rate of 5 µL/h were filled with 2 mL of 38-mg/mL DS solution in 70% ethanol for a total dose of 4.5 mg/day. The pumps were implanted subcutaneously in 5 intact female cynomolgus monkeys for 1 menstrual cycle each. The pumps were replaced every 2 weeks according to their nominal duration time. During control cycles that preceded and followed treatment cycles, the animals were implanted with osmotic pumps containing only 70% ethanol. During all cycles, blood was collected 3 days/week for radioimmunoassays (RIA) of DS, estradiol, progesterone (P), FSH, and LH. Urine was collected daily for RIA of pregnanediol glucuronide (PDG) and conjugated estrone. Materials for monkey LH and FSH RIA were obtained from the National Hormone and Pituitary Agency, University of Maryland, as a grant from the NIH, NIDDK.

All serum hormones measured for each monkey were done within a single assay. For each animal, arithmetic means were calculated for a given hormone or metabolite separately for the 2 phases of the menstrual cycle. The first day of the luteal phase (LP) was defined as the first day of increased pregnanediol excretion following the urinary estrone peak. Peak periovulatory values of estradiol or gonadotropins were not included in the calculation of the mean hormone values for the follicular phase (FP). Similarly, mean FP estrone excretion does not include the midcycle peak values. Except for estradiol and FSH, all the results of RIA measurements did not differ significantly between the 2 control cycles. For this reason, they were combined together to serve as a control for statistical analysis. Paired data for each monkey (control vs. DS administration) were analyzed using a 2-tailed t-test. Numerical data are expressed as the arithmetic means ± SE.

Results

DS administration elevated its levels in serum by 270% ± 72% (P < 0.01; Table 37.1). Other serum hormone levels are presented in Table 37.2. Resultant hyperandrogenaemia suppressed estradiol levels by 57% ± 7% in FP and 61% ± 6% in LP (P < 0.02). In FP of the cycle that followed DS administration, estradiol concentrations were still suppressed by 70% ± 12% in comparison to FP of the preceding control cycle (P < 0.02). Consistent with decreased negative estradiol feedback, FSH levels were increased during DS administration by 44% ± 1% in FP (P < 0.0001) and 32% ± 3% in LP (P < 0.001) and also in the FP of the cycle following DS administration by 18% ± 4% (P < 0.05). DS administration resulted in the suppression of LH levels in serum by 20% ± 1% in FP (P < 0.05) and 31% ± 3% in LP (P < 0.005) as well as of progesterone levels by 67% ± 9% in LP (P < 0.005).

Pregnanediol excretion in urine was also decreased by 50% ± 9% in LP (P < 0.01; Table 37.3). Estrone excretion in urine was increased during DS

TABLE 37.1. Concentrations of DS in the serum of monkeys (µg/mL).

	Monkey				
	A	B	C	D	E
Control cycles	151	173	234	289	283
During DS infusion	449	1082	936	576	927

TABLE 37.2. Serum hormone levels in follicular (FP) and luteal (LP) phases.

| | Monkey | | | | |
| | A | B | C | D | E |
	FP/LP	FP/LP	FP/LP	FP/LP	FP/LP
Estradiol (pg/mL)					
Control cycle	42/51	66/28	84/46	38/25	31/20
During DS admin.	13/14	18/10	40/12	15/13	21/11
After DS admin.	5/—	7/—	29/—	7/—	23/—
FSH (ng/mL)					
Control cycle	23/24	20/17	21/15	25/20	25/16
During DS admin.	33/32	29/24	30/21	35/27	37/21
After DS admin.	29/—	25/—	24/—	30/—	26/—
LH (ng/mL)					
Control cycles	46/55	42/55	51/66	47/62	74/64
During DS admin.	39/42	33/40	41/40	38/44	57/41
Progesterone (ng/ml)					
Control cycles	—/12	—/12	—/14	—/9	—/12
During DS admin.	—/3	—/1	—/8	—/2	—/6

TABLE 37.3. Urinary pregnanediol (PDG) and estrone excretion.

| | Monkey | | | | |
| | A | B | C | D | E |
	FP/LP	FP/LP	FP/LP	FP/LP	FP/LP
PDG (µg/day)					
Control cycles	—/6.7	—/3.1	—/5.2	—/5.3	—/6.3
During DS admin.	—/2.3	—/1.0	—/4.0	—/2.1	—/4.0
Estrone (µg/day)					
Control cycles	2.3/2.3	0.4/0.5	1.0/1.0	2.1/1.3	0.5/0.5
During DS admin.	2.8/2.8	0.6/0.7	1.5/1.3	2.2/2.1	0.9/1.0

administration by 41% ± 13% in FP and 41% ± 7% in LP (both P < 0.02; Table 37.3.

DS did not affect the menstrual cycle, nor did FP length. However, in the cycle that followed DS administration, the length of the LP was decreased by an average of 4 days in comparison to the length of the LP in the control cycle preceding DS administration (P < 0.02; not shown).

Discussion

The physiologic effects of steroid hormones are time dependent. That is, in the course of time, the molecular mechanism responsible for the observed response may vary. An example would be that of the fast and delayed negative-feedback effects of glucocorticoids on ACTH secretion (5). Steroid hormones may also have opposing effects over short versus longer periods of exposure, such as the positive- and negative-feedback actions of estradiol on gonadotropin secretion (6). In our study, we investigated the effects of subacute exposure to increased androgen concentrations on the hormones of the pituitary-ovarian axis. Elevated FSH levels in this study seem to be the result of decreased levels of serum estradiol and the resulting decreased negative feedback on FSH secretion. Decreased estradiol in the presence of elevated FSH suggests that the mechanism by which estradiol is suppressed by subacute exposure to DS is peripheral and not central. The decrease in serum estradiol may be due to decreased ovarian secretion or, more likely, to increased metabolic clearance. The reason that we favor the latter is that excretion of estrone was not decreased in the cycle after DS treatment, whereas estradiol levels remained suppressed.

In addition, it is well established that androgens decrease the concentration of sex-hormone binding globulin (SHBG)(7), a result of which is increased clearance of estradiol. Increased estrone excretion during DS administration is probably a result of increased aromatization of exogenous androgens. In contrast to estradiol, the production rate of progesterone was suppressed in the LP during DS infusion, as indicated by the decrease in excretion of pregnanediol. The mechanism of this suppression seems to be mainly central since LH levels were depressed by about 1/3 during DS administration. Decreased LH serum concentrations in this study evidently reflect negative androgen feedback on its secretion. The underlying mechanism of this phenomenon—reduced frequency of pulsatile LH release—has been demonstrated in the ovariectomized monkey (8).

Since inhibin secretion in the LP is LH dependent (9), decreased LH secretion during DS infusion may decrease inhibin secretion, which could lead to the elevated FSH levels observed. However, the most plausible explanation for the dissociation between FSH and LH secretion observed in our study is the differential sensitivity to negative estradiol and androgen feedback. FSH is known to be more sensitive to alterations in estradiol concentrations since its levels rise or fall more rapidly and consistently than LH does in women before menopause (10) or on replacement estrogen therapy (11). In contrast, LH levels may be more sensitive to negative androgen feedback. Androgen has been shown to decrease GnRH pulse frequency in female macaques (8), and because of its considerably shorter half-life, LH would be expected to be more affected than FSH.

The results of this study indicate that disturbances of the pituitary-ovarian axis can still persist after normalization of subacute hyperandrogenaemia, as documented by disturbed estradiol and FSH levels and a significantly shortened LP in the cycle that followed DS administration. They also document

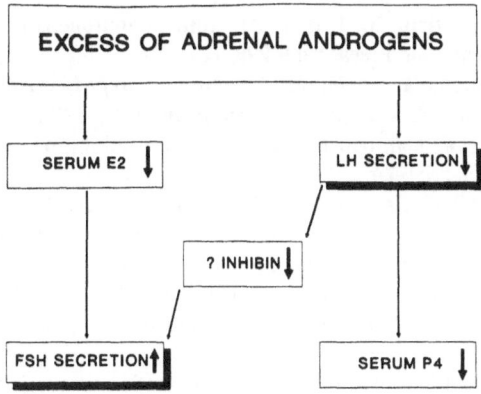

FIGURE 37.1. Modulation of the pituitary-ovarian axis by subacute exposure to increased levels of adrenal androgens. (E2 = estradiol; P4 = progesterone.)

that subacute exposure to an excess of adrenal androgens did not lead to endocrine changes associated with *chronically* elevated androgen levels of, for example, polycystic ovary syndrome. Whether chronic administration of DS would eventually lead to increased LH and decreased FSH is not known.

Summary

Within the period of 1 menstrual cycle, the elevation of serum DS levels 2.7-fold by constant infusion of DS decreased serum estradiol despite significantly elevated levels of serum FSH. Serum LH was decreased, apparently as a result of a direct effect of androgens on LH secretion. The decrease in serum progesterone levels observed in the presence of this degree of adrenal androgen excess may be sufficient to impair fertility. Figure 37.1 is a graphical representation of the findings of the study.

Acknowledgments. Supported in part from a grant from the NIH, HD-21921.

References

1. DeVane GW, Czekala NM, Judd HL, Yen SSC. Circulating gonadotropins, estrogens, and androgens in polycystic ovarian disease. Am J Obstet Gynecol 1975;121:496-500.
2. Cassorla FG, Chrousos GP. Congenital adrenal hyperplasia. In: Becker KL, ed. Principles and practice of endocrinology and metabolism. Philadelphia: JB Lippincott 1990:604-13.

3. Parker LN. Hirsutism. In: Parker LN. Adrenal androgens in clinical medicine. New York: Academic Press, 1989:298-319.
4. Parker LN. Adrenal androgen metabolism. In: Parker LN. Adrenal androgens in clinical medicine. New York: Academic Press, 1989:3-29.
5. Keller-Wood ME, Dallman MF. Corticosteroid inhibition of ACTH secretion. Endocr Rev 1984;5:1-24.
6. Nakai Y, Plant TM, Hess DL, Keogh EJ, Knobil E. On the sites of the negative and positive feedback actions of estradiol in the control of gonadotropin secretion in the rhesus monkey. Endocrinology 1978;102:1008-14.
7. Maruyama Y, Aoki N, Suzuki Y, et al. Sex-steroid binding protein (SBP), testosterone oestradiol and DHEA in prepuberty and puberty. Acta Endocrinol 1987;114:60-7.
8. Dubey AK, Plant TM. Testosterone administration to ovariectomized monkeys (*Macaca mulatta*) reduces the frequency of pulsatile luteinizing hormone secretion. Biol Reprod 1985;32:1109-15.
9. McLachlan RI, Cohen NL, Vale WW, et al. The importance of luteinizing hormone in the control of inhibin and progesterone secretion by the human corpus luteum. J Clin Endocrinol Metab 1989;68:1078-85.
10. Lenton EA, Sexton L, Lee S, Cook ID. Progressive changes in LH and FSH and LH:FSH ratio in women throughout reproductive life. Maturitas 1988;10:35-43.
11. Geola FL, Frumar AM, Tataryn IV, et al. Biological effects of various doses of conjugated equine estrogens in postmenopausal women. J Clin Endocrinol Metab 1980;51:620-5.

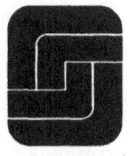

38

Basal Gonadotropins in Regularly Menstruating Women: Age-Related Changes in Follicle Stimulating Hormone (FSH) and Luteinizing Hormone (LH) Prior to the Perimenopause

N.A. Ahmed-Elabbiary, E.A. Lenton, I.D. Cooke, and D. Wright

The traditional marker of reproductive senescence in women is the menopause, characterized by the loss of menstrual or fertility cycles at midlife. The female climacteric is based primarily on the loss of ovarian function. It has been suggested that a gradual rise in FSH levels appears to be the first detectable endocrine manifestation of reproductive aging (1). However, most investigators reported a rise in FSH and, later, LH levels after the age of 40 years (2, 3) or even after the age of 45 (4). In these reports, investigators reported this rise in FSH as a marker of the menopausal transition that consequently reflects "a state of partial ovarian failure," which proceeds the actual menopause and loss of reproductive functions. Unlike women, healthy old men do experience a rise in FSH and LH later in life, but to a lesser degree than do postmenopausal women, despite the absence of gonadal failure or changes in plasma testosterone (T) (5, 6).

In this study, we tried to find if women, like men, also experience an age-related increase in gonadotropins in the absence of gonadal failure and independent from the "expected" perimenopausal rise of gonadotropins. To answer this question, it would be ideal to set up longitudinal studies of single individuals over the course of several years. However, this is unlikely to be practical, particularly because of subjects' compliance and because a study that relies on human volunteers of necessity has to reach a compromise between the ideal and the practical. Thus, a cross-sectional approach was used in this study.

Subjects and Methods

Subjects

The study population consisted of normal women aged 20–44 years who had regular menstrual cycles of 23–35 days' duration (7, 8) during the previous year. Apart from occasional cases who were overweight on the Garrow Chart, they all had normal general physical and gynecological examinations, and none had overt signs of endocrine or other abnormalities with the exception of a few cases of primary dysmenorrhea. None of them had hormonal contraception or had conceived for 6 months prior to this study. They all had normal thyroid function tests, normal plasma prolactin (9), and evidence of ovulation as demonstrated by the biphasic basal body temperature chart and at least one occasion of a midleuteal serum progesterone of >30 mmL/L (10). Also, they all had a hysterosalpingography, and diagnostic laparoscopy, and all of their partners had at least one semen analysis that was interpreted according to the WHO criteria (11). This population was a mixture of women referred to the University Research Clinic for AID treatment and women with tubal or unexplained infertility.

Methods

Daily venous blood samples (10 mL) were collected each morning (between 0800 and 1100 h) beginning on the 4th day (day 4) of spontaneous menstrual bleeding. The whole blood was separated within 30–60 min, and the plasma was stored at –20°C until assayed. All samples from each woman were assayed in a single hormone assay run. Table 38.1 documents the timing of each observation in an "ideal" 28-day cycle. Follicular (abdominal) ultrasound examinations (U/S) were commenced on day 7 to day 8 (occasionally earlier in women with shorter cycles) and were performed daily until 48 h after follicular rupture had occurred. Ovulation was diagnosed by rapid shrinkage or disappearance of the follicle in < 48 h of the LH surge. The appearance of fluid in the pouch of Douglas or on the endometrial ovulation

TABLE 38.1. Timing of FSH, LH, and ovarian U/S monitoring in "ideal" 28-day cycle.

Investigation	Day of cycle													
	4	5	6	7	8	9	10	11	12	13	14	15	16	17
Plasma FSH	X	x	x											
Plasma LH	x	x	x	x	x	x	x	x	x	x	x	x	x	x
Ovarian U/S				x	x	x	x	x	x	x	x	x	x	x

ring was considered to be supportive evidence only. Ultrasound scans were performed on subjects who had a full bladder using a Kretz Cambison 320 sector scanner with a 3-mHz output.

Measurements of plasma FSH and LH were performed using monoclonal antibody-based immunoradiometric assays (Miaclone) from Sereno Diagnostic Ltd, Surrey, UK. The sensitivity and interassay coefficient of variations were 0.3 U/L and 3.9% for LH and 0.3 U/L and 6.8% for FSH. The 1st IRP (68/40) and the 2nd IRP (78/549) were used in LH and FSH assays, respectively.

Statistical Analysis

For the purpose of this study, basal FSH was defined as day 4, day 5, or day 6 plasma FSH values, and basal LH was defined as the mean of 4 consecutive (days 4–7) LH measurements to reduce any sampling error due to LH pulsatility.

It has been shown that the frequency distribution of FSH and LH values does not follow a normal curve; however, it does follow a lognormal distribution (14). Day 4, day 5, and day 6 FSH and basal LH values were log transformed, and probability plots were used to define the geometeric mean and 95% confidence intervals (which includes 95% of the population). This technique has been previously described for gonadotropin and steroid concentrations (14) and for follicular and luteal phase lengths (7, 8). An "approximate straight line" on the probability plot is a good indication of the normality of the hormone distribution (15). Student's t-test and simple regression analysis were applied on log-transformed values. All data were corrected back to arithmetic units for graphic display.

Results

Endocrine and ovarian U/S data of 30 women were suggestive of anovulation or polycystic ovary syndrome (LH:FSH 2.5) and were excluded from further analysis.

General Population Characteristics

The mean age of women included in the study (n = 398) was 33.5 ± 4.8 years (mean ± SD). Follicular and luteal phase lengths were 13.4 ± 2.7 and 13.6 ± 2.0, respectively.

Basal FSH and LH Concentrations

Table 38.2 shows the geometric means (G-mean) and 95% confidence intervals (CI) of basal FSH and LH concentrations. There was a strong

TABLE 38.2. G-mean and 95% CI of basal FSH and LH.

Hormone	G-mean	95% CI
Basal (day 4) FSH	7.2	4.4–10.0
Basal (day 5) FSH	6.9	4.2–9.6
Basal (day 6) FSH	6.7	3.9–9.4

TABLE 38.3. The r- and P-values between day 4, day 5, and day 6 FSH concentrations.

Regression analysis	r	P
Day 4 to 5	0.91	0.0001
Day 4 to 6	0.81	0.0001
Day 5 to 6	0.88	0.0001

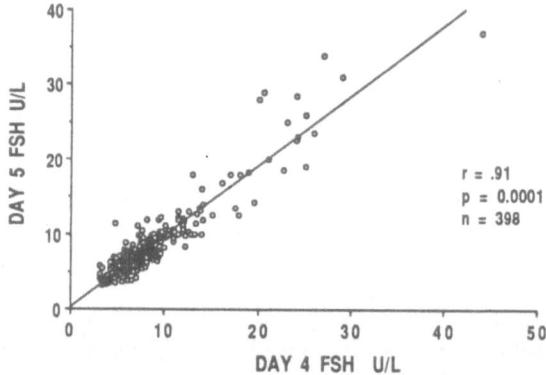

FIGURE 38.1. Correlation between day 4 and day 5 plasma FSH concentrations.

positive significant correlation between day 4, day 5, and day 6 FSH values (Fig. 38.1 and Table 38.3). There was also a positive significant correlation (r = 0.401; P = 0.0001) between basal LH and basal (day 4) FSH concentrations (Fig. 38.2).

Effect of Age on Basal Gonadotropin Concentrations

To examine the effect of age on basal FSH and LH concentrations, the population (n = 398) was divided into 9 age groups. Women aged 27–40 were divided into 7 groups of 2-year bands; however, there were relatively fewer women aged <27 (n = 30) or >41 (n = 30), and these women were grouped into 2 groups: 20–26 and 41–44. Using simple regression analysis, for all women there was a significant positive correlation (r = 0.468; P = 0.0001) between day 4 FSH concentration and age (Fig. 38.3) and a

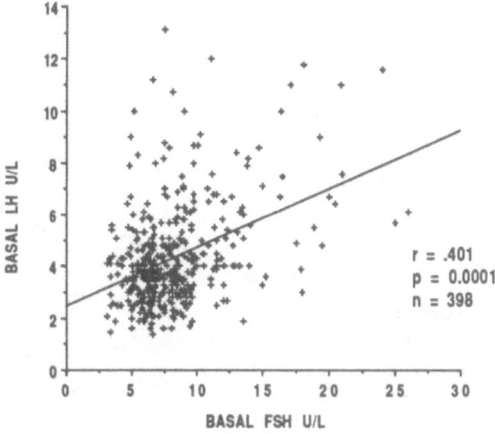

FIGURE 38.2. Relation between basal FSH and basal LH.

weaker but significant correlation (r = 0.225; P = 0.0001) between age and basal LH.

Figures 38.4 and 38.5 show the G-mean (and error of the mean) for basal (day 4) FSH and basal LH values in the 9 age groups. The number of women in each age group is given at the base of each column.

Effect of Age on Basal FSH Concentrations

From Figure 38.4, it is clear that there is a gradual, steady increase in FSH values with age and that this increase started from age 27–28. This increase

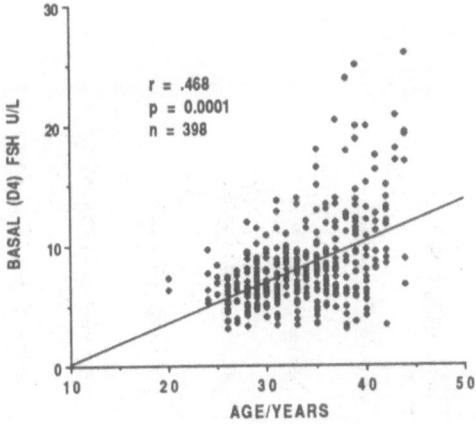

FIGURE 38.3. Relationship between age and basal FSH.

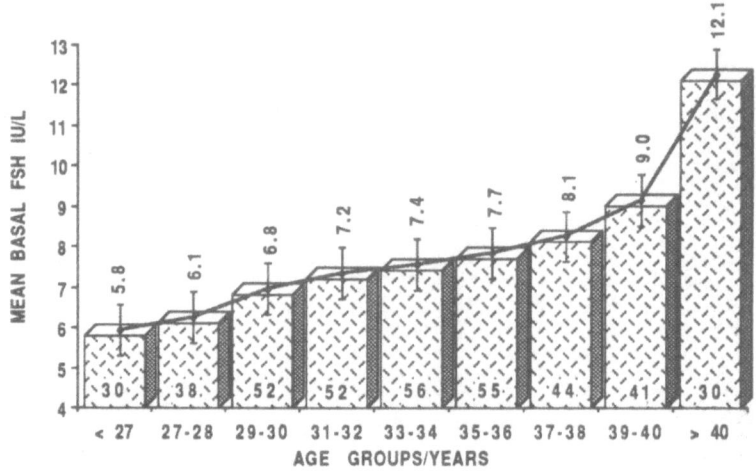

FIGURE 38.4. Changes in plasma FSH concentrations as a function of age.

in FSH values became quite significant (P = 0.0001) at age 29–30 when compared with younger women (20–28). Similarly, women aged 20–30 (n = 120), representing over 30% of the study population, had significantly lower FSH values (P = 0.002) than women aged 30–32. Table 38.4 shows the t-test results (P values) when FSH values of different age groups were compared.

The increase in FSH values with age was relatively gradual until age 37–38 when there was a steeper increase, with a further more marked increase after the age of 40 that most likely represents the well documented perimenopausal increase of FSH concentrations.

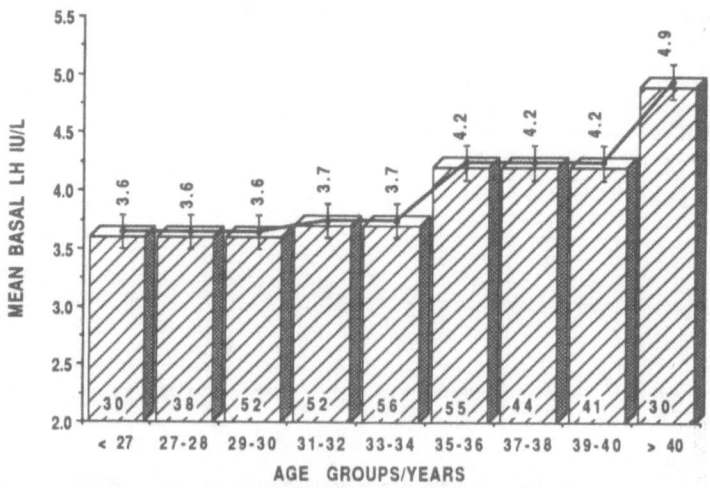

FIGURE 38.5. Changes in basal plasma LH concentrations as a function of age.

TABLE 38.4. Results of t-test (P-values) when FSH values of different age groups were compared.

Age group (years)	Comparison with the preceding 2 groups	Comparison with all younger women (P)
<27		
27–28	NS	NS
29–30	a	0.0001
31–32	b	0.0020
33–34	c	0.0020
35–36	d	0.0100
37–38	e	0.0200
39–40	f	0.0020
> 40	g	0.0010

NS = not significant.

a: P = 0.001 and 0.03 when compared with age groups <27 and 27–28, respectively.

b: P = 0.0007 and 0.04 when compared with groups 27–28 and 29–30, respectively.

c: P = 0.007 and NS when compared with age groups 29–30 and 31–32, respectively.

d: P = NS when compared with age groups 31–32 and 33–34, respectively.

e: P = 0.01 and NS when compared with age groups 33–34 and 35–36, respectively.

f: P = 0.001 and NS when compared with age groups 35–36 and 37–38, respectively.

g: P = 0.0001 when compared with any age group.

Effect of Age on Basal LH Concentrations

Figure 38.5 shows that basal LH concentrations were similar in all age groups until age 35–36 when LH values increased (P = 0.0001). This increase was maintained in age groups 37–38 and 39–40 and was followed by a further increase in LH values in women >40 yrs (P = 0.0001). Table 38.5 shows the P-values when basal LH concentrations were compared between the study subpopulations.

Effect of Age on LH Values During the LH Surge

Figure 38.6 shows that LH concentrations during the midcycle LH surge increased slightly more in older (>34) than in younger (<34) women, but this increase was not statistically significant.

TABLE 38.5. Results of t-test (P-values) when basal LH values were compared between the study subpopulation.

Subpopulation (years)	Compared with (years)	P
35–40	20–34	0.0001
>40	20–34	0.0001
>40	35–40	NS

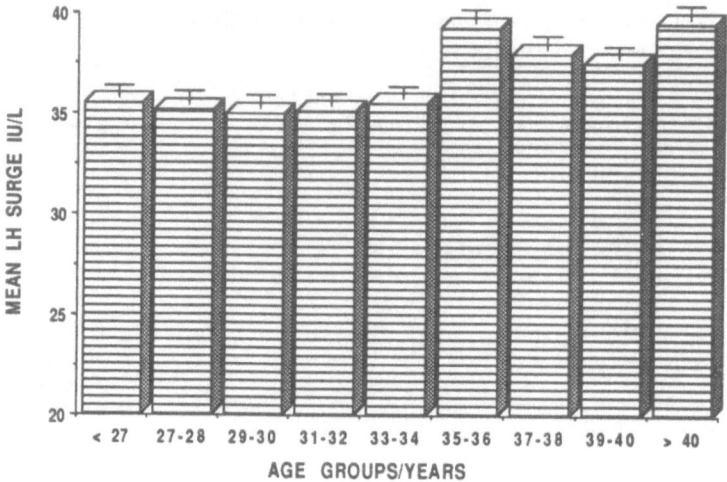

FIGURE 38.6. Plasma LH concentrations during the midcycle surge in different age groups.

Within-Group FSH-LH Relationship

As already discussed, there was a positive correlation between basal FSH and LH (r = 0.401; P = 0.0001). The same positive correlation existed within all age groups, but was weaker in the younger (<34) versus the older (>34) age groups (Table 38.6). This probably reflects the concomitant increase in both basal LH and FSH concentrations in older age groups (>34). Figure 38.7 shows the correlation between both gonadotropins in the 3 oldest age groups (37–44).

Discussion

In this study, mean values and ranges of basal FSH and LH using the relatively new radioimmunometric assays were presented and the phenom-

TABLE 38.6. The r- and P-values between basal LH and FSH within age groups.

Age group (years)	r	P
20–34	0.126	NS
35–36	0.201	NS
37–38	0.450	0.0030
38–39	0.550	0.0003
>40	0.790	0.0001

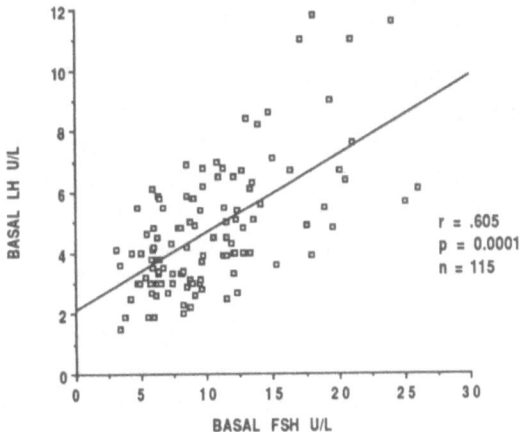

FIGURE 38.7. Relationship between basal FSH and basal LH in women aged 37–44.

enon of age-related increase in gonadotropins was investigated. Despite the fact that hormonal data from an infertile population are used in this study to assess such a critical relationship as the gradual increase in gonadotropins with age, we are confident that it is valid to use these hormone profiles as representative of the normal population because basal gonadotropin values were found to be similar in both regularly menstruating ovulatory infertile women and normal women (16, 17), as well as in the conceiving and nonconceiving cycles of previously infertile women (18).

In the present study, there was a strong positive correlation between day 4, day 5, and day 6 FSH values, suggesting that one single FSH measurement would be representative of the early follicular phase FSH profile. This finding was also suggested by Pepperell et al. (19), as they found that single plasma samples invariably provided a valid estimate of the current mean plasma FSH and LH in ovulatory cycles.

Lenton et al. (18) found that except during the midcycle surge, plasma FSH concentrations are highest during the early to midfollicular phase. Thus, any age-related changes in FSH concentrations could be most pronounced during that stage of the cycle (2). As this study has shown that day 4 FSH values were the highest of the 3 consecutive days' measurements, it is consequently suggested that one single (preferably day 4) FSH measurement would be truly representative of the early follicular phase FSH concentration and most likely to reflect any age-related changes in this hormone. The positive correlation between basal gonadotropins found in this study has also been described by others (19), as well as the correlation between both hormones during the midcycle peak (18).

Age-Related Rise in Gonadotropins

The present study suggests a positive significant correlation between age and basal FSH levels ($r = 0.468$; $P = 0.0001$) and a positive but weaker correlation between age and basal LH values. This is supported by the findings of Metcalf et al. (3), who also reported similar positive correlation between age and both FSH and LH in women aged 22–48, as well as of Ryes et al. (1), who found a positive correlation between age and FSH, but not LH. This supports our hypothesis of an age-related increase in FSH values and probably in LH values as well.

Most previous studies investigating the changes in gonadotropin concentrations with age emphasized the perimenopausal and menopausal rise in FSH and LH (1, 2, 4, 20). Sherman and Korenman (4) claimed that there was not a marked increase in gonadotropin concentrations until age 46, but in their study, they compared hormonal data of quite a small number of subjects ($n = 10$, 6, and 5; aged 18–30, 40–41, and 46–50, respectively). Ryes et al. (1) studied regularly menstruating and ovulating women ($n = 58$) and reported significant increase in FSH levels in women aged 40–44. Similarly, Lenten et al. (2) and Lee et al. (20) reported a significant increase in FSH values in women >41, which was followed later (2–3 years prior to menopause) by a rise in LH levels. In these studies, investigators reported the rise in gonadotropin in perimenopausal women due to the partial ovarian failure (3) preceding the menopause. These studies did not establish that there is a specific age-related increase in gonadotropin levels distinct from the changes associated with the start of menopausal transition.

This study suggests that an age-associated increase in FSH concentration starts quite early in reproductive life (29–30 years) (Fig. 38.4) and that this increase is steady and continues during the 3rd decade until age >40 when there is a further, more marked increase that is likely to be due to the menopausal transition reported by other workers (1, 2, 4, 20). However, LH levels did not show any increase until age 35–36, with a further increase in women >40 (Fig. 38.5). Similar findings have been reported, as Ryes et al. (1) found an increase of FSH accompanied by normal LH and estradiol in some normally ovulating women aged 34–39 years, Lee et al. (20) found a significant difference in FSH values between women aged 24–35 and women >36, and Metcalf et al. (3) suggested an age-related rise in FSH in women >40.

Men and women differ in that in women sex hormone production is intimately linked to the presence of gametes. As the number of oocytes is fixed at birth and are lost at a relatively constant rate, gonadal failure is the inevitable result (21). The number of oocytes in the mammalian ovary declines exponentially from birth until the menopause (22). In 1952 Baker (22) suggested that by the time of the menopause, only 1% of the original oocyte reserve remains in the ovary. A recent report (23) suggested the virtual absence of follicles in the postmenopausal ovary, a lower estimate of follicles in regularly menstruating perimenopausal women (1000–2500), and an accelerated rate of follicular depletion in the last decade of menstrual life. Thus, the finding of an age-related rise in gonadotropins should not be unexpected in view of the gradual reduction of oocyte reserve with age and in view of a similar finding in men in the absence of gonadal failure (5, 16).

The phenomenon of an age-related rise in gonadotropins is probably due not only to ovarian aging and a reduced number of follicles, but also to granulosa cell (GC) aging. It has been shown that cultured GC from women >40 had markedly reduced mitotic frequency, reduced DNA synthetic ability, reduced in vitro production of E_2, and reduced gonadotropin binding activity (24). In addition, the same phenomenon—that is, an age-related rise in FSH—has also been reported in rodents (25, 26). De Paslo and Chappel found increased circulating immunoreactive FSH levels on the estrus in rats 5 months and older, compared to levels measured in 2- to 3-month old rats. They also found that the increased FSH levels in virgin females preceded the age-related disruption of the estrus cycle,while plasma LH levels did not change until the age of 9 months (25). It has been suggested that the age-associated increase in circulating FSH levels on estrus may be attributed to an enhanced basal secretion of FSH from the pituitary gland (26).

The etiology of the perimenopausal rise in FSH (and later, LH) is still debatable. Sherman and Korenman (4) advocated that reduced inhibin secretion as a consequence of the number of follicles declining with age would contribute to the perimenopausal rise in FSH. The same view was held by Vagenakis (27). However, Metcalf and Livesey (3) felt that decreased inhibin secretion is unlikely to explain the rise in FSH levels with age in their regularly menstruating ovulating subjects. Recently, it has been shown that inhibin was undetectable in the circulation of postmenopausal women (28). If the age-related increase in FSH is due to decreased inhibin consequent to gradual depletion of follicles, then it must be demonstrated that there is also a concomitant age-related decrease in inhibin levels in the absence of ovarian failure. There is little doubt that the ovarian exhaustion of follicles is the pacemaker of reproductive senescence in women. However, there is some evidence that the hypothalamus may also be involved (29), and it has been suggested that the sensitivity of the hypothalamo-pituitary axis to falling estrogen levels increases with age (3).

The demonstration of an age-related rise in gonadotropins raises two questions: (1) Is there any cause-effect relationship between the age-related rise in gonadotropins and fertility, as it has already been demonstrated that the drop in fecundity begins before age 35 (30), well before the expected perimenopausal changes; and (2) what should be the future definition of the perimenopause—should it include the woman's age, menstrual regularity, her plasma FSH concentration, or perhaps the number of follicles remaining in her ovary? In summary, this study presented some evidence of an age-related rise of FSH very early in reproductive life followed by a rise in LH at age 35–36. These findings represent some reproductive markers in the sequence that extends from before birth to advanced ages. Thus, the phenomena of reproductive ontogeny and senescence are best seen as a contiuum in which functional changes reflect varying influences from ovaries to endocrine loci.

References

1. Ryes FI, Winter JSD, Faiman. Pituitary-ovarian relationship preceding the menopause. Am J Obstet Gynecol 1977;129:557-64.
2. Lenton EA, Sexton L, Lee S, Cooke ID. Progressive changes in LH and FSH and LH: FSH ratio in women throughout reproductive life. Maturitas 1988;10:35-43.
3. Metcalf MF, Livesey JH. Gonadotrophin excretion in fertile women: effect of age and the onset of the menopause. J Endocrinol 1985;105:357-62.
4. Sherman BM, Korenman SG. Hormonal characteristics of the human menstrual cycle throughout reproductive life. J Clin Invest 1975;55:699-706.
5. Sparrow D, Bosse R, Row JW. The influence of age, alcohol consumption and body build on gonadal function in men. J Clin Endocrinol Metab;51:508-12.
6. Neaves WB, Johnson L, Porter JC, Parker CR, Pett CS. Leydig cell numbers, daily sperm production and serum gonadotrophin levels in aging men. J Clin Endocrinol Metab 1984;59:756-63.
7. Lenton EA, Landgren BM, Sexton L, Harper R. Normal variation in the length of follicular phase of the menstrual cycle. Br J Obstet Gynaecol 1984;91:681.
8. Lenton EA, Landgren BM, Sexton L. Normal variation in the length of the luteal phase of the menstrual cycle: identification of the short luteal phase. Br J Obstet Gynaecol 1984;91:685-9.
9. Lenton EA, Sulaiman R, Sobowale O, Cooke ID. The human menstrual cycle: plasma concentrations of prolactin, LH, FSH, oestradiol and progesterone in conceiving and non-conceiving women. J Reprod Fert 1982;65:131-9.
10. Hall MGR. Ovulation failure and induction. In: Studd J, ed. Progress in obstetrics and gynaecology. London: Churchill Livingston, 1982.
11. Belsey MA, Eliasson R, Gallegos AJ, Moghissi K, Paulsen C, Prasad M. Laboratory manual for the examination of human semen and semen-cervical mucus interaction. Singapore: Press Concern, 1980.
12. O'Herlihy C, Crespigny L, Robinson H. Ultrasound monitoring of ovulation. In: Behrmen SJ, et al, eds. Progress in infertility. Boston: Little, Brown, 1988:479-97.
13. Richie WG. Ultrasound in the evaluation of normal and induced ovulation. In: Wallach EE, Kempers RD, eds. Modern trends in infertility and conception control. Chicago: Yearbook Medical Publications,1988.
14. Kletzky OA, Nakamura RM, Thorneycroft IH, Mishell DR. Log normal distribution of gonadotrophins and ovarian steroid values in the normal menstrual cycle. Am J Obstet Gynecol 1975;126:688-94.
15. Dudley BAC. Mathematical and biological inter-relations. New York: Wiley and Sons, 1977:21:51.

16. Lenton EA, Adams M, Cooke ID. Plasma steroid and gonadotrophin profiles in ovulatory, but infertile women. Clin Endocrinol (Oxf) 1978;8:241-55.
17. Coats JRT, Dodson K, MacNaughton MC. Hormone profiles in normally menstruating and infertile women. Eur J Obstet Gynecol Reprod Biol 1974; (4/1 suppl):S169-74.
18. Lenton EA, Sulaimon R, Sobowale O, Cooke ID. The human menstrual cycle: plasma concentrations of prolactin, LH, FSH, oestradial and progesterone in conceiving and non-conceiving women. J Reprod Fertil 1982;65:131-9.
19. Peperell RJ, De Kretser DM, Rennie GC. Plasma gonadotrophin levels in ovulatory and non-ovulatory patients. Br J Obstet Gynaecol 1976;83:68-76.
20. Lee SJ, Lenton EA, Sexton L, Cooke ID. The effect of age on the cyclical patterns of plasma LH, FSH, oestidial and progesterone in women with regular menstrual cycles. Hum Reprod 1988;3:851-5.
21. Honey AF. The "physiology" of climacterism. Clin Obstet Gynecol 1986;29(2): 397-406.
22. Baker TG. Primordial germ cells. In: Austin CR, Short RV, eds. Germ cells and fertilization. 1972:1-13.
23. Richardson SJ, Senikas V, Nelson JF. Follicular depletion during the menopausal transition: evidence for accelerated loss and ultimate exhaustion. J Clin Endocrinol Metab 1987;65:1231-7.
24. Uno Y. Aging phenomenon of granulosa cells in the human ovary. Hokkaido Igaku Zasshi 1987;62:558-63.
25. De Paolo LV, Chappel SC. Alteration in the secretion and production of follicle stimulating hormone precede age-related lengthening of oestrus cycles in rats. Endocrinology 1986;118:1127-33.
26. De Paolo LV. Increases in the basal secretion rate of follicle stimulating hormone (FSH) accompany age-associated changes in serum FSH levels on oestrus. Proc Soc Exp Biol Med 1988;189:168-72.
27. Vagenakis AG. Endocrine aspects of menopause. Clin Rheumatol 1989;8 (suppl 2):48-51.
28. McLachlan RI, Robertson DM, Healey DL, De Kresten DM, Burgen HG. Plasma inhibin levels during gonadotrophin induced ovarian hyperstimulation for IVF: a new index of follicular function. Lancet 1986;1:1233.
29. Finch CE, Felicio LS, Mobbs CV, Nelson JF. Ovarian and steroid influences on neuroendocrine aging process in female rodents. Endocrinol Rev;5:467-97.
30. Federation CECOS, Schwartz D, Mayaux MJ. Female fecundity as a function of age. Results of artificial insemination in 2193 multiparous women with 9200 spermic husbands. New Engl J Med 1982;306:404-6.

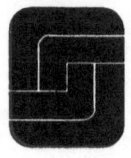

39

Effect of the LH:FSH Ratio in the Late Luteal Phase on Follicular Growth of the Next Menstrual Cycle

K. Aisaka, H. Tsuzuki, S. Kaneda, Y. Toriya, M. Nojima, K. Kokuho, and K. Yoshida

It is well known that gonadotropins play important roles in the development of ovarian follicles. Recently, the accuracy for measuring various hormones has been improved by using the specific purified monoclonal antibodies (MCA) (1, 2). It has also been pointed out that the growth of the main follicle begins during the late luteal phase of the last menstrual cycle (3, 4). The present study was performed to elucidate whether the serum gonadotropin levels in the late luteal phase affected follicular growth in the following menstrual cycle.

Subjects and Methods

The subjects were 11 volunteer women whose biphasic basal body temperature (BBT) charts showed high phases of more than 13-days' duration. They were from 22 to 32 years old (27.4 ± 4.6 years old, mean ± SD), and their menstrual cycles were from 28 to 30 days. All the subjects had taken endocrinological examinations to eliminate various endocrinological disorders (such as occult or latent hyperprolactinemia [5–7], polycystic ovarian disease [8, 9], etc.). Then, serum levels of LH and FSH were measured in duplicate samples in the late luteal phase by immunoradiometric assays using standards of WHO 1st International reference preparation (1st IRP) 68/40 for LH and WHO 2nd IRP human pituitary gonadotropin (2nd IRP-hPG) 78/549 for FSH with the specific purified MCA (1, 2). The intra- and interassay coefficients of variation of both assays were below 10%. The sensitivity of the LH assay was 1.0 mIU/mL and that of the FSH assay was 0.5 mIU/mL. Blood samplings were also done in the follicular and periovulatory phase of the following menstrual cycles, and serum levels of LH and FSH were examined in the same ways. Follicular development in the following cycle was observed by transvaginal ultrasonography as precisely as possible.

Then, the subjects were divided into two groups. In group A, the diameter of the main follicle was more than 20 mm (n = 6). In group B, the diameter of the main follicle was less than 20 mm (n = 5). Serum levels of LH and FSH and the LH: FSH ratio in each menstrual phase were compared between these two groups. Serum levels of estradiol (E) and progesterone (P) were also measured in the midluteal phase of the following cycles as an index of luteal function. The significances of these values on follicular development and the following luteal function are discussed next. Student's t-test was used for statistical comparison of the two groups, and P < 0.05 was chosen to indicate statistical significance.

Results

There was no significant change in serum gonadotropin levels between groups A and B in the late luteal phase of the last menstrual cycle (LH:3.3 ± 0.7 vs. 3.9 ± 0.5; FSH:6.1 ± 1.3 vs. 4.8 ± 0.9 mIU/mL, respectively, mean ± SD). However, the LH:FSH ratio in this phase showed a significant increase in group B compared to that of group A (A:0.56 ± 0.14; B:0.84 ± 0.14; P < 0.02) (Fig. 39.1).

There was also a significant inverse correlation between the maximum follicular diameter and the LH:FSH ratio in the late luteal phase of the last menstrual cycle (y = −10.261x + 26.355; r = −0.730; P < 0.02) (Fig. 39.2). No significant changes in serum levels of LH and FSH and the LH:FSH

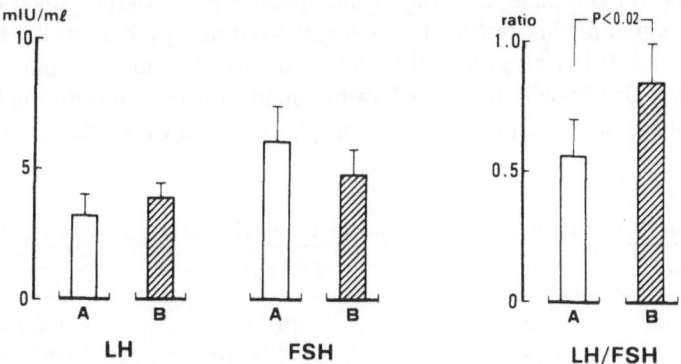

FIGURE 39.1. Changes of serum LH and FSH levels and the LH:FSH ratio in the late luteal phase of the last menstrual cycle.

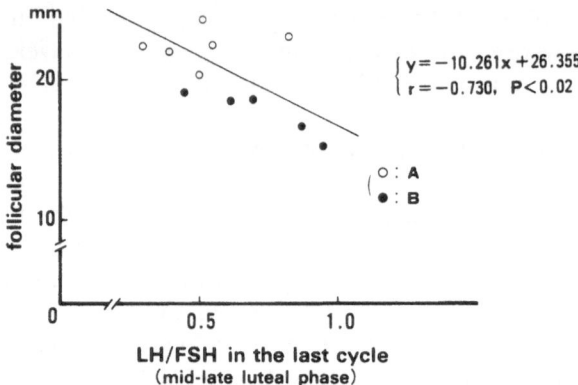

$$y = -10.261x + 26.355$$
$$r = -0.730, \quad P < 0.02$$

FIGURE 39.2. Correlation between maximum follicular diameter and LH:FSH ratio in the late luteal phase of the last menstrual cycle.

ratio were observed in any phases of the following menstrual cycle (Table 39.1). Serum E and P levels in the midluteal phase of the following cycles in women of group A tended to be higher than those of group B(E:252.4 ± 36.5 vs. 214.6 ± 41.2 pg/mL; P:12.5 ± 2.0 vs. 11.0 ± 2.9 ng/mL, respectively).

From these results, it was suggested that the FSH-predominant state in the late luteal phase of the menstrual cycle might be preferable for follicular maturation in the following menstrual cycle and might also affect luteal function of the following cycle. The clinical course of the same case is shown in Figure 39.3.

Discussion

Research on follicular maturation has made rapid progress since clinical application of in vitro fertilization and embryo transfer programs has become widespread. It is well known that follicular growth is mainly controlled by FSH. It is also known that growth of the main follicle begins during the late luteal phase of the last menstrual cycle (3, 4). As shown in the results, there

TABLE 39.1. Serum LH and FSH and the LH:FSH ratio in the following cycle.

Phase	LH (mIU/mL)	FSH (mIU/mL)	LH:FSH ratio
Follicular	A: 3.4 ± 0.7	9.0 ± 1.5	0.36 ± 0.12
	B: 3.5 ± 0.7	8.1 ± 1.2	0.43 ± 0.15
Ovulatory	A: 34.9 ± 8.6	15.7 ± 3.8	2.24 ± 0.81
	B: 35.5 ± 9.1	16.2 ± 4.2	2.20 ± 0.77

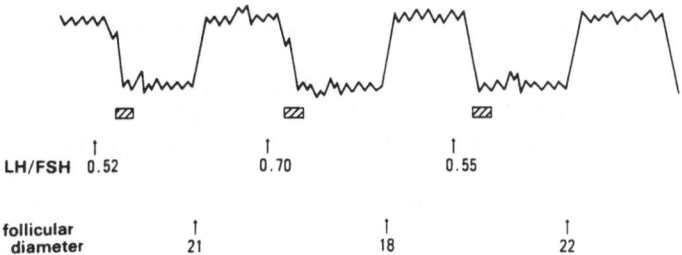

LH/FSH 0.52   0.70   0.55

follicular
diameter   21   18   22

FIGURE 39.3. Follow-up of the same case (28 years old, 28–29 days of the menstrual cycle).

was a significant inverse correlation between the LH:FSH ratio in the last menstrual phase and the follicular diameters that were observed in the following menstrual cycles. There were no significant changes in the serum levels of LH and FSH or in the LH:FSH ratio in the follicular and the periovulatory phases of the following menstrual cycles. These results seemed to indicate that the FSH-predominant state was necessary for the follicular growth, especially in the early stage of follicular development.

The pulsatile patterns of LH and FSH were not examined in this study. Further study must be done on this point. However, the physiological significance of the FSH-predominant state in the late luteal phase of the last menstrual cycle for follicular growth was proven even with the single-point blood sampling used in this study. From these results, it is concluded that follicular growth in the next menstrual cycle is predictable by the LH:FSH ratio in the late luteal phase of the last menstrual cycle.

References

1. Research Committee for the immunoradiometric assays of LH and FSH in Japan(Rep. Aono T). Multicentric clinical studies on immunoradiometric assays for measurement of serum LH and FSH using the pituitary gonadotropin standards. Clin Endocrinol(Tokyo) 1989;36:1087-97.
2. Jaakkola T, Ding YQ, Lehtinen PK, et al. The ratios of serum bioactive/immunoreactive LH and FSH in various clinical conditions with increased and decreased gonadotropin secretion. J Clin Endocrinol Metab 1990;70:1496-505.
3. Hodgen GD. The dominant ovarian follicle. Fertil Steril 1982;38:281-8.
4. Scott RT, Jr, Hodgen GD. The ovarian follicle: life cycle of a pelvic clock. Clin Obstet Gynecol 1990;33:551-62.
5. Ben-David M, Schenker JG. Transient hyperprolactinemia: a correctable cause of idiopathic female infertility. J Clin Endocrinol Metab 1983;57:442-4.
6. Mori H, Aisaka K, Matsuoka R, et al. The mechanism of induction of ovulation

by bromocriptine in euprolactinemic anovulation. Foria Endocrinol Jap 1985;61: 38-47.

7. Aisaka K, Ando S, Kokuho K, et al. Effects of transient or occult hyper-prolactinemia on luteal function. Foria Endocrinol Jap 1986;62:117-25.

8. Futterweit W. Polycystic ovarian disease. New York: Springer-Verlag, 1984: 97-111.

9. Aisaka K, Kaneda S, Tsuzuki H, et al. Comprehensive approach to clinical background and effect of bromocriptine administration in the patients of endocrinological polycystic ovarian disease. Foria Endocrinol Jap 1990;66:101-12.

40

Secretion Pattern of FSH in Patients Suffering from Chorionic Gonadotropin-Producing Tumors

P. BERGER, S. MADERSBACHER, R. KLIEBER, AND G. WICK

Intrinsic human follicle stimulating hormone (hFSH) activity (FSA) of human chorionic gonadotropin (hCG) has been proposed for many years (1). FSA was demonstrated in extracts of pregnancy urine and crude or highly purified hCG preparations. Whether FSA is due to cross-contamination of these hormone preparations with hFSH or represents "true" FSA is still a matter of debate. Studies employing immunoprecipitation techniques with polyclonal antisera suggest that the latter is more likely (2). These studies have been carried out using hormone standard preparations of various origin. So far, no investigations have been performed with pregnancy- and tumor-derived sera containing high concentrations of hCG.

The biochemical similiarity of hCG to the other human glycoprotein hormones is the basis for the proposed intrinsic effect of excess amounts of hCG: All four glycoprotein hormones are composed of two subunits (designated α and β) that are noncovalently linked to form the holohormone.

Our laboratory has previously produced a large panel of monoclonal antibodies (MCA) against hCG and hFSH (3, 4), enabling us to develop immunoenzymometric assays (IEMA) with predictable specificities as well as to study hormone-receptor interactions (5). Here, we describe an observation made in patients suffering from hCG-producing testicular cancer: We found a highly significant inverse correlation between hCG and hFSH serum levels that might have its basis in the FSA of hCG.

Subjects and Methods

Serum Samples and Hormones

Serum samples (n = 195) from patients suffering from seminomatous (n = 1) and nonseminomatous (n = 12) testicular cancer were collected over observation periods of 6–12 months. Prior to the radioreceptor assays (RRA), these sera were dialyzed against 0.05-M Tris-HCl (pH 7.4) for 16 h at 4°C. hCG (highly purified) was kindly provided by V.C. Stevens (Ohio State University, Columbus, OH); hFSH-I-3 (NIADDK), hLH-I-1 (NIADDK), and rat FSH (rFSH-I-7) were generously supplied by the National Pituitary Agency (Baltimore, MD).

Hormone Quantification

hFSH and hCG were measured by MCA-based 2-site IEMA according to a method published previously (6). The pair of MCA applied in the IEMA for hFSH was chosen on the basis of specificity and epitope compatibility, as described elsewhere (3). hCG was quantified using a solid-phase-bound MCA specific for the conformationally (c) intact holohormone (c-MCA, code: INN-hCG-45) and a second horse-radish peroxidase-labeled detection MCA (code: INN-hCG-22) that recognizes free and combined hCGß (β-MCA). Estradiol (E_2) was determined by a commercially available RIA (DRG-Instruments GmbH, Marburg, F.R.G.).

Radioreceptor Assay (RRA)

Decapsulated testes from adult Sprague-Dawley rats were cut into small pieces and homogenized in 10-mL ice-cold 0.05-M Tris-HCl with an Ultra turrax tissue homogenizer (3 × 5 sec), followed by 3 washing steps (3200 × g, 20 min, 4°C). The pellet was diluted to 100- or 200-mg tissue wet weight (tww) per mL 0.05-M Tris-HCl supplemented with 1% bovine serum albumin (BSA) and 30-mM $MgCl_2$.

The RRA for hCG with radioiodinated hLH-I-1 was described previously (5). The RRA for hFSH was performed with slight modifications. Aliquots of the testis homogenate (250 µL, 200-mg tww/mL) were incubated with 50-µL hormone standard or serum (diluted in 0.05-M Tris-HCl/1% BSA), and 100 µL of [^{125}I]rFSH (250,000 cpm/tube) for 16 h at 20°C.

Immunoabsorption of Sera

In order to analyze the basis of the FSA in serum, patients' sera were preincubated with MCA either specific for the free and the combined β-subunit of hCG (β-MCA, code: INN-hCG-2) (6) or for the intact hFSH molecule (c-MCA, code: INN-hFSH-117) (3). The ascites-derived MCA were purified by ammonium-sulfate precipitation and subsequently dialyzed in parallel to the patients' sera. Prior to the RRA, 100 µL of the MCA preparations (1-mg IgG/mL) were incubated with 50 µL serum (diluted 1:10) for 1 h at room temperature on an orbit shaker.

Results

Assay Characteristics

The sensitivities of the IEMAs for hCG and hFSH were 16 pg/mL and 10 pg/mL, respectively. The crossreactivities of both IEMAs with respect to other glycoprotein hormones were less than 0.01%. When spiking hFSH samples with 5-μg hCG/mL, we found no detectable response in the IEMA for hFSH. Intra- and interassay coefficients of variation for both IEMAs were less than 12%.

Inverse Correlation of hCG and hFSH Serum Levels

The correlation of serum levels of hFSH and hCG was analyzed by means of longitudinal follow-up studies (observation period: 6–12 months, ~25 sera/patient). In all cases investigated (n = 13), hCG was highly elevated ($>10^8$ pg/mL) before polychemotherapy was initiated, whereas hFSH was undetectable at that time (<10 pg/mL) in all but one of the patients, who had very low hFSH levels of about 30 pg/mL. Under successful polychemotherapy, hCG levels declined to physiological concentrations (<240 pg/mL, 2 mIU/mL), and hFSH reached normal or even elevated levels (100–9000 pg/mL, 1–90 mIU/mL).

A statistically highly significant negative correlation between hCG and hFSH was observed ($P < 0.001$) in all cases. When hCG concentrations were higher than 10^5–10^6 pg/mL, hFSH was undetectable. Figure 40.1 exemplifies the inverse correlation of hCG and hFSH levels in patient F.R.

17β-Estradiol and hCG

To analyze steroidogenesis at changing hCG concentrations, E_2 was measured in the sera of 3 patients. A statistically significant positive correlation between hCG and E_2 was observed ($P < 0.01$), whereas hFSH was negatively correlated to E_2 ($P < 0.01$) in all cases (Fig. 40.1).

RRA for hCG

The ability of tumor-derived hCG to interact with the LH/CG receptor (LH/CG-R) was studied by RRA using rat testes homogenates. The hCG standard and the patients' sera exhibited parallel displacement curves. Immunoreactive holo-hCG as determined by IEMA was 20% higher than the levels calculated by RRA. Immunoabsorption of the sera and the hormone standard with an MCA specific for the β-subunit of hCG (code: INN-hCG-2) caused a 99.5% decrease in signal, indicating that 99.5% of hCG could be neutralized. The anti-hCGβ-MCA (INN-hCG-2) itself did not interfere with [^{125}I]hLH receptor binding.

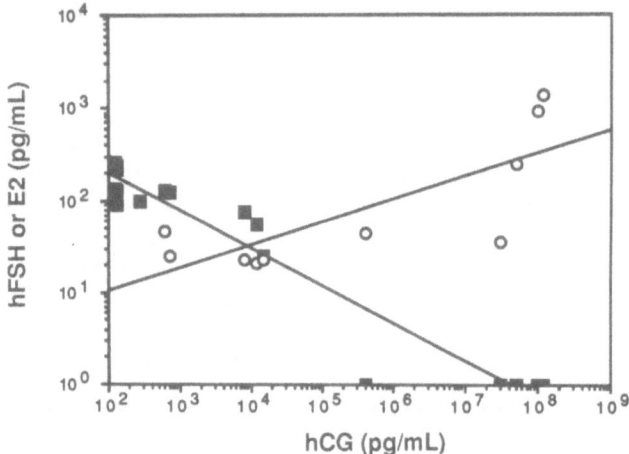

FIGURE 40.1. Correlation of 17β-estradiol (open circle) and hFSH levels (closed square) with hCG levels in the sera collected from patient F.R. who suffered from choriocarcinoma. hFSH levels were negatively correlated to hCG (P < 0.001; r = 0.96) as determined by linear regression analysis, whereas 17β-estradiol levels were positively correlated (P < 0.01; r = 0.78). hCG levels fell during polychemotherapy by a factor 10^6.

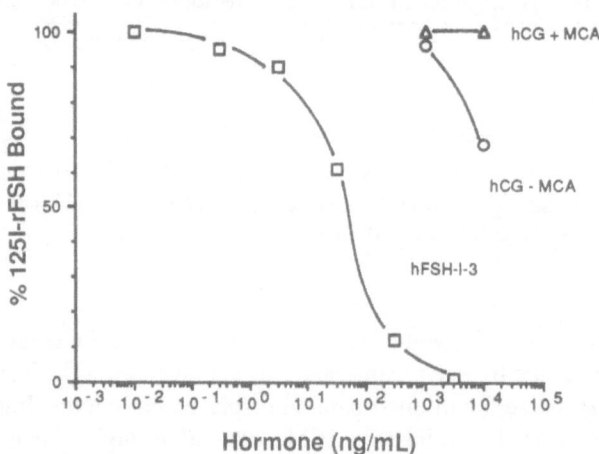

FIGURE 40.2. Effective block of FSA in the serum of the patient F.R. (open circle) by an MCA (open triangle) directed against hCGβ (INN-hCG-2). The FSA of tumor-derived hCG is about 0.1% in terms of hFSH-I-3 (open square) on a w/w basis; serum levels of hCG were determined by IEMA.

hFSH-Like Activity of Tumor-Derived hCG

FSA of tumor-derived hCG was analyzed by the RRA for hFSH (Fig. 40.2). The ability of hCG to block binding of $[^{125}I]$rFSH to its receptor was found to be 0.1% in terms of the hFSH standard, suggesting that the intrinsic FSA of tumor-derived hCG is 1000-fold less than that of hFSH. This ability could be totally blocked by adding a β-MCA specific for hCG (INN-hCG-2).

The anti-hFSH-MCA (INN-hFSH-117) was shown to block 3 μg/mL of the hFSH standard, but had no effect on the tracer, $[^{125}I]$rFSH. This is in agreement with the results obtained in the IEMA for hFSH that these sera do not contain detectable hFSH.

Discussion

Our results clearly indicate that hCG is responsible for the in vitro FSA in sera of testicular cancer patients as this intrinsic activity could be effectively blocked by an hCGβ-MCA. In order to exclude interactions of the MCA with the tracers, the RRA setups had to be carefully designed: in the RRA for hCG, the MCA for hCG neutralization (INN-hCG-2) did not interfere with either the $[^{125}I]$hLH tracer (even in a 20,000-fold molar excess) or with hFSH, as shown in the RRA for FSH. The MCA used in the hFSH-RRA (INN-hFSH-117) is both hormone and species specific (3) and, therefore, recognizes neither $[^{125}I]$rFSH nor hCG, but neutralizes the hFSH standard very well.

As determined by RRA, FSA of tumor-derived serum hCG is about 0.1% of hFSH, which is in the same range as previously shown for hormone standards (2). Recalculating the patients' hCG serum levels ($>10^8$ pg/mL) in terms of FSA, these sera have an apparent activity of $~10^4–10^5$ pg/mL, corresponding to 100–1000 mIU hFSH/mL, and, therefore, by far exceed physiological values.

What are the mechanisms underlying the statistically highly significant negative correlation of hCG and hFSH levels observed in all patients? The possibility of an assay artifact in the 2-step IEMA for hFSH by means of blocking the capture MCA with high concentrations of serum hCG (hCG is present in a 10^8-fold molar excess to hFSH in these sera!) and therefore producing false-negative results can be ruled out as (a) both anti-hFSH-MCA used in the hFSH-IEMA do not crossreact with hCG as shown in 1- and 2-site RIA and ELISA (3), (b) spiking the hFSH standard with 5-μg hCG/mL does not alter the signal of the IEMA, and (c) no bioactive hFSH was detected in these sera.

A second explanation could be the induction of inhibin production in

Sertoli cells (SC) caused by the FSA of hCG, which then suppresses pituitary hFSH secretion (7). The calculated FSA of hCG in these sera would, at least in vitro, be effective in stimulating inhibin release from Sc (8). However, in patients suffering from hCG-producing tumors, only an FSH-independent inhibin secretion could be observed (9), and exogenous hCG administration is not able to stimulate inhibin production in postpubertal male individuals (10).

A third possible mechanism could be the suppression of hFSH secretion via FSA-induced E_2-synthesis, although no conclusive studies on FSH suppression by E_2 in males are available (11). The highly elevated E_2 values (10- to 20-fold as compared to physiological male values) would favor this theory.

In summary, we have shown by immunoabsorption studies a specific FSA of hCG in sera of patients suffering from testicular tumors. These findings demonstrate an additional intrinsic activity of tumor-derived hCG besides the well-known in vitro TSH-like actvity (12). This FSA might be responsible for the observed negative correlation of hCG and hFSH serum levels in testicular cancer patients.

References

1. Albert A. Follicle stimulating activity of human chorionic gonadotropin. J Clin Endocrinol Metab 1969;29:1504-9.
2. Siris ES, Nisula BC, Catt KJ, et al. New evidence for intrinsic follicle-stimulating hormone-like activity in human chorionic gonadotropin and luteinizing hormone. Endocrinology 1978;102:1356-61.
3. Berger P, Panmoung W, Khashabi D, Mayregger B, Wick G. Antigenic features of human follicle stimulating hormone delineated by monoclonal antibodies and construction of an immunoradiometric assay. Endocrinology 1988;123:2351-9.
4. Kofler R, Berger P, Wick G. Monoclonal antibodies against hCG, I. Production, specificity and intramolecular binding sites. Am J Reprod Immunol 1982;160:212-6.
5. Schwarz S, Berger P, Nelboeck E, et al. Probing the receptor interaction of glycoprotein hormones with monoclonal antibodies. J Recept Res 1988;8:437-53.
6. Berger P, Klieber R, Panmoung W, Madersbacher S, Wolf H, Wick G. Monoclonal antibodies against the free subunits of human chorionic gonadotropin. J Endocrinol 1990;125:301-9.
7. De Jong FH. Inhibin. Physiol Rev 1988;68:555-607.
8. Morris PL, Vale WW, Cappel S, Bardin CW. Inhibin production by primary Sertoli cell-enriched cultures: regulation by follicle-stimulating hormone, androgens, and epidermal growth factor. Endocrinology 1988;122:717-25.
9. Fingschedt U, Mann K, Clemm C, Nieschlag E. Elevated inhibin levels in patients with malignant teratomas [Abstract]. In: Proc 72nd annu meet Endocr Soc. Atlanta: Endocrine Society, 1990:167.

10. McLachlan RI, Finkel DM, Bremner WJ, Snyder PJ. Serum inhibin concentrations before and during gonadotropin treatment in men with hypogonadotropic hypogonadism: physiological and clinical implication. J Clin Endocrinol Metab 1990;70:1414-9.
11. McNeilly A. The control of FSH-secretion. Acta Endocrinol 1988;288:31-40.
12. Mann K, Schneider N, Hörmann R. Thyrotropic activity of acidic isoelectric variants of human chorionic gonadotropin from trophoblastic tumors. Endocrinology 1986;118:1558-66.

41

Progesterone Effects on FSH Secretion in Estrogen-Treated Normal Men

A. MANCINI, P. ZUPPI, C. FIUMARA, M.L. FABRIZI, T. IACONA,
L. SAMMARTANO, E. MENINI, AND L. DE MARINIS

The phenomenon of *positive feedback* between estrogens and luteinizing hormone (LH), originally thought to be exclusive to females on the basis of experimental studies in rodents (1, 2), has been shown to be present in male primates, including humans (3–6). The interactions between steroids and follicle stimulating hormone (FSH) have been less thoroughly investigated. In vivo studies have only been concerned with the regulation of FSH in pre- or post-menopausal women (7–9).

In order to investigate the modulatory effect of steroids on FSH secretion in vivo in males, we have tested a group of patients with carcinoma of the prostate. We administered estradiol, previously shown to exhibit only a suppressive effect on FSH (10, 11), then added progesterone (P) at different times after the onset of estradiol treatment.

Materials and Methods

We have studied 22 patients with carcinoma of the prostate after they had given an informed consent. They were aged 51–75 (mean 65.2) and were on no hormone medication. They were divided into 3 groups.

Group 1 (n = 6)

Estradiol benzoate (E_2B) in oil (Progynon B Schering, Schering Pharmaceutical, Bloomfield, NJ) was administered daily in a dose of 1.5 mg/day I.M. every 24 h (at 0800 h) for 6 days. Blood samples were collected every 24 h during the daily hormone administration (at 0800 h). Moreover, on day 4 (after 72 h of E_2B treatment), blood samples were collected for a period of 12 h, at 2-h intervals, to investigate the circadian hormone variation in the middle of the estrogen treatment.

Group 2 (n = 8)

The patients of this group underwent the same administration of estrogen as group 1. In addition, 72 h after the initiation of E_2B treatment, 10 mg of P I.M. (Gestone Pabyrn, GB) was administered. Blood samples were collected every 2 h for 12 h after the P-administration.

Group 3 (n = 8)

The patients of this group underwent the same administration of estrogen as group 1. In addition, 96 h after the initiation of E_2B treatment, 10 mg of P I.M. (Gestone Pabyrn, GB) was administered. Blood samples were collected every 2 h for 12 h after P-administration.

Methods

Blood samples were collected in heparinized tubes and centrifuged, and the plasma was frozen immediately after each study. Plasma PRL , LH, and FSH were assayed in each sample. Testosterone (T) and 17 β-estradiol (E_2) were assayed in the samples collected at 0800 h on the day before and on the 6th day of E_2B treatment. All samples were assayed in duplicate by RIA methods. The intraassay variations for these assays were 4% for PRL, 5.5% for LH, 5% for FSH, 10% for T, and 10% for E_2. To avoid interassay variations, all samples from a serial study were measured in a single assay. The normal range for these hormones in our laboratory is 5–20 ng/mL for PRL, 5–15 mIU/mL for LH, 5–20 mIU/mL for FSH, 4–8 ng/mL for T, and 20–60 pg/mL for E_2. Statistical analysis was performed using Student's t-test for paired data for assessing significance within a single group of subjects and analysis of covariance for assessing significance among groups of subjects.

Results

Daily basal levels of LH, FSH, and PRL in the 3 groups of patients are shown in Table 41.1. As expected, estrogen treatment exerted an inhibition on FSH secretion, a stimulation of PRL secretion, and a biphasic effect on LH secretion—that is, an initial LH decrease until 48 h of E_2B treatments followed by a return toward basal levels or to levels exceeding the basal ones after 72–96 h. The FSH variations, in samples obtained at 2-h intervals on the day of P-administration (in groups 2 and 3) and after 72 h in group 1 are shown in Figure 41.1, expressed as the mean percentage variation in comparison with basal levels (100%). While a progressive FSH decline was observed in group 1 subjects treated with estrogen alone, a positive effect on FSH secretion was observed in group 2 between 2 and 4 h after P-administration. In group 3, a similar phenomenon—that is, an increasing

TABLE 41.1. Mean (±SEM) daily plasma levels of LH, FSH, and PRL during estradiol treatment in the 3 groups of subjects tested.

	LH (mIU/mL)					
	0 h	24 h	48 h	72 h	96 h	120 h
Group 1	12.2	5.9	5.6	7.5	12.7	7.9
	±1.0	±1.0	±0.6	±1.5	±1.7	±0.5
Group 2	6.0	4.7	4.6	5.4	5.3	—
	±1.2	±0.6	±1.0	±1.3	±0.7	—
Group 3	26.3	13.9	13.8	18.2	35.3	23.1
	±3.7	±1.9	±3.0	±6.7	±10.7	±7.8
	FSH (mIU/mL)					
	0 h	24 h	48 h	72 h	96 h	120 h
Group 1	10.5	7.8	6.7	6.4	6.2	5.2
	±1.2	±1.3	±1.1	±1.0	±0.9	±1.1
Group 2	6.2	5.2	4.2	4.2	3.6	—
	±0.9	±0.8	±0.8	±0.7	±0.5	—
Group 3	19.2	15.1	13.5	12.8	15.9	11.6
	±3.5	±3.1	±2.7	±4.2	±5.4	±2.7
	PRL (ng/mL)					
	0 h	24 h	48 h	72 h	96 h	120 h
Group 1	9.1	8.7	8.1	10.0	23.3	20.7
	±3.03	±4.3	±3.5	±3.1	±7.9	±6.1
Group 2	5.3	6.7	8.2	7.7	15.3	—
	±0.9	±0.9	±0.9	±1.2	±2.5	—
Group 3	8.6	9.4	11.7	14.9	13.9	14.8
	±1.4	±1.3	±1.9	±0.9	±1.0	±2.3

effect of P—was observed later, 8–10 h after the administration of the steroid. Estrogen levels were significantly increased during the E_2B treatment, while T-levels were suppressed in the same period. Steroid levels are reported in Table 41.2.

Discussion

These data indicate that the acute administration of P in estrogen-pretreated normal men can exert a positive-feedback action on FSH secretion, which appears to be rapid after 72 h of E_2B administration and delayed after 96 h of E_2B administration. The feedback effects of P on gonadotropins have been extensively studied in normal women (7) and gonadectomized and post-

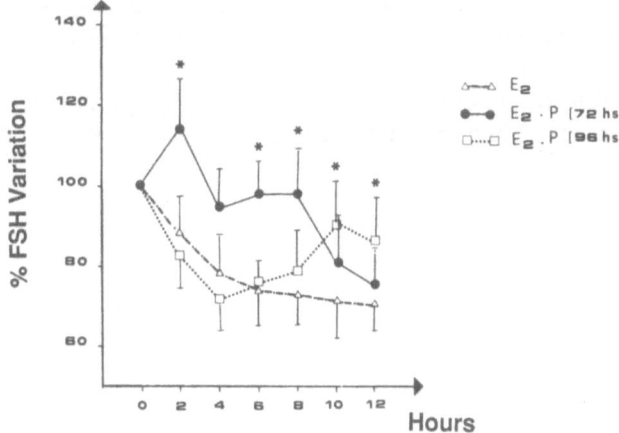

FIGURE 41.1. Mean (±SEM) percentage FSH variation after P-administration (at 72 h for group 2 or at 96 h for group 3) and during estrogen treatment (at 72 h for group 1, control). (*P < 0.05, the significance of difference when compared with group 1 values.)

menopausal estrogen-primed women (12–14). The concomitant effects on LH, FSH, and PRL suggest a central mechanism(s) to explain these phenomena. However, both the neural noradrenergic mechanisms and modulation of pituitary responsiveness to GnRH seem to be involved (9). Our results, extending our previous observations (10), suggest that similar mechanisms occur in intact men (nonorchiectomized men with carcinoma of the prostate) after a short (3 days) estrogen pretreatment. The fall in T-levels, which is induced by exogenous estradiol administration, could play a role in eliciting these effects. Moreover, the duration of estrogen pretreatment seems to be crucial for the pattern of gonadotropin response to acute P-administration.

In conclusion, these data confirm the biphasic effects of E_2-administration

TABLE 41.2. Mean (±SEM) plasma steroid levels at the start and at the end of estradiol treatment in the 3 groups of subjects tested. ([a]P < 0.05, compared with basal, or 0-h, levels.)

	Estradiol (pg/mL)		Testosterone (ng/mL)	
	0 h	120 h[a]	0 h	120 h[a]
Group 1	51.3 ± 0.9	1137.6 ± 632.1	6.7 ± 1.4	2.8 ± 0.9
Group 2	54.3 ± 15.5	839.3 ± 337.4	6.1 ± 0.5	4.1 ± 1.7
Group 3	77.5 ± 2.5	870.0 ± 229.1	4.3 ± 0.5	3.4 ± 1.7

on LH secretion in intact adult humans males. While E_2 alone showed an inhibitory effect on FSH secretion, the addition of P also induced a positive action, resulting in a clear FSH peak in some of the patients tested. In human males, peripheral steroids can exert effects on gonadotropin secretion similar to those observed in normal pre- and postmenopausal women.

Acknowledgments. This work has been partially supported by Foundation Paola Pavone.

References

1. Barraclough CA. Modification in the CNS regulation of reproduction after exposure of prepuberal rats to steroid hormones. Recent Prog Horm Res 1966;22: 503-39.
2. McLusky NJ, Naftolin F. Sexual differentiation of the central nervous system. Science 1981;211:1294-303.
3. Karsch FJ, Weck RF, Butler WR, et al. Induced LH surges in the rhesus monkey: strength-duration characteristics of the estrogen stimulus. Endocrinology 1973; 92:1740-7.
4. Kulin HE, Reiter EO. Gonadotropin and testosterone measurements after estrogen administration to adult men, prepuberal and puberty boys, and men with hypogonadotropinism: evidence for maturation of positive feedback in the male. Pediatr Res 1976;10:46-51.
5. Barbarino A, De Marinis L. Estrogen induction of luteinizing hormone release in castrated adult human males. J Clin Endocrinol Metab 1980;51:280-6.
6. Barbarino A, De Marinis L, Mancini A. Estradiol modulation of basal and gonadotropin-releasing hormone-induced gonadotropin release in intact and castrated men. Neuroendocrinology 1983;36:105-11.
7. Shaw RW, Butt WR, London DR. The effect of progesterone on FSH and LH response to LHRH in normal women. Clin Endocrinol (Oxf) 1975;4:543-50.
8. Lasley BL, Wang CF, Yen SSC. The effects of estrogen and progesterone on the functional capacity of the gonadotrophs. J Clin Endocrinol Metab 1975;4:820-6.
9. Nicoletti A, Filipponi P, Fedeli L, et al. Progesterone positive feedback on gonadotropin release in estrogen-primed postmenopausal women: central nervous system and pituitary as possible sites of action. J Clin Endocrinol Metab 1981;53:135-8.
10. Barbarino A, De Marinis L, Mancini A. Presence of positive feedback between estrogens and luteinizing hormone in normal and hypogonadal men: evidence against a perinatal hypothalamic imprinting. In: Caria Mendes J, Neto MC, Castro e Almeida ME, eds. Actas do V Congresso da Societad Europeia de Andrologia. Lisbon: European Anthropological Association, 1988:381-8.
11. Chang RJ, Jaffe RB. Progesterone effects on gonadotropin release in women pretreated with estradiol. J Clin Endocrinol Metab 1978;47:119-25.

12. Odell WD, Swerdloff RS. Progestagen-induced luteinizing and follicle-stimulating hormone surge in post-menopausal women: a simulated ovulatory peak. Proc Natl Acad Sci USA 1968;61:529-36.
13. Nillius SJ, Wide L. Effects of progesterone on the serum levels of FSH and LH in postmenopausal women treated with oestrogen. Acta Endocrinol (Copenh) 1971; 67:362-7.
14. Rakoff JS, Yen SSC. Progesterone induces acute release of prolactin in estrogen primed ovariectomized women. J Clin Endocrinol Metab 1978;47:918-21.

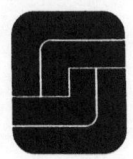

Author Index

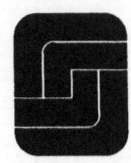

Subject Index

Acetylcholine, 233
ACTH, 232, 303–305, 372
Activin, 7, 9, 14, 29, 31, 167–175, 257, 262, 269
Adenosine monophosphate, cyclic, 11, 13–15, 124, 125, 131, 137, 145–153, 156–163, 173, 175, 180–187, 191, 196, 199, 202–204, 217–221, 231–233, 237–242, 247, 249, 313, 356–361
    -dependent protein kinase, *see* Protein kinase A
    response element, 109–112, 117, 147, 148, 151–153, 175, 247, 249
Adenylate cyclase, 12–14, 123, 124, 129, 133, 137–139, 145, 173, 180, 208, 218, 231, 233, 237, 356, 361
Adrenal androgen, 369–373
Agarose gel electrophoresis, 15, 169, 346; *see also* SDS gel electrophoresis
Age-related gonadotropin levels, 375–386
Alpha-melanocyte stimulating hormone, 232, 304
Amenorrhea, 265, 266, 275–291; *see also* Chronic anovulatory syndrome
Androgen, 10, 14, 15, 149, 188, 208, 231, 232, 234, 246–251, 265, 266, 328, 359, 369–373; *see also* particular androgens
    adrenal, 369–373
Androgen binding protein, 15, 221–225, 232, 238, 239, 246–251
Androstenedione, 179, 208, 340
Antiovarian antibodies, 277, 284–291

AP-1 transcription factor, 96, 102, 103
Apolipoprotein E, 178–188
Aromatase activity, 10, 14, 44, 46, 126, 145, 149–151, 153, 208, 209, 328, 330, 333
Autoimmune disorders, 276, 277, 282–291
Azoospermia, 50, 257

Bird, 54–63, 83
Blood-testis barrier, 217, 225–227
Breast cancer, 115, 278

Calcium/calcium ion, 13, 220, 233, 237, 356
cAMP, *see* Andenosine monophosphate, cyclic
cAMP-dependent protein kinase, *see* Protein kinase A
Cancer, 115, 251, 278, 323–328, 393–398, 400–404; *see also* tumor cell lines
Carbohydrate structure of glycoprotein hormones, *see* Oligosaccharide
CAT, *see* Chloramphenicol acetyl transferase
Catecholamine, 3, 5
Central nervous system, 1–6, 42, 45, 46, 61
c-fos, 95–104, 239
Chicken, 57, 58, 149
Chicken pox, 278
Chloramphenicol acetyl transferase, 110–117, 147, 153, 169, 172, 173, 357–361
Cholera toxin, 13, 97, 180–183, 199